PATIENT EDUCATION

A Practical Approach

Edited by

Richard D. Muma, MPH, PA-C
Assistant Director and Assistant Professor
Department of Physician Assistant
School of Health Sciences
College of Health Professions
Wichita State University
Wichita, Kansas

Barbara Ann Lyons, MA, PA-C
Associate Professor
Department of Physician Assistant Studies
School of Allied Health Sciences
The University of Texas Medical Branch
Galveston, Texas

Teresa A. Newman, BS, PA-C
Physician Assistant
Fort Worth, Texas

Barbara A. Carnes, PhD, RN, CS
Assistant Professor
Department of Mental Health/Management Nursing
School of Nursing
The University of Texas Medical Branch
Galveston, Texas

and

Illustrations by
John Todd Louis
Galveston, Texas

APPLETON & LANGE
Stamford, Connecticut

96 97 98 99 00 / 10 9 8 7 6 5 4 3 2 1

Prenctice Hall International (UK) Limited, *London*
Prentice Hall of Australia Pty Limited, *Sydney*
Prentice Hall Canada, Inc., *Toronto*
Prentice Hall Hispanoamericana, S.A., *Mexico*
Prentice Hall of India Private Limited, *New Delhi*
Prentice Hall of Japan, Inc., *Tokyo*
Simon & Schuster Asia Pte. Ltd., *Singapore*
Editora Prentice Hall do Brasil Ltda., *Rio de Janeiro*
Prentice Hall, *Upper Saddle River, New Jersey*

Library of Congress Cataloging-in-Publication Data
Patient education : a practical approach / edited by Richard D. Muma
 . . . [et al.] ; and illustrations by John Todd Louis.
        p.   cm.
    Includes index.
    ISBN 0-8385-2039-1 (pbk. : alk. paper)
    1. Patient education.   I. Muma, Richard D.
    [DNLM: 1. Patient Education—methods.   W 85 P2976 1996]
R727.4.P375   1996
615.5′07—dc20
DNLM/DLC
for Library of Congress   95-35463
                                                                                                      CIP

Acquisitions Editor: Cheryl L. Mehalik
Production Editor: Todd Miller
Designer: Mary Skudlarek

PRINTED IN THE UNITED STATES OF AMERICA

ISBN 0-8385-2039-1

90000

9 780838 520390

Contents

Management 108
Life-style Changes 109
Addison's Disease..............................110
General Characteristics....................110
Signs, Symptoms, and Diagnosis 110
Management 111
Life-style Changes 111
Cushing's Syndrome 112
General Characteristics....................112
Signs, Symptoms, and Diagnosis 112
Management 112
Life-style Changes 113

11. Gastrointestinal Disorders.....................115
Hepatitis 115
General Characteristics....................115
Signs, Symptoms, and Diagnosis 115
Management 118
Life-style Changes 118
Pancreatitis 119
General Characteristics....................119
Signs, Symptoms, and Diagnosis 119
Management 119
Life-style Changes 120
Irritable Bowel Syndrome 121
General Characteristics....................121
Signs, Symptoms, and Diagnosis 121
Management 121
Life-style Changes 121
Diverticulosis....................................122
General Characteristics....................122
Signs, Symptoms, and Diagnosis 122
Management 122
Life-style Changes 122
Peptic Ulcer Disease 123
General Characteristics....................123
Signs, Symptoms, and Diagnosis 123
Management 123
Life-style Changes 123
Hiatal Hernia.....................................124
General Characteristics....................124
Signs, Symptoms, and Diagnosis 124
Management 124
Life-style Changes 124

12. Renal Disorders.................................125
Renal Calculi 125

General Characteristics....................125
Signs, Symptoms, and Diagnosis 125
Management 127
Life-style Changes 127
Acute Glomerulonephritis....................128
General Characteristics....................128
Signs, Symptoms, and Diagnosis 128
Management 128
Life-style Changes 129
Pyelonephritis 130
General Characteristics....................130
Signs, Symptoms, and Diagnosis 130
Management 130
Life-style Changes 131
Cystitis 132
General Characteristics....................132
Signs, Symptoms, and Diagnosis 132
Management 132
Life-style Changes 133
Urinary Incontinence 134
General Characteristics....................134
Signs, Symptoms, and Diagnosis 134
Management 136
Life-style Changes 138

13. Neurologic Disorders..........................139
Seizure Disorders...............................139
General Characteristics....................139
Signs, Symptoms, and Diagnosis 139
Management 139
Life-style Changes 139
Stroke 141
General Characteristics....................141
Signs, Symptoms, and Diagnosis 141
Management 141
Life-style Changes 143
Headaches 144
General Characteristics....................144
Signs, Symptoms, and Diagnosis 144
Management 144
Life-style Changes 145
Alzheimer's Disease............................146
General Characteristics....................146
Signs, Symptoms, and Diagnosis 146
Management 146
Life-style Changes 147

Contributors

Tammy Becker, PA-C
Physician Assistant
Temple, Texas

J. Dennis Blessing, PhD, PA-C
Associate Professor
Department of Physician Assistant Studies
School of Allied Health Sciences
The University of Texas Medical Branch
Galveston, Texas

Patricia A. Bunton, MA, PA-C
Academic Coordinator
Department of Physician Assistant
School of Health Sciences
College of Health Professions
Wichita State University
Wichita, Kansas

Roberto Canales, PA-C
Lecturer
Department of Physician Assistant Studies
School of Allied Health Sciences
The University of Texas Medical Branch
Galveston, Texas

Barbara A. Carnes, PhD, RN, CS
Assistant Professor
Department of Mental Health/Management
School of Nursing
The University of Texas Medical Branch
Galveston, Texas

Collier M. Cole, PhD
Associate Professor
Department of Physician Assistant Studies
School of Allied Health Sciences and
Clinical Associate Professor
Department of Psychiatry and Behavioral Sciences
School of Medicine
The University of Texas Medical Branch
Galveston, Texas

Janice G. Curry, PA-C
Physician Assistant
Division of Infectious Diseases
Department of Internal Medicine
School of Medicine
The University of Texas Medical Branch
Galveston, Texas

Debra D. Davis, PA-C
Physician Assistant
Department of Family Medicine
Wichita Clinic
Wichita, Kansas

Jeffrey W. East, PA-C
Physician Assistant
Division of Infectious Diseases
Department of Internal Medicine
School of Medicine
The University of Texas Medical Branch
Galveston, Texas

John Fuchs, Jr, PharmD
Coordinator of Clinical Services
Department of Pharmaceutical Care
The University of Texas Medical Branch
Galveston, Texas

Joey D. Hobbs, PA-C
Physician Assistant
Crossroads Family Medicine Rural Health Clinic
Leonard, Texas

Heather Walters Hull, RN, MSN, ARNP, PNP
Site Coordinator
Family Nurse Practitioner Program
School of Nursing
College of Health Professions
Wichita State University
Wichita, Kansas

Marvis J. Lary, PhD, PA-C
Chairperson
Department of Physician Assistant
School of Health Sciences
College of Health Professions
Wichita State University
Wichita, Kansas

Barbara Ann Lyons, MA, PA-C
Associate Professor
Department of Physician Assistant Studies
School of Allied Health Sciences
The University of Texas Medical Branch
Galveston, Texas

Catherine S. Marsh, RN, RMT
Registered Nurse and
Massage Therapist
The University of Texas Medical Branch
Galveston, Texas

Bernadette M. Montgomerie, RN
Registered Nurse
Division of Infectious Diseases
Department of Internal Medicine
School of Medicine
The University of Texas Medical Branch
Galveston, Texas

Richard D. Muma, MPH, PA-C
Assistant Director and Assistant Professor
Department of Physician Assistant
School of Health Sciences
College of Health Professions
Wichita State University
Wichita, Kansas

Teresa A. Newman, PA-C
Physician Assistant
Fort Worth, Texas

Stephen D. Newman, MD
Cardiologist
Department of Cardiology
John Peter Smith Hospital
Fort Worth, Texas

David P. Paar, MD
Assistant Professor
Division of Infectious Diseases
Department of Internal Medicine
School of Medicine
The University of Texas Medical Branch
Galveston, Texas

Sandee Roquemore, PA-C
Physician Assistant
Galveston, Texas

Doris J. Rosenow, PhD, RN
Assistant Professor
Department of Adult Health
School of Nursing
The University of Texas Medical Branch
Galveston, Texas

Albert F. Simon, MEd, PA-C
Program Director
Physician Assistant Program
Saint Francis College
Leretto, Pennsylvania

Karen S. Stephenson, MS, PA-C
Assistant Professor
Department of Physician Assistant Studies
School of Allied Health Sciences
The University of Texas Medical Branch
Galveston, Texas

Angela Wegmann, PA-C
Physician Assistant
Peoples Community Clinic
Austin, Texas

Preface

After the student clinician learns how to diagnose disease states and develop treatment plans, it is important for her or him to discuss with patients specific health care information related to their illness. The student should be able to discuss with patients the pathophysiology of disease states, symptoms and progression of disease, treatment modalities including drugs, nutrition, and exercise, and counsel those patients who are experiencing emotional reactions to their illness. *Patient Education: A Practical Approach* addresses these issues.

This book is important and timely in light of the recent health care reform movement. Since prevention is emphasized, greater care will be placed on educating patients; specifically, this means focusing on methods that will lead to improved patient understanding of diseases, increased adherence to medical regimens, and early recognition of problems by the patient.

Although all health care providers will play a role in educating patients, this book is aimed toward midlevel practitioner students and professionals: advanced practice nurses and physician assistants. These practitioners have been identified as key players in the delivery of primary care and patient education.

A strength of this book is that it provides the clinician with useful and practical patient education information on many primary-care diseases. All parts of the book provide step-by-step information, whether it be learning the approach to patient education, selecting patient education materials, or reviewing one of several primary care diseases.

Patient Education is divided into 19 chapters. Chapter 1 introduces the general approach to patient education. It is here that the student can learn the required components of a patient education session which includes discussion of disease, treatment options, prevention, compliance, and psychosocial issues. Chapter 2 discusses methods to "fine tune" the approach one may take when educating patients. Subjects such as age, family issues, socioeconomic status, ethnicity, and death are discussed. Chapter 3 is reserved for a discussion of ways to select patient education material. This includes information on personalizing patient educational material and the use of computers to do so. Chapter 4, entitled "Behavior Modification," discusses issues such as diet, exercise, high-risk sexual behaviors, smoking, prevention, and wellness and how all of these topics can be incorporated into the patient education session. Chapter 5 addresses the issue of medication nonadherence. A step-by-step approach gives the clinician a methodology for recognizing and managing noncompliance in patients. Chapter 6 discusses how one can incorporate patient education into clinical practice. Chapters 7 through 19, constitute the clinical focus of the book; they include more than 70 medical conditions organized by body system. Each system section contains the most frequently seen diseases or medical conditions and includes illustrations for patient teaching.

Part III contains patient education handouts that can be photocopied and given to the patient. Additionally, the handouts as well as a blank template for customization are included on an easty-to-use 3.5 inch computer disk for those who wish. The files are in WordPerfect 5.1® format. Finally, in Appendix 2 there is a brief overview of alternative medicine. The purpose of this section is not to discuss in detail the specific types of alternative therapies, but rather give the reader a general picture of alternative practices and why patients choose them.

This book can be used in nursing, physician assistant, and medical curricula when medical interviewing, physical examination, and clinical medicine courses are completed. Ideally the book should be used in a separate patient education course; however, patient education content may be integrated into other courses throughout the curriculum of study.

Most chapters offer references to current reviews and studies on the corresponding topic for the individual who wishes to pursue any topic in greater detail.

The overall goal of this book is to provide the health care student or clinician with concise, up-to-date information on patient education and various primary care diseases to enable the optimal care of patients.

Richard D. Muma
Barbara Ann Lyons
Teresa A. Newman
Barbara A. Carnes

Acknowledgments

We acknowledge the input of our students who have helped shape the contents of this book, the cooperation of our contributing authors, and the continuing support of our colleagues. We would like to thank our editor, Cheryl Mehalik of Appleton & Lange, for her interest in the book and her helpfulness throughout the production of the manuscript.

PATIENT EDUCATION

A Practical Approach

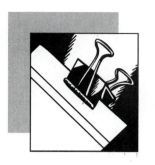

Part One
Patient Education

An Approach to Patient Education

Collier M. Cole

Introduction

As the 21st century approaches, it is an understatement to observe that the health care field is increasingly complex and diversified. In recent years there have been dramatic changes in the number of providers, advances in medical technology and the understanding of disease, and striking developments in various methods to treat these problems. The bottom line, or raison d'etre, of these advancements in health care delivery is to be able to provide better patient treatment toward the goal of effecting a healthy outcome. The chief means to accomplish this goal is through an interactive educational process. Whether it involves asking an individual simply to take medication or to make substantial life-style changes to promote better health, providers must be able to effectively communicate, educate, and motivate the patient.

Various approaches to patient education have been outlined over the years and are currently used in the training of health care providers.[1-7] All emphasize the importance of providing accurate information and encouraging patients to assume more responsibility for their own treatment. Many of the techniques employed to accomplish such education share common characteristics. For example, explanations need to be given in simple terms, avoiding jargon that might be confusing. Also, the health care provider must assess the patient's understanding of the information in case further explanation is necessary to clarify questions or reduce confusion. Careful attention must also be given to patients' emotional responses to a particular diagnosis or treatment method, as these reactions can have significant impact on outcome.

Effective patient education should be duly recognized as an integral building block in the entire health delivery process, of equal importance to clinical and technological advancements in the field. For example, Greenberg noted how important this two-way communication process is and how its impact can be felt way beyond the immediate medical problem being treated.[8] He suggested that good patient education will:

- *enable patients to assume greater responsibility for their own health care;*
- *improve their ability to manage acute as well as chronic illnesses;*
- *provide opportunities to choose healthier life-styles and practice preventive medicine;*
- *improve compliance with medication and treatment regimens;*
- *increase satisfaction with care and thus reduce the risk of liability;*
- *attract patients to your practice; and*
- *lead to a more efficient, cost-effective health care system.*

A Model for Patient Education

Recognizing the importance of patient education is the first step. Then follows the actual learning of techniques involved in the communication-interview process in order to be able to effectively educate and motivate patients to be active participants in their own health care, rather than passive responders. Thus, specific courses that teach medical interviewing and patient education skills are necessary. The format may include lectures for the purpose of describing the "content" of the medical interview (eg, topics to be covered) and the "process" of the interaction (eg, use of specific interviewing techniques). In addition, opportunities should be available to practice these interviewing skills through small-group role play with simulated patients recruited from the community who are trained to act very much like real patients. Simulated patients should report various health symptoms and express the variety of emotional reactions that often accompany such health problems. Another method is the use of a checklist, which can aid in learning how to put the interview together and cover both content and process aspects of the interaction. Figure 1–1 displays the various elements involved in this checklist.

One can easily adapt this model to accommodate whatever disease problem needs to be reviewed with the patient. Following is a brief discussion of the elements listed, which can serve as a refresher for conducting the interview.

1. Opening the Interview

- Putting the patient at ease
- Use of social amenities
- Eye contact
- Professional demeanor
- Layout of interview plan

Opening the patient education interview, like opening any communicative interchange, can be enhanced by using several short phrases that serve as social amenities. These can include such remarks as, "Any problems getting into the office today?" or "Hope you haven't had to wait long," or "Are you enjoying the nice weather today?" All of these serve to "break the ice" and set the stage for the social interaction about to follow. Furthermore, they can be of clinical importance in that they allow the interviewer to quickly assess the patient's general attitude. A smile and pleasant response communicates a mood far different from another one in which the patient simply grunts or stares back. This latter communication may suggest pain or discomfort, a "let's get down to business" attitude, or perhaps underlying fear at what may be about to happen. Other essential ingredients of the interview involve using good eye contact and maintaining a professional demeanor (eg, neat appearance, concerned and attentive attitude, appropriate note-taking).

Finally, in setting the stage for the interview, giving the patient some sense of what is going to occur (eg, a layout) is essential for the soon-to-follow educational process. Just as in a classroom situation where an outline of a lecture can help a student follow the material, so can a layout for the health education interview assist the patient. For example, one might say, "What I would like to do today is explain our findings to you and what we have come up with as a diagnosis. Then I would like to describe the treatment plan we have developed for you and respond to any questions you may have about it. Does that sound okay?"

2. Discussion of the Disease

- Report lab findings
- Give diagnosis
- Assess what patient knows
- Assess patient's initial feelings and attitudes
- Explain pathophysiology
- Vocabulary appropriate to patient
- Correctness of information
- Assess patient's final understanding

One can make the transition from the opening interchange to this section with a remark such as, "Now let's talk about our findings." This is the opportunity to report on lab work, x-rays, or other medical procedures completed so that a patient clearly understands what he or she was being tested for and what the results suggest. As noted earlier, using clear explanations with no jargon is essential.

After summarizing the laboratory and physical findings gathered during the patient's first appointment, it is now time to give a diagnosis, which might begin, "After reviewing the lab findings and your physical examination, we have concluded that you have a problem called. . . ." It is best then to ask the patient, "What do you know about this condition?" This will allow the interviewer to quickly identify any myths or misinformation the patient currently holds, as well as any particular fears the individual may have about the diagnosis (eg, perhaps a relative had a similar diagnosis and experienced continuing problems). Clearly such issues will need to be addressed during the course of the education interview.

The importance of assessing the patient's attitudes and feelings regarding a diagnosis cannot be overemphasized. This should be done early on in the interview and again toward the end. One might, for instance, say, "How do you feel now about learning that you have this sort of problem?" Being able to provide support and reassurance to a patient apprehensive

STUDENT _____ RATER _____ DATE_____

Instructions: Rate the student's performance in each of the following areas. Where appropriate, mark the narrative descriptors in the left column. Circle one number in the right column for each category.

Weak   Outstanding

1. OPENING THE INTERVIEW

    Putting the patient at ease _____   Use of social amenities _____
    Eye contact _____   Professional demeanor _____
    Layout of plan _____

    1   2   3   4   5   6   7   8   9
    Notes: _____
    _____
    _____

2. DISCUSSION OF DISEASE

    Assesses what patient knows _____   Assesses patient's attitudes/feelings _____   Reports lab findings _____   Explains pathophysiology _____   Vocabulary appropriate to patient _____
    Correctness of information _____   Assesses patient's final understanding _____

    1   2   3   4   5   6   7   8   9
    Notes: _____
    _____
    _____
    _____
    _____
    _____

3. TREATMENT

    Presents complete plan _____   Presents treatment goals _____
    Explains side effects/complications _____   Treatment individualized to patient _____   Assesses patient compliance _____   Correctness of information _____   Assesses patient's final understanding _____

    1   2   3   4   5   6   7   8   9
    Notes: _____
    _____
    _____
    _____
    _____

4. ASSESSMENT OF PATIENT'S UNDERSTANDING OF DISEASE AND TREATMENT

    Assesses patient's overall understanding of disease and treatment _____
    Assesses patient's attitudes _____   Allows for questions _____
    Flexible in presentation _____

    1   2   3   4   5   6   7   8   9

    Notes: _____
    _____
    _____

5. APPROPRIATE USE OF COUNSELING TECHNIQUES

    Tried to clarify patient's statement _____   Reassurance and empathy _____   Appropriate use of silence _____   Appropriate vocabulary _____   Use of open-ended questions _____   Facilitative behavior _____   Use of notes _____   Use of educational aids _____
    Flexible _____   Good use of probes _____   Good transitions _____
    Appropriate pacing _____   Good use of summaries _____   Overall physical appearance _____   Nonverbal language _____   Appropriate use of patient's background _____   Makes clear the next step for patient _____   Asking for questions _____

    1   2   3   4   5   6   7   8   9
    Notes: _____
    _____
    _____
    _____
    _____
    _____
    _____
    _____
    _____
    _____

6. OVERALL EFFECTIVENESS OF CONDUCTING PATIENT COUNSELING

    Rapport building _____   Discussion of disease (pathophysiology) _____
    Treatment program _____   Assessment of patient's understanding of disease and treatment _____   Use of counseling techniques _____

    1   2   3   4   5   6   7   8   9
    Notes: _____
    _____
    _____

7. COMMENTS AND SUGGESTIONS FOR IMPROVEMENT: _____

_____

_____

_____

_____

Figure 1–1. Patient Education Rating Form

about his or her condition is an integral part of the treatment process and can help to ensure compliance with later treatment directives.

At this point in the interview, it is now valuable for the health care provider to explain the pathophysiology of the disease process. Such information should be provided in simple, straightforward terminology and it can often be facilitated by the use of diagrams or analogies that are more comprehensible. Providing such information both verbally and visually may contribute to a more complete understanding. Once the explanation has been provided, it is critical to check out the patient's comprehension and understanding of his or her condition. To do so, one might ask, "I would like you to explain back to me, very briefly, your understanding of this problem." Any misinformation can then be corrected to ensure full and accurate awareness of the situation.

3. Treatment

- Present treatment goals
- Present complete treatment plan
- Treatment individualized to patient
- Explain side effects or complications of medication
- Correctness of information
- Assess patient's compliance
- Assess patient's final understanding

Following the pathophysiology discussion, one now needs to review the specific treatment plan that has been designed for this particular patient. To move into this section one might say, "Now let's talk about how we're going to treat this problem." It's best to start off by highlighting the overriding goals of the treatment plan. For example, common goals can be to alleviate pain, reduce and eliminate the disease process, ensure satisfactory functioning, and maintain a satisfying quality of life-style. Then one might go on to say, "To accomplish these goals, we've developed a three-step treatment plan for you." This would be the opportunity to identify and explain fully the specific steps in the treatment plan (eg, medication, exercise, weight reduction, smoking cessation, or whatever is appropriate for the defined condition). It should be noted that it is particularly helpful if the interviewer identifies the number of steps in the treatment plan, whether three or four or more. Doing so can provide a framework, which tends to be less confusing for the patient and aids in acquiring a full picture of

what is being asked, rather than what so often happens when a health care provider tries to explain a treatment plan by saying, "And next . . . , and next . . . , and next. . . ." Facilitating the treatment explanation by providing handouts or diagrams and encouraging a question-and-answer dialogue can maximize the effectiveness of this interactive process (see Patient Information Sheets).

When medication is being discussed as a treatment step, it is of special importance that one be very clear about the uses and side effects of such medication, including any potential interactions with other drugs or food as well as proper methods of storing the medication. Reviewing such important considerations and providing package inserts or other data sheets regarding a medication that a patient can take home are vital to increasing compliance and avoiding unnecessary problems (see Chapter 5).

As one might expect, certain aspects of a treatment plan will likely be easier for a patient to follow than others. For example, it may be easier for an individual to take medication than to try to make substantial changes in his or her life-style. One can always expect some resistance and difficulty when trying to effect the latter changes. In order to make some assessment of how a patient is going to handle the prescribed treatment plan, it can be prudent to ask probing questions such as, "Which of these treatment steps will be the easiest for you to follow?" and "Which will be the most difficult?" In some instances, it may be more practical to try to encourage the patient to accomplish those treatment steps that are easiest to comply with and save the more difficult ones to address for a later interview. Otherwise, one may run the risk of turning off the patient completely, and he or she may not return for any follow-up.

At the conclusion of this section it is once again important to assess the patient's final understanding of what needs to be done. This might be accomplished by a request such as, "I would like you to repeat for me now the treatment steps involved in your plan." By so doing, one can ensure that the patient comprehends the treatment program and is prepared to go forward with the prescribed plan.

4. Summarizing the Interview

- Assess patient's overall understanding of disease and treatment
- Allow for questions

- Assess patient's attitudes and feelings toward disease and treatment
- Provide handouts
- Schedule follow-up visit

Upon completion of discussing both pathophysiology and treatment, it is helpful to assess the patient's overall understanding. This can be done by asking, "Are there any questions now about your condition or about the treatment plan we've developed?" This would provide the patient the final opportunity to raise issues that may be unclear as well as allow the interviewer to evaluate final comprehension and gauge compliance. In addition, this would be the time for the interviewer to ask, "Now that you are aware of your condition and the treatment steps you need to follow, how do you feel about this whole process?" Again, it is critical to ensuring an eventual positive outcome to assess how the patient feels about the situation. Underlying fears or doubts about being able to follow the treatment plan need to be addressed. Typically, a patient may be overwhelmed by what has been presented and may feel that he or she is not going to be able to handle the necessary steps in treatment. This is often a point at which the health care professional can demonstrate empathy, offering support and encouragement. For example, one might say, "I know this is a lot to deal with right now, but I want to assure you that I will be here to support you throughout this process." This sort of reassurance can be timely and helpful to the patient about to leave and embark upon making changes. In addition, providing various materials that the patient can take home for further study and for sharing with family can be quite helpful. Finally, scheduling a follow-up appointment and making sure the patient will be able to attend at the appointed time brings the interview to conclusion.

5. Appropriate Use of Interviewing Techniques
- Tries to clarify patient's statements
- Reassurance and empathy
- Appropriate use of silence
- Appropriate vocabulary
- Use of open-ended questions
- Facilitative behavior
- Use of notes
- Use of educational aids
- Flexible in presentation

- Good transitions
- Appropriate pacing
- Good use of summaries
- Professional in appearance and demeanor
- Appropriate use of nonverbal language
- Appropriate use of patient's background
- Makes clear the next step for patient
- Asks for questions
- Closure and follow-up

The above techniques are basic to any good interview process. It is critical to use appropriate vocabulary to make sure a patient fully understands the nature of the disease as well as the treatment being prescribed. In addition, patients should be encouraged to express their thoughts and feelings, and this can be accomplished with such techniques as facilitation, eye contact, use of silence, and open-ended as well as direct questions. The key to a successful interchange involves flexibility on the part of the interviewer. It may be important to vary from the didactic, informational aspects of the interview to pay attention to a patient's need for reassurance and empathy. Moving through the interview in a well-paced fashion and using smooth transitions from section to section makes the entire interview more understandable to the patient as he or she tries to absorb all the information being offered. Finally, the use of audiovisual aids or handouts can be critical to ensuring that a patient fully comprehends his or her medical problem as well as what needs to be done to address it.

Specific Suggestions for Enhancing the Patient Education Process

1. Pay Attention to Using Good Interviewing Techniques. Helping patients to successfully deal with medical problems involves being able both to educate and to motivate for change. This requires use of skillful interpersonal techniques. One needs to be attuned to both verbal and nonverbal aspects of the interaction. With time and practice, one will develop a sense of when it's best to be silent and listen to a patient and when to provide specific educational information or support. Being prepared and organized ahead of time (eg, having lab work on the chart, pulling together handouts, having a written-out treatment plan specifically for the patient) will facilitate the entire process and likely improve understanding and compliance.

2. Present Information Through Several Channels. Do not simply rely on direct verbal communication to ensure a patient's understanding. For some people, verbal learning is not as successful as visual learning. That is, some individuals may understand and retain information better if they are able to look at a handout, chart, or follow an examination of an x-ray. Also, some patients may benefit from the opportunity to meet and talk with others who have dealt with a certain problem or are currently undergoing treatment for a particular medical condition. Such peer support can be a very effective tool in motivating an individual to comply with treatment.

3. Always Supplement the Educational Process with Handouts. The patient education process can be overwhelming, as so much information may need to be covered. It is therefore recommended to provide patients with brochures, handouts, medication inserts, an outline of the treatment plan, or other materials that will permit later perusal to reinforce what was covered during the actual interview.

4. Involve Families or Significant Others Where Possible. Remember that the patients are part of a larger family system. Most often these family members are very concerned about the health of their loved one, and involving them in the treatment process can be very useful. Indeed, such involvement may in some cases ensure compliance with a treatment plan. Ask how the patient is going to explain a particular health problem to his or her family. Invite family members to attend a follow-up appointment so that they, too, can hear about the situation and learn how they can help.

5. Be Sure to Raise the Sensitive Issues. There are certain subjects that tend to be highly sensitive, and some patients may have underlying concerns or fears that they may not openly voice. Such topics as sexuality or death and dying fall into this category. Because these topics may produce embarrassment or feelings of despondency, a patient may be reluctant to inquire about them. Therefore, it is critical for the health care professional to initiate such discussion

when it is clearly pertinent to the treatment plan (eg, medications that might interfere with sexual functioning, the need for a patient to recognize that the treatment options for a particular condition may be only palliative). Raising these issues signals that it is all right to talk about more sensitive matters and allows the patient to openly express his or her underlying fears and concerns.

6. Be Attuned to Emotional Reactions. As noted above, patients experience emotional reactions to learning of a particular illness and the need to follow a course of treatment. Providing comprehensive health care requires exploring these emotional topics. Whether the patient is expressing fear, anger, anxiety, or depression, unless the health care professional inquires about such reactions and takes steps to address them, treatment outcome may be in jeopardy. Allowing for ventilation of feelings and offering support are viewed as an integral part of the patient education process.

7. Don't Feel that Once the Topic is Covered it is Completely Resolved for the Patient. For some individuals, providing education about a disease or treatment plan will be enough to motivate them to go forward and carry out what has been prescribed. For others, however, there may be lingering confusion or questions after this interview that will need to be addressed at a later time. In addition, certain aspects of the treatment plan that are more difficult for a patient to deal with (eg, making life-style changes such as smoking cessation or weight reduction) will need to be reviewed and reencouraged at a later appointment. It is always prudent to review a patient's treatment plan at each subsequent follow-up visit, offering praise for the accomplishments and noting areas for additional attention.

8. It's Okay to Say, "I Don't Know." It is not uncommon for a health care professional to be asked a question that he or she is unprepared for and for which a ready answer is not immediately available. Rather than trying to stumble through a lame explanation or using technical jargon in an effort to cover up, it is always recommended that the interviewer simply respond with, "I don't know." Realistically, one may not have the answer to certain questions, and it is best to acknowledge this fact. The interviewer might go on to say something like, "I really don't know the answer to that question, but let me look into it and I'll get back to you with an answer."

Conclusion

It is hoped that the model and suggestions offered in this chapter on how to approach the patient education interview will serve as a "refresher" for the reader. While this is certainly not the only approach to use, it is one that is comprehensive and addresses both process and content aspects of the interview. It is expected that each health care provider will develop his or her own style of interacting with patients, perhaps altering this model to fit his or her specific needs.

As the reader goes through this text, he or she should imagine how each particular problem might be adapted to the framework presented here.

References

1. Bates B. *A Guide to the Physical Examination and History*. 5th ed. Philadelphia, Pa: JB Lippincott Co; 1991.
2. Guckian, J, ed. *The Clinical Interview and Physical Examination*. Philadelphia, Pa: JB Lippincott Co; 1987.
3. Enelow A, Swisher S. *Interviewing and Patient Care*. 3rd ed. New York, NY: Oxford University Press; 1985.
4. Sherilyn-Cormier L, Cormier W, Weissen R. *Interviewing and Helping Skills for Health Professionals*. Monterey, Calif. Wadsworth Health Sciences Division; 1984.
5. Henderson G. *Physician-Patient Communication*. Springfield, Ill: Charles C Thomas; 1981.
6. Bernstein L. *Interviewing: a Guide for Health Professionals*. 3rd ed. New York, NY: Appleton-Century-Crofts; 1980.
7. Stevenson I. *The Diagnostic Interview*. 2nd ed. New York, NY: Harper & Row, 1971.
8. Greenberg L. Build your practice with patient education. *Contemp Pediat*. September 1989;85–106.

2

Factors Influencing Patient Education

Richard D. Muma

Introduction

There are many parts to the concept of health, including how one thinks about disease and its cures. Health care in the United States is based primarily on treating acute, well-advanced disease processes, using an infectious disease paradigm. However, the causes of poor health and serious disease processes are no longer associated with a single infectious microbe but instead are linked to a multiplicity of factors, particularly behavioral and cognitive habits along with specific social and physical environments. Patients often react to illness and its management in ways learned from others, according to their cultural norms, and according to their own perception of the severity of the illness. Before engaging in a patient education session, one must realize that every patient responds differently and several variables or factors play a role in that response. Some of those factors identified for discussion in this chapter include age, ethnicity, family issues, socioeconomic status, and the chronicity of illness.

Age

Although an obvious consideration, age is not always reflected in patient education materials and is often overlooked in the patient education counseling session. One must remember the range of care starts with infants and ends with the elderly. Let us start with children. They are not small adults, and their wants, needs, thinking processes, and emotional and physical status differ from those of an adult. For example, small children often view hospitalization as a punishment, not as means of getting well.[1] This belief is further reinforced when parental figures make such statements as, "If you go outside without shoes on you may get sick and have to go see the doctor." This type of belief often leads to false perceptions about clinicians and to a child's difficulty in accepting medical advice or treatment. Infants, although not directly involved in patient counseling sessions, have special needs and respond to touch and nonverbal communication.[1] As children grow older, however, one must keep in mind the current fads, language, and norms that exist. For example, teenagers often believe themselves to be experts in every area and, in some cases, do not heed advice. Furthermore, certain instructions given to teenagers regarding prevention of illness may not be "cool" or in line with the thinking of their peer group.

Adults are more mature and have different concerns from adolescents. For instance, young adults (ages 20 to 40) are at a point in life where multiple activities (eg, college, relationships, children) keep them busy.[1] These patients need practical approaches to education; approaches that are not time-consuming and unrealistic in relation to their lives. As adults grow older (ages 40 to 60) they become more conscious of the possibility of health problems and in most cases are willing to follow a patient education prescription. However, some may lack self-confidence, which can cause avoidance of the risk of failure in learning anything new.[1] Adults over the age of 65 are similar to middle-aged adults in their willingness to learn new ideas, but the provider must be aware of the individuals' past experiences, involve them in the learning process, and motivate them to learn.[1] Elderly patients may feel that it is hardly worth the effort to learn new information and skills, since they think their life is nearing the end.[1]

Ethnicity

Before we discuss ethnicity, it is important to define the adjective, *ethnic. Ethnic* is defined in the 1982 version of the *Amer-*

ican Heritage Dictionary of the English Language as follows: of or pertaining to a social group that claims or is accorded special status on the basis of complex, often variable traits including religious, linguistic, ancestral, or physical characteristics. Ethnicity is simply defined as the condition of belonging to a particular ethnic group.[2] Examples of ethnic groups in the United States include African American, Asian, Caucasian, Hispanic, and Native American. There are at least 106 ethnic groups and more than 170 Native American groups in the United States.[3] Ethnic groups should not be confused with minority groups, as the latter are seen as different from the majority group of which they are part. However, some ethnic groups are also classified as minorities, eg, African Americans in the United States. One can see that the phenomenon of ethnicity is complex, ambivalent, paradoxical, and elusive.[4] As clinicians, it is important to be aware of the ethnic backgrounds of patients. The differences in language and culture each group exhibits will certainly influence the way patient education is communicated.[5] For example, some feel HIV prevention literature is not communicated effectively to African American populations. HIV programs are hampered because of the presence of culturally specific attitudes and beliefs, including those pertaining to the roles of males and females.[5]

Family

Although consideration of the individual is important in patient education, the patient's family is also of central importance if teaching is to be effective.[6] How a family functions influences the health of its members as well as how an individual reacts to illness. Including the family members and significant others in patient education sessions will facilitate adherence, understanding of the disease process, and confidence needed to perform specific skills. Hence, the health professional should capitalize on what family members can do for the patient and work with them in encouraging the patient in tasks that may be difficult. For example, when educating a patient with diabetes mellitus who requires insulin injections, involvement of the family in teaching sessions demonstrating insulin injections will most likely improve compliance. Family members can also serve as troubleshooters when the patient has difficulty performing complex tasks. However, not all patients have family or significant others available for support. This is frequently seen in cases of HIV infection. Patients are often isolated from others after their diagnosis is made known.

These patients are often on complex medical regimens involving the use of intravenous catheters. Unavailable support sometimes leads to poor care, missed doses, and increased morbidity and mortality.

The health professional can do much to facilitate the effectiveness of patient teaching by fostering discussion among significant others. A professional who has continued contact with the patient and his or her significant others may check on the progress of the patient when necessary and identify any new problems that may interfere with optimal care.

Socioeconomic Status

The socioeconomic status of patients should be carefully considered when initiating education sessions. Individuals in lower socioeconomic groups are less likely to seek treatment, if they seek treatment they tend to access health care later in the course of their illness, and they die sooner than individuals in higher socioeconomic classes. Hence, the clinician should be aware of the patient's personal income, living arrangements, and employment status but also have an increased awareness of the patient's health. Lower socioeconomic status has been linked to the development of disease states, the most noted being coronary artery disease.[7,8] For example, the provider clearly cannot erase poverty and improve access to health care for all; however, he or she can exert a positive impact on lower socioeconomic groups by working with their members to promote healthier life-styles.[5] Some individuals often do not know what resources are available. The provider should point individuals to local resources that provide services and, if not possible, attempt to arrange for those services for the patient.

Chronicity of Disease

Finally, illnesses that are acute present differently from those that are chronic and will cause a variety of reactions among patients. Health care providers must be aware of those illnesses that require extra emotional support and possible psychiatric intervention when preparing for patient education sessions. Furthermore, it is not enough to simply inform a patient of his or her medical condition without time for an initial reaction. Patients require time to react to a new diagnosis. The perceived seriousness and natural course of a disease will help determine how a patient will respond. For instance, the patient diagnosed with acute pharyngitis may feel really terrible during the illness but knows that it is a curable disease and usually self-limiting. Hence, this patient may have fewer emotional problems and require less counseling. Whereas the patient diagnosed with stage IV breast cancer, in which the long-term prognosis is known to be poor, will have an emotional response that may need further intervention involving a psychiatrist, social worker, or nursing care.

References

1. Anderson C. *Patient Teaching and Communication in an Information Age.* Albany, NY: Delmar Publishers; 1990:76–102.
2. *The American Heritage Dictionary of the English Language.* New York, NY: Dell Publishing Co; 1982:247.
3. Thernstrom S. *Harvard Encyclopedia of American Ethnic Groups,* p. vii. Cambridge, Mass: Belknap Press of Harvard University; 1980.
4. Senior C. *The Puerto Ricans: Strangers Then Neighbors.* Chicago: Quadrangle Books; 1965:21.
5. Lyons BA, Valentine P. Prevention. In: Muma RD, Lyons BA, Borucki MJ, et al, eds. *HIV Manual for Health Care Professionals.* Norwalk, Conn: Appleton & Lange; 1994:257.
6. Falvo DR. *Effective Patient Education.* Rockville, MD: Aspen Publications; 1985:99–109.
7. Marmot MG, Adelstein AM, Robinson N, et al. Changing social-class distribution of heart disease. *Br Med J.* 1978; 2:1109–1112.
8. Morgenstern H. The changing association between social status and coronary heart disease in a rural population. *Soc Sci Med.* 1980;14A:191–201.

3

Selecting and Evaluating Sources of Patient Education Materials

Barbara Ann Lyons

Patient education draws on a broad-based set of materials that can help explain a spectrum of topics. On some occasions, the patient education process is short and quite focused, while at other times it is long and detailed. An example of a brief encounter is the education of a patient on an acute medical problem, like a viral sore throat, which has few sequelae and will respond without particular treatment. For such a medical problem, usually a brief discussion of palliative treatments (ie, saline gargles and throat lozenges) is all that is needed. On the other hand, patient education needs to be more detailed for a condition of longer duration, such as pregnancy or a chronic disease state like diabetes. In these two conditions, there are continual changes that occur and many behaviors to explain. One would need to use several techniques and allow sufficient time to explain both types of problems.

Types of Instructional Materials

There are many types of instructional aids that can be used with patients. The first major category is printed material. Fact sheets are usually single-page sheets used to distill information about a disease or treatment (see Chapter 20). These fact sheets give the major points of information and are useful for the patient to use as guidelines at home. The advantages of fact sheets are that they are short and can easily keep the attention of the patient. The single-page fact sheet can be of low cost to procure or reproduce and can be modified with individual instruction for each patient. Individualization can be accomplished by having an area at the bottom of the sheet for personal instruction or by having the fact sheets on computer,

with the opportunity to fill in specifics before printing. Single-sheet handouts are easy to keep in a file drawer or folder in the examining room for easy access. For offices with computer capability in the examining rooms, the sheet can be printed at the time of need, obviating the need for storage of preprinted materials.

Disadvantages of the fact sheet include that they may be too short to be very detailed and may not answer some of the patient's questions, especially if the disease process or its treatment is very complex. It is possible that fact sheets may be more expensive if reproduced from rented or leased computer software than if they are produced by the clinic personnel. If a computer and printer are required for reproduction of fact sheets, it would add to the cost. If a computer system is already in place, the added cost, is minimal when the fact sheets are designed by clinic personnel.

Another type of printed material is pamphlets, which are usually small in size and concern a particular disease or treatment. Advantages of pamphlets are that they are short and may be provided at no cost by pharmaceutical companies or low cost by professional societies. These materials are professionally designed, edited, and printed. Pharmaceutical companies frequently provide patient education pamphlets describing the pathophysiology and treatment of conditions that the drugs they sell are intended to treat. For example, a pharmaceutical company that sells a major antihypertensive drug may provide materials about hypertension and its treatment.

Disease-specific and professional societies may sell, at a low cost, pamphlets about the disease or condition that is their cause. For example, the American Cancer Society provides materials about specific tumors as well as about prevention of cancer. Another type of society is a group of health professionals who have a particular medical interest. The American Ophthalmology Association provides pamphlets about diseases of the eye in general as well as specific eye disease entities, like macular degeneration and diabetic retinopathy.

Health departments may also provide pamphlets for local use concerning problems in a particular community. These pamphlets may reflect the diversity of the local population and may be in languages other than English. These materials are usually free of cost, but they may not be as professionally produced, may not use glossy paper, and may include no photographs.

One of the disadvantages of pamphlets is that they cannot usually be personalized for a particular patient. Some pamphlets are intended to sell or accompany particular drugs and may give undue emphasis to that drug treatment regimen or pharmaceutical company, while others give balanced views of the options available. It is wise to review all materials for suitability to one's patient population.

Books are another level of printed material and include fuller information about a disease or condition, with consideration given to explicit, detailed discussion of the topics. These books may be provided by the clinician's practice or recommended for the patient to purchase. Some books may be provided free of charge by pharmaceutical companies or at low cost by professional or disease-oriented associations.

One advantage of a book is that more detail is available concerning the disease or condition. The increased level of detail may reduce requests for further information, since the patient can refer to the resource rather than contact the medical care provider. For example, an obstetrician's practice may provide a small paperback about pregnancy and related issues that explains basics of related problems and states measures to be taken, as well as when further input by the health care provider is warranted.

Disadvantages include high cost, as books are usually more expensive than fact sheets or pamphlets. Reading level may also be higher than for the less detailed forms of printed information. Since much more information is presented, there is more opportunity for information to be at variance with the clinician's beliefs. Books are not as easily updated as shorter forms of printed materials and, of course, are not personalized for a particular practice setting or patient.

Magazines are another form of printed material. Magazines contain articles that usually highlight a new breakthrough in the diagnosis or treatment of a disease or condition, making the topic newsworthy. Magazine articles usually contain up-to-date information and make information widely available to the general public. Magazine articles may not have a medical point of view, which may be a disadvantage. Articles may be of use at or near the time of publication, but they are not updated on a regular basis and therefore may be of limited value as they become less current. A noteworthy article can usually be reproduced with permission of the publisher.

Some practices keep special anatomic pictures in the examining rooms to help clinicians explain common problems. For example, anatomic ear diagrams are used in many practices where otitis media is a common disorder. As necessary, the clinician can point out the anatomic problem as the condition is being discussed. Some practices have added chalkboards to examining rooms so that spontaneous drawings can be made by the health care provider or patient educator. Some clinicians resort to drawings on paper to help describe the problem.

Audiovisual materials do not require patients to have reading ability. Several types of audiovisuals may be used. Audiotapes are inexpensive, and audiocassette players are generally available in most patient populations. Audiotapes can be easily updated in a practice setting. They may be easily duplicated and are sometimes provided by drug companies or other sources. Reading ability is not required unless they are accompanied by written materials. Audiotapes have a cost; however, they are generally less expensive than books, but more expensive than the other printed materials.

Videotapes are becoming a popular option for distributing patient education information. Videos on various medical topics are produced and distributed by pharmaceutical companies, hospitals, and offices. For example, companies that produce prenatal vitamins and infant formula produce and distribute, through pediatrician offices, a videotape on the technique of breast-feeding. Many patients have videocassette recorders (VCRs) in their homes, which makes this technique very effective. This method is especially helpful for demonstrating skills, since the video can be replayed and stopped at the will of the viewer so that skills can be practiced. Some practice settings have VCRs in the waiting room or in a viewing room so that videos can be viewed at the practice setting and questions can be answered after the video is viewed. This method is effective since it takes advantage of more than one route for imparting information. It is also independent of reading level. Cost may be a drawback for some. It is cheapest to lend the video to the patient for home viewing, with subsequent return to the practice when finished. A more expensive approach is to set-up a VCR viewing area in the practice setting; however, this requires designated space for viewing, tape storage, VCR equipment, equipment maintenance, and security measures. If a lending library is used, there are personnel costs for keeping track of materials. Other more advanced forms of technology such as interactive video, computer-assisted instruction, laser disk technology, Internet access, and medical television programs increase costs even more. Synchronized slide-tape programs use older technology and may be a less expensive option.

Finally, classes and self-help groups offered by health care workers and other professionals can present information regarding a particular subject (ie, diabetes and nutrition). These sessions may be presented in a classroom, workshop, or small group. An advantage of this approach is that information can be shared easily, with immediate reinforcement. The cost associated with this format may be prohibitive in some practices and for some patients, but some insurance companies may reimburse this type of medical expense.

Sources of Instructional Material

Patient education materials can be found through many sources. Pharmaceutical and medical equipment companies often provide disease or condition information related to the drugs or other products the company sells. Materials vary greatly, as described earlier. The materials can be procured by contacting the company or its representative. Current addresses and telephone numbers can be found in the *Physicians' Desk Reference.*

Professional organizations can be a source of balanced education materials. The American College of Obstetrics and Gynecology, American Academy of Dermatology, American Medical Association, and the American Academy of Pediatrics are cases in point (Table 3–1).

The United States Government is the source for many low-cost, balanced patient education materials (Table 3–2). Basic information can be procured through its consumer education division in Pueblo, Colorado. Other information can be gained through contacting specific sections of the government that lead research efforts for specific diseases. For example, the National Heart, Lung, and Blood Institute provides information on heart and lung diseases, whereas the National Cancer Institute provides information on cancers. Both have materials related to changing behaviors and prevention.

Some medical journals provide articles that have information specifically designed for patients and can either be duplicated or purchased for distribution. This information is often written by leading experts in the medical field and reports cutting-edge material and the latest advances in medicine.

The popular press provides many types of patient information. Local newspapers and magazines like *The New York Times, Time, US News and World Report, Newsweek,* and other monthly publications like *Men's Health* and *Women's Day* provide information in health columns and occasionally as cover story material. Other magazines, like *Consumer Reports*, may provide special medical reports in the magazine and then as reprints. Other publishers use magazines to impart information, such as Lamaze and childbirth information.

Food and food product vendors may be the source for a variety of materials related to food issues. Types of information that may be obtained include diet instruction sheets, recipes, low-calorie or low-sodium or low-cholesterol diets, information on the relationship between diet and disease, and information on feeding infants. Types of products that often have information with them include sugar substitutes, decaffeinated products, low-fat and low-cholesterol foods, dietary supplements, baby food, and infant formula. The information may be displayed with the food or food product and may contain a patient incentive, including coupons and rebates.

Disease-specific foundations and societies are also a good place to find balanced information on a disease or condition (Table 3–3). Examples include the American Heart Association, Arthritis Foundation, National Kidney Foundation, American Diabetes Association, and the American Cancer Society. Many types of information are available to help patients and their families understand and live with the disease or condition.

Factors for Evaluation

It is important to pick the appropriate tool for the job. Ideally, a clinician should have many different kinds of patient education materials available to accommodate every patient's

TABLE 3–1. LIST OF PROFESSIONAL ORGANIZATIONS

American Academy of Allergy
and Immunology
611 E Wells St
Milwaukee, WI 53202
(414) 272-6071

American Academy of Dermatology
930 N Meacham
Schaumburg, IL 60173
(708) 330-0230

American Academy of Family Physicians
8880 Ward Pkwy
Kansas City, MO 64114
(816) 333-9700

American Academy of
Orthopaedic Surgeons
222 S Prospect Ave
Park Ridge, IL 60068-4058
(708) 823-7186

American Academy of Pediatrics
141 Northwest Point Blvd
Elk Grove Village, IL 60009
(708) 228-5005

American Academy of Neurology
2221 University Ave SE
Ste 355
Minneapolis, MN 55414
(612) 623-8115

American Academy of
Home Care Physicians
4550 W 77th St
Edina, MN 55435
(410) 730-1623

American Burn Association
c/o Cleon Goodwin, MD
1205 Manhattan Ave
Suite 304
Brooklyn, NY 11222
(800) 548-2876

American Cancer Society
1599 Clifton Rd, NE
Atlanta, GA 30329
(404) 320-3333

American College of Emergency Physicians
PO Box 619911
Dallas, TX 75261-9911
(214) 550-0911

American College of Gastroenterology
4900-B S 31st St
Arlington, VA 22206-16656
(703) 931-4520

American College of Obstetricians
and Gynecologists
409 12th Street SW
Washington, DC 20024-2188
(202) 638-5577

American College of Physicians
Independence Mall W
Sixth St at Race
Philadelphia, PA 19106-1572
(215) 351-2400

American College of Radiology
1891 Preston White Dr
Reston, VA 22091
(703) 648-8900

American College of Surgeons
55 E Erie St
Chicago, IL 60611
(312) 664-4050

American Diabetes Association
1660 Duke St
Alexandria, VA 22314
(703) 549-1500

American Federation of Home and Health
1320 Fenwick Ln, Ste 100
Silver Spring, MD 20910
(301) 588-1454

American Gastroenterological Association
6900 Grove Rd
Thorofare, NJ 08068
(609) 848-9218

American Geriatrics Society
770 Lexington Ave
New York, NY 10021
(212) 308-1414

American Heart Association
7320 Greenville Ave
Dallas, TX 75231
(214) 750-5335

American Hospital Association
840 N Lake Shore Dr
Chicago, IL 60611
(312) 280-6000

American Lung Association
1740 Broadway
New York, NY 10019
(212) 315-8700

American Medical Association
515 N State St
Chicago, IL 60610
(312) 464-4623

American Neurological Association
2221 University Ave SE, Ste 350
Minneapolis, MN 55414
(612) 623-2401

American Orthopaedic Society
222 S Prospect
Park Ridge, IL 60068
(708) 698-1628

American Psychiatric Association
1400 K St NW
Washington, DC 20005
(202) 682-6000

American Public Health Association
1015 15th St NW
Washington, DC 20005
(202) 789-5600

American Society on Aging
833 Market St, Rm 511
San Francisco, CA 94103
(415) 882-2910 or (800) 537-9728

American Society of Internal Medicine
2011 Pennsylvania Ave, Ste 800
Washington, DC 20006
(202) 835-2746

American Thoracic Society
1740 Broadway
New York, NY 10019-4374
(212) 315-8700

American Urological Association
11512 Allecingie Pkwy
Richmond, VA 23235
(804) 379-1306

Arthritis Foundation
1314 Spring St NW
Atlanta, GA 30309
(404) 872-7100

Association of Reproductive
Health Professionals
409 12th St SW
Washington, DC 20024-2125
(202) 863-2475

Asthma and Allergy Foundation of America
1125 15th St NW
Ste 302
Washington, DC 20005
(202) 466-7643

Infectious Disease Association of America
1200 19th Ave NW, Ste 300
Washington, DC 20036-2401
(202) 857-1139

Gerontological Association of America
1275 K St NW, Ste 350
Washington, DC 20005-4006
(202) 842-1275

National Hospice Organization
1901 N. Moore St, Ste 901
Arlington, VA, 22209
(703) 243-5900

TABLE 3–2. FEDERAL AGENCY TELEPHONE NUMBERS

The White House
(202) 456-1414

Centers for Disease Control and Prevention
(404) 639-3311

Department of Health and Human Services
(202) 690-0257

Food and Drug Administration (FDA), main number
(301) 443-1544

Other FDA numbers
Breast Implant Inquiries
(800) 332-3541
Center for Biologics Executive Secretariat
(301) 594-1800
Center for Devices and Radiological Health
(301) 443-4690
Center for Drug Evaluation and Research
(301) 594-1012
Freedom of Information
(301) 443-6310
General Consumer Inquiries
(301) 443-3170
Mandatory Medical Device Reporting
(301) 427-7500
Medical Advertising
(800) 238-7332
MedWatch (24-Hour service for reporting problems with drugs, devices, biologics [except vaccines], medical foods, dietary supplements.)
(800) 332-1088
Office of Health Affairs, Medicine Staff (Information on FDA activities)
(301) 443-5470
Office of Orphan Products Development (Information on products for rare diseases)
(301) 443-4718
Office of Public Affairs (Interviews/press inquiries on FDA activities)
(301) 443-1130
Seafood Hot Line (24-Hour service, prerecorded message/request information [English/Spanish])
(800) 332-4010
USP Medication Errors (For reporting of medication errors or near-errors to help avoid future problems through improvement on product names and packaging)
(800) 233-7767
Vaccine Adverse Event Reporting (24-Hour service)
(800) 822-7967
Veterinary Adverse Drug Reaction Program
(301) 594-0749

Health Care Financing Administration
(202) 690-6726

Health Resources and Services Administration
(301) 443-2216

Indian Health Service
(301) 443-1083

Institute of Medicine
(202) 334-2169

National Academy of Sciences
(202) 334-2000

National Institutes of Health (NIH), main number
(301) 496-4000

Other NIH numbers
Clinical Center
(301) 496-4114
Division of Computer Research and Technology
(301) 496-5703
Fogarty International Center for Advanced Study in the Health Sciences
(301) 496-1415
National Cancer Institute
(301) 496-5615
National Center for Nursing Research
(301) 496-8230
National Center for Research Resources
(301) 496-5793
National Eye Institute
(301) 496-2234
National Heart, Lung, and Blood Institute
(301) 496-5166
National Institutes on Aging
(301) 496-9265
National Institute on Alcohol Abuse and Alcoholism
(301) 443-3885
National Institute of Allergy and Infectious Disease
(301) 496-2263
National Institute of Arthritis and Musculoskeletal and Skin Diseases
(301) 496-4353
National Institute of Child Health and Human Development
(301) 496-3454
National Institute on Deafness and Other Communication Disorders
(301) 402-0900
National Institute of Dental Research
(301) 496-3571
National Institute of Diabetes and Digestive and Kidney Diseases
(301) 496-5877
National Institute on Drug Abuse
(301) 443-6480
National Institute of Environmental Health Sciences
(919) 541-3201
National Institute of General Medical Sciences
(301) 594-2172
National Institute of Mental Health
(301) 443-3673
National Institute of Neurological Disorders and Stroke
(301) 496-9746
National Library of Medicine
(301) 496-6221

National Science Foundation
(202) 357-1110

Substance Abuse and Mental Health Services Administration
(301) 443-3783

US Public Health Service
(202) 690-7694

TABLE 3–3. NATIONAL HEALTH ORGANIZATIONS

Adoption of Special Kids, Aid to (AASK
  America)
  (415) 543-2275

AIDS Clinical Trials Information Service
  (800) TRIALS-A

AIDS Hotline, National
  (800) 342-AIDS

AIDS Information Clearinghouse, National
  (800) 458-5231

Aging, National Center for Vision and
  (800) 334-5497

Aging, National Institute on
  (800) 222-2225

Al-Anon Family Group Headquarters, Inc
  (800) 344-2666

Alcohol and Drug Abuse, National
  Council on
  (800) 622-2255

Alcohol and Drug Information, National
  Clearinghouse for
  (800) 729-6686

Alcoholism, American Council on
  (800) 527-5344

Alcoholism, National Council on
  (800) 622-2255

Alzheimer's Association
  (800) 272-3900

Alzheimer's Disease Education and
  Referral Center
  (800) 438-4380

Alzheimer's & Related Disorders Center
  (800) 621-0379

Amyotrophic Lateral Sclerosis Association
  (800) 782-4747

Anemia Foundation, Inc, Cooley's
  (800) 522-7222

Arthritis Consulting Services
  (800) 327-3027

Arthritis Foundation
  (800) 283-7800

Asthma and Allergy Foundation of America
  (800) 7-ASTHMA

Autism Hotline, National
  (304) 525-8014

Back Pain Hot Line
  (800) 247-2225

Blind, American Council of the
  (800) 424-8666

Blind, American Foundation for the
  (800) 232-5463

Blind Children's Center
  (800) 222-3566

Blind, Guide Dog Foundation for the
  (800) 548-4337

Blind, Job Opportunities for the
  (800) 638-7518

Blind, Recordings for the
  (800) 221-4792

Blinded Veteran's Association
  (800) 669-7079

Blindness, National Society to Prevent
  (800) 331-2020

Burn Association, American
  (800) 548-2876

Cancer Communications, Office of
  (800) 422-6237

Cancer Foundation, The Candlelighters
  Childhood
  (800) 366-2223

Cancer Information and Counseling Line,
  AMC
  (800) 525-3777

Cancer Institute, National
  (800) 4-CANCER

Cancer Research, American Institute for
  (800) 843-8114

Cancer Society, American
  (800) ACS-2345

Child Abuse and Family Violence, National
  Council on
  (800) 222-2000

Civil Rights, Office for, US Dept of HHS
  (800) 368-1019

Cleft Palate Foundation
  (800) 242-5338

Cocaine, 800
  (800) 262-2463

Colitis, The National Foundation
  for Ileitis and
  (800) 343-3637

Craniofacial International Foundation,
  Children's
  (800) 535-3643

Cystic Fibrosis Foundation
  (800) FIGHT-CF

Deafness Research Foundation
  (800) 535-3323

Deaf Program,
  Captioned Films/Video for the
  (800) 237-6213

de Lange Syndrome Foundation, Cornelia
  (800) 753-2357

Depressive Illness, National Foundation for
  (800) 248-4344

Depressive and Manic Depressive
  Association, National
  (800) 82-NDMDA

Diabetes Association, American
  (800) 232-3472

Diabetes Foundation, Juvenile
  (800) JDF-CURE

Down Syndrome Congress, National
  (800) 232-NDSC

Down Syndrome Society, National
  (800) 221-4602

Drug Abuse, National Council on Alcohol
  and (Hope Line)
  (800) 622-2255

Drug Abuse, National Institute of
  (800) 729-6686

Drug Information and Referral Line,
  National
  (800) 662-HELP

Dyslexia Society, Orton
  (800) 222-3123

EAR Foundation
  (800) 545-4327

Easter Seal Society, National
  (800) 221-6827

Endometriosis Association
  (800) 992-3636

Epilepsy Foundation of America
  (800) 332-1000

Epilepsy Information Service
  (800) 642-0500

Epilepsy Library, National (EFA)
  (800) EFA-4050

Eye Care Project, National
  (800) 222-3937

Facial Reconstruction,
  National Foundation for
  (212) 263-6656

Family Violence, National Council on
  Child Abuse and
  (800) 222-2000

Headache Foundation, National
  (800) 843-2256

Head Injury Foundation, National
  (800) 444-NHIF

Hearing Aid Helpline
  (800) 521-5247

Hearing Information Center
  (800) 622-3277

Hearing Institute, Better
  (800) 327-9355

Heart Association, American
  (800) 242-8721

Hemophilia Foundation, National
  (800) 42-HANDI

Hospice International, Children's
  (800) 242-4453

Hospice Organization, National
  (800) 658-8898

Huntington's Disease Society of America
  (800) 345-HDSA

Ileitis and Colitis, The National
  Foundation for
  (800) 343-3637

(continued)

TABLE 3–3. NATIONAL HEALTH ORGANIZATIONS *(continued)*

Impotence Information Center (800) 843-4315	Healthy Mothers, Healthy Babies Coalition (800) 673-8444	Scleroderma Foundation, United (800) 722-4673
Incontinence, Simon Foundation for (800) 23-SIMON	Multiple Sclerosis Society, National (800) 344-4867	Sickle Cell Disease, National Association for (800) 421-8453
Infants With Disabilities and Life-Threatening Conditions, National Information Clearinghouse (800) 922-9234	Myasthenia Gravis Foundation (800) 541-5454	SIDS Alliance (800) 221-SIDS
Kidney Foundation/Fund, American (800) 638-8299	Neurofibromatosis Foundation (800) 323-7938	Speech-Language-Hearing Association, American (800) 638-TALK
Kidney Foundation, National (800) 622-9010	Organ Donation, The Living Bank (800) 528-2971	Spina Bifida Association (800) 621-3141
Kidney Patients, American Association of (800) 749-2257	Osteoporosis Foundation, National (800) 223-9994	Spinal Cord Injury Association, National and Hot Line (800) 962-9629
Leukodystrophy Foundation, United (800) 728-5483	Ostomy Association, United (800) 826-0826	STD Hot Line, National (800) 227-8922
Liver Foundation, American (800) 223-0179	Paralysis Association, American (800) 225-0292	Stroke Association, National (800) 787-6537
Lung Association, American (800) LUNG-USA	Parkinson's Disease Association, American (800) 223-APDA	Stroke Connection (800) 553-6321
Lung Line (National Jewish Center for Immunology and Respiratory Medicine) (800) 222-LUNG	Parkinson's Educational Program (800) 344-7872	Stuttering, National Center for (800) 221-2483
Lupus Foundation of America (800) 558-0121	Parkinson Foundation, National (800) 327-4545	Tourette's Syndrome Association (800) 237-0717
Lupus Society, American (800) 331-1802	Rare Disorders, National Organization of (800) 999-6673	Tuberous Sclerosis Association, National (800) 225-NTSA
Lymphedema Network, National (800) 541-3259	Rehabilitation Information Center, National (800) 346-2742	Vietnam Veterans and Their Families, National Information System for (800) 922-9234
Mental Health Association, National (800) 969-6642	Rehabilitation Technology, Center for (800) 726-9119	Vision and Aging, National Center for (800) 334-5497
Mentally Ill, National Alliance for the (800) 950-NAMI	Retinitis Pigmentosa Foundation, National (800) 683-5555	Visiting Nurse Association of America (800) 426-2547
	Reyes Syndrome Foundation, National (800) 233-7393	

needs. This is prohibitive in most practice settings, however. Therefore, each situation should be evaluated and the right amount of information should be presented. Some materials, especially those provided by for-profit businesses, may contain a significant product slant. All materials should be evaluated closely so that the message presented is as close to what the clinician wants to impart as possible. With any printed text, the material may not be presented at the appropriate level of language for the patient or be in the primary language of the patient. English is the primary language used in most written materials. Occasionally, and now more frequently than in years past, materials in Spanish are available. If it is necessary to have materials in different languages, practice-generated materials should be translated by a professional so that information is accurately relayed. The cost of any patient education method would need to be determined and fitted into the practice budget.

Conclusion

In conclusion, one should not attempt to totally educate a patient with a chronic disease or condition at the time of diagnosis. Patients may not hear more than the diagnosis at that time and need time to adjust psychologically to the diagnosis. Often patient education is an ongoing process.

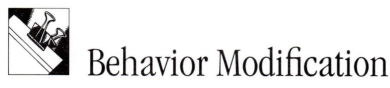

4

Behavior Modification

J. Dennis Blessing

Introduction

Behavior modification is likely to be the most difficult therapeutic modality a clinician will use. Behavior modification may be as necessary for those individuals with no discernible disease states and who are asymptomatic as for individuals with obvious disease and health problems. Behavior modification can be simply defined as changes in life-style that

1. *improve physical, social, and mental well being*
2. *prevent, delay, or lessen the effects of poor health habits*
3. *reduce, minimize, or lessen the effects of disease states*
4. *reduce the likelihood of developing some disease states.*

Personal behaviors, especially those developed over a lifetime or that are due to addictive substances, can be difficult to change. Many behaviors are deeply ingrained in an individual's personal, social, and cultural identity and activities of daily living. Patients and providers are frustrated by behavior modification modalities for many reasons, eg, changes in life-style, changes in enjoyable activities, long response time, and high failure or recidivist rates. Most patients will understand and agree with the need for behavior modification but will not try or will be unable to achieve goals.

Behavior modification success depends on many factors. The first and foremost of these are that the individual must be willing, ready, motivated, and committed to making the modification(s). Coupled with these characteristics is the need for self-regulation with support, encouragement, and guidance from family, friends, and care providers. Finally, the patient and provider must recognize that personal habits developed over long periods of time are ingrained in daily living and will take daily effort and time to change. For example, weight is rarely gained over a short period and should not be lost rapidly over a short period. Eating behaviors are ingrained and are often associated with many pleasurable activities. Another example is tobacco use. Not only is nicotine an addictive substance, but its use is associated with social activities and glamorized in advertisements. Many smokers can stop for varying periods of time, especially after going through a cessation program. However, there is high return to smoking within 1 year by most who complete cessation programs.

For care providers it is important to expect failures and setbacks in behavior modification plans. It is more important to not let these setbacks frustrate and anger the provider and have those emotions interfere with the care, support, and encouragement of the patient. Providers should also be willing to commit time to working with patients. Patient education, particularly when it involves behavior modifications, takes time, repetition, and frequent follow-up. For a busy, active office, special times may need to be set aside for patient education sessions, such as in the evenings. Also, it must be realized that patient education sessions may not be covered by third-party payers. That does not lessen the obligation of the care provider to include behavior modification and patient education as part of the health care services that are necessary for the needs of patients.

Regardless of the behavior modification being attempted, there are some general guidelines to be followed.

1. The Individual Must be Ready and Committed to Making the Change. For some individuals there may be a precipitating event, eg, the smoker who wants to quit after a respiratory infection. For some individuals the motivation may be the result of patient education from their care provider. Patients must be informed of the consequences and risks of poor health behaviors. They must also understand the benefits of behavior modification.

2. A Course of Action Must be Designed with Specific, Reasonable, Obtainable Goals and Time Lines. The plan must be adaptable to the patient and not just a handout from some source. There are many good diet plans, but to hand an overweight patient a plan and say "Follow this" is not adequate.

3. Time Must be Committed to the Patient for Instructions, Discussion, Follow-up, Support, and Encouragement. The care provider must be as committed to this as the patient.

4. The Patient Must be Supported and Encouraged by Family, Friends, and Care Providers. At times this may mean including other individuals in patient sessions, such as the wife who cooks for an overweight husband. There is tremendous benefit to the emotional well-being of the patient when he or she believes that someone is interested and cares for him or her.

5. Support Groups May be Very Beneficial. This can include such activities as smoking cessation classes, alcohol support groups, weight loss support groups, etc. Many of these groups are reputable and contribute to successful behavior modification. Before recommending a support group, the provider should be sure it meets the needs of the patient. Avoid recommending groups that proclaim rapid changes and successes, boast of unusually high success rates, or make other dubious claims and are unfamiliar to you.

6. The Provider Should be Prepared to Deal with Setbacks. These will occur. Patients should be encouraged to realize that when a setback occurs, efforts should be directed to returning to the behavior modification plan. For

some problems, new goals and new plans may need to be designed.

7. Providers Must be Willing to Seek Help or Refer Those Patients Who Need Specific Interventions. Providers must also recognize their limitations and refer elsewhere in the best interest of the patient. An example is family counseling for the alcoholic's family. Ultimately, the provider should always act and respond in the best interest of the patient. If you cannot deal with a patient's problem, find someone who can.

Most health care providers will have to commit themselves to extra effort in order to deal with behavior modification. Many of the skills needed are not learned in school. Paradigms, techniques, and philosophies change. Extended time and patient contact is necessary. Reimbursement can be a problem. However, the successful care provider will be the one who meets these challenges and can influence healthy behaviors in his or her patients.

Diet

Americans are becoming more health and diet conscious than ever before. Mass media advertising is replete with an emphasis on healthy living, exercise, and weight control programs. People recognize that being overweight is unhealthy and contributes to major health problems. Despite this knowledge and society's influence, and with large numbers of people dieting, failure rates are high.

When a patient is being counseled on dieting and weight loss, consideration should be given to the amount of weight to be lost; concurrent medical problems, particularly diabetes mellitus; and the setting of obtainable weight loss goals and time lines for meeting those goals. Many patients will be interested in commercial weight loss programs, medically directed weight loss programs, or use of appetite suppressants. Consideration should be given to the risks and benefits of any diet program or plan, and these should be explored fully with the patient. For most care providers, it is beneficial to refer the patient to a dietitian for consultation. For some individuals, referral for medically supervised weight loss programs will be necessary. This should be done carefully, with referrals only to well-established clinicians with proven programs.

The dieting patient needs frequent follow-ups with a health care provider or dietitian. Weight loss should not be rapid, and the patient must understand that a diet will be a lifelong process. There will be setbacks and intervals when loss will not occur. The patient must be reassured that this is natural and encouraged not to abandon his or her efforts. Adjuncts to dieting should also be included. The major beneficial adjunct is exercise. There is almost no medical condition that does not improve with exercise, even if the exercise is limited to walking. For the very sedentary dieter, walking is excellent beginning exercise, and a program should be initiated.

Care providers have access to a large volume of diet and exercise references. These should be used extensively in developing programs for dieters. Support groups or involvement of family can be very beneficial and should be encouraged by the provider. No matter which diet or program of weight loss is chosen, the care provider is instrumental in its selection, institution, and follow-up.

Exercise

There are very few absolute contraindications to exercise. The benefits of exercise are well documented. These benefits have been incorporated into disease prevention programs, health promotion and wellness programs, and have been demonstrated to be therapeutic adjuncts for a large number of disease conditions. A few examples of problems that benefit from exercise are obesity, cardiovascular disease, hypertension, stress, osteoporosis, and general and cardiovascular fitness. Almost all people can do some type of exercise.

When one is choosing or designing an exercise program, attention must be paid to several factors. The care provider should identify the reasons for exercise, eg, an adjunct to weight loss. An exercise program should be chosen that fits the individual based on age, physical limitations, health conditions, and personal goals. Some individuals may be very sedentary and need a program that fits professional and life-style activities. Others may need programs that address very particular needs, such as the inclusion of range of motion for certain joints, whereas others may desire to become competitive athletes. Providers must assess the beginning exercise tolerance before designing an exercise program. Evaluation must include an assessment of the individual's ability to do a program. This assessment may involve a history and physical examination or include stress tests and other evaluation modalities.

No matter what program or type of exercise is chosen, most individuals should begin with short duration, low inten-

sity, and few repetitions. Increases in each of these three areas should be slow and within the capabilities of the patient, without putting the patient at undue risk or compromising personal safety. The care provider should consult reference materials that outline and explain the best methods for individuals based on their needs and conditions. Most exercise references will include methods of monitoring patient progression (Table 4–1).

It is important for the provider to emphasize that exercise is necessary. There are multiple benefits. One doesn't have to be an athlete or be competitive. Exercise can be pleasurable. The statement "No pain, no gain" is not true. Exercise can be done alone or in groups. It can be accomplished within daily activities. It should, however, be done on a regular basis, and every little bit helps.

Smoking

Cigarette smoking is a major cause of morbidity and mortality in the United States. It is a highly addictive behavior that has physical and psychological components. It may be the most difficult behavior to modify. There are no low- or moderate-use levels. One either smokes or one does not. Total cessation is the only acceptable health choice. Many smokers quit, and the majority relapse, usually in less than a year.

There are a number of smoking cessation programs and medical practices that offer cessation programs. Well-planned, -directed, and -delivered cessation programs with support groups tend to have better success rates. Some cessation programs employ techniques using nicotine gum (2 mg/piece) or nicotine patches. The gum is chewed in place of smoking, but no more than 30 pieces per day can be used. The most common amount of gum used is 10 to 12 pieces. The gum should not be used for more than 6 months and use should decrease over a 2-to 3-month period.

The nicotine patches are relatively new but seem to offer a reasonable option for treating physical addiction. There are a number of brands available, and different companies offer different support systems for users of their products. The usual approach is to use patches with a relative high dose of nicotine for 4 weeks, then patches with a medium dose for 4 weeks, and patches with a low dose for 4 weeks. A common dosing pattern for the patches is 21 mg, 14 mg, and 7 mg. There are differences among brands. The care provider should consult package information, support information, and the *Physician's Desk Reference* for product information. Support should

TABLE 4-1. CATEGORIZATION OF ACTIVITY LEVELS THAT CAN SERVE AS GUIDE TO PRESCRIBING DOSE AND PROGRESSION OF PHYSICAL ACTIVITY[1]

Level[2]	Criteria (Mode, Duration, Frequency, Intensity)	Examples of Activities
Level 5: vigorously active[3]	One or more dynamic activities that work large muscle groups 20 min or more per session Three or more sessions per week 65% or more of maximum heart rate or somewhat hard to hard perceived exertion	Running/jogging, fast walking, swimming, bicycling, vigorous calisthenics, aerobic dance, aerobic work-outs, aerobic sports[4]
Level 4: moderately active	One or more dynamic activities that work large muscle groups 15 min or more per session One to three sessions per week 50–65% of maximum heart rate or somewhat hard perceived exertion	Running/jogging, fast walking, swimming, bicycling, calisthenics, continuous stair climbing, weight training, dancing, nonaerobic sports[5]
Level 3: mildly active	Activity that limbers body and moderately contracts large muscle groups 30–60 min per day total Daily Fairly light to somewhat hard perceived exertion	Walking, frequent stair climbing, calisthenics, weight training, heavy gardening, heavy housekeeping, major home repairs
Level 2: minimally active	Activity done during normal daily routine that limbers body and lightly contracts muscles 15–30 min per day Daily Very light to fairly light perceived exertion	Walking, occasional stair climbing, light gardening, light housekeeping, light home repairs
Level 1: sedentary	Essentially no physical activity above minimum demands of daily living Little or no perceived exertion	Watching television, working at desk, riding in car, taking elevator, eating

[1] Reproduced, with permission, from Simons-Morton BG, Pate RR, Simons-Morton DG: Prescribing physical activity to prevent disease. *Postgrad Med* 1988,83;(1):165.
[2] Patients can be prescribed activity one level above their current activity level, with gradual progression to the highest level attainable.
[3] Based on the prescription for cardiorespiratory conditioning recommended by the American College of Sports Medicine.
[4] Examples include roller skating, cross-country skiing, and soccer.
[5] Examples include tennis, basketball, baseball, and downhill skiing.

be given in every way possible to patients trying to stop smoking.

Regardless of the method chosen for smoking cessation, some general steps should be taken prior to beginning the cessation effort. Care providers should educate patients to the benefits of cessation and the risks of continuation. Patients should be helped to understand why and when they smoke. The patient's significant others should be included in the patient's effort so they can provide support during times of increased "urges." A number of behavioral techniques can help patients through stress periods. These include aversion techniques (such as smelling wet ashes kept in a bottle), attention-occupying techniques (such as walking), and substitution techniques (such as holding something in the hand or mouth). A number of references and information are available on smoking cessation. If a provider is going to direct cessation programs for patients, it is necessary to be-

come very knowledgable about such programs and the interventions used (Table 4–2). This is particularly true for understanding the use of drugs, nicotine gum, and the nicotine patches. In many instances, formal cessation programs run by experienced health care professionals may be the best choice. Ultimately the decision to stop smoking must be made by the patient. However, even the most determined patient may not succeed.

High Risk Sexual Behaviors

Human immunodeficiency virus (HIV) infection and resultant acquired immune deficiency syndrome (AIDS) are increasing at alarming rates. This is particularly true for people in younger age groups and for heterosexuals. It is very important that all individuals be counseled about HIV transmission and its prevention. This must be done in a professional, prudent manner with care and concern for the patient's well-being.

TABLE 4-2. SMOKING CESSATION TIPS FOR PATIENTS

1. Ask about smoking at every opportunity. Use questions such as "Do you smoke?," "How much?," "How soon after waking do you have your first cigarette?," "Are you interested in stopping smoking?," "Have you ever tried to stop before?," "If so, what happened?"
2. Advise all smokers to stop smoking. State your advice clearly, for example: "As your physician, I must advise you to stop smoking now." Personalize the message to quit. Refer to the patient's clinical condition, smoking history, family history, personal interests, or social roles.
3. Assist the patient in stopping.
   a. Set a quit date. Help the patient pick a date within the next four weeks, acknowledging that no time is ideal. Consider signing a stop-smoking contract with patients.
   b. Provide self-help materials.
   c. Consider prescribing nicotine gum or a nicotine patch, especially for highly addicted patients (those who smoke one pack a day or more or who smoke their first cigarette within 30 minutes of waking).
   d. If the patient is not willing to quit now, provide motivating literature.
4. Arrange follow-up visits.
   a. Call or write the patient within 7 days after initial visit, reinforcing the decision to stop and reminding the patient of the quit date.
   b. Arrange a follow-up visit within 1–2 weeks after the quit date. At this time, ask about the patient's smoking status to provide support and help prevent relapse. Relapse is common; if it occurs, encourage the patient to try again immediately.
   c. Schedule a second follow-up visit in 1–2 months. For patients who have relapsed, discuss the circumstances of the relapse and other special concerns.

From Glynn TJ, Manley MW: *How to help your patients stop smoking. A National Cancer Institute manual for physicians.* National Cancer Institute, 1989. Publication No. DHHS (PHS) 89-3064.

Many providers and patients are reluctant to discuss matters considered very personal and private, especially if sexual activity is involved. Discussion of HIV and AIDS and other sexually transmitted diseases should be approached in a manner similar to a discussion of any patient problems. Reassurance about patient confidentiality may need to be reinforced.

There is much about HIV and AIDS that is still unknown. For this very reason, it is incumbent on the care provider to be as knowledgable as possible. It is dangerous to assume that a patient is not at risk if a sexual history and an evaluation of risk factors are not taken. It is even more dangerous to allow false beliefs to continue and not be corrected or challenged. Patients must understand that high-risk behaviors exist within all ethnic, racial, and socioeconomic groups. Those individuals who engage in high-risk behaviors and do not recognize or believe they are at risk are probably at greatest risk. It is the duty of every care provider to educate every patient about risk factors and how to reduce those risks.

Currently, it is recognized that HIV transmission can occur with heterosexual activity, homosexual activity, intravenous drug use through sharing needles, blood transfusions, from mother to infant, and accidental exposure to contaminated needles, instruments, etc. Each of these risk behaviors and risk factors can be controlled and avoided. There is a large volume of information and references on risk factors, prevention, conversions, prognosis, treatment, and research. It is im-

perative that care providers be up-to-date and knowledgable about current data and recommendations concerning HIV and AIDS (see Chapter 16). The Centers for Disease Control and Prevention provides information resources and can be an excellent reference for patients and health care providers. Many community agencies are active in public information and provide educational materials, as well as support groups. Care providers should be familiar with community resources and use them as necessary.

Unprotected intercourse, particularly with or between individuals in high-risk groups, is a major risk factor for HIV exposure. Patients need to understand that no one is immune and that HIV can be contracted from a single exposure. Individuals at greatest risk are those who have multiple partners, do not use condoms and engage in anal intercourse. Latex condoms can be effective if used correctly. However, many individuals, particularly men, have misconceptions about condoms. Gender, cultural, and social beliefs may influence condom use and acceptability. An example is the statement, "Real men don't use condoms!". These ingrained beliefs are difficult to change, but offering clear, concise, and accurate information is the best approach to use. Individuals must understand that everyone is at risk, there is no immunization, and currently, there is no cure (Table 4–3).

Ultimately, providers must make HIV and AIDS education a part of every patient's care and knowledge. This must be done in a nonjudgmental fashion; free of personal bias; with

TABLE 4-3. "SAFER SEX" PRACTICES SUGGESTED FOR REDUCING THE RISK OF SEXUALLY TRANSMITTED DISEASES

The most effective strategies are sexual abstinence or the maintenance of a mutually monogamous sexual relationship. In other cases, the following practices should be observed:

- Always use a latex condom during sexual intercourse. The application of spermicides and the use of diaphragms by women may also decrease risk.
- Avoid multiple partners, anonymous partners, prostitutes, persons with multiple partners, persons who use intravenous drugs, and those not known to be seronegative for human immunodeficiency virus (HIV).
- Avoid sexual contact with persons who have a genital discharge, genital warts, genital herpes lesions, or evidence of hepatitis B surface antigen.
- Do not practice anal intercourse. Avoid all sexual activities that could cause cuts or tears in the lining of the rectum, vagina, or penis.
- Avoid oral-anal sex to prevent enteric lesions.
- Avoid genital contact with oral herpetic lesions.
- Persons at increased risk should be especially careful to avoid mouth contact with the penis, vagina, or rectum.
- Persons who use intravenous drugs should receive treatment and should never use unsterilized or shared injection equipment.
- Persons at increased risk should have a periodic examination for sexually transmitted diseases.

SAFE SEXUAL ACTIVITIES
Massage
Hugging
Body rubbing (dry)
Kissing (dry)
Masturbation (on healthy skin)
Hand-to-genital touching or mutual masturbation

POSSIBLY SAFE SEXUAL ACTIVITIES (these activities are completely safe if both partners are known to be uninfected)
Kissing (wet)
Oral sex on men wearing latex condoms
Oral sex on women (who are not menstruating or experiencing a vaginal infection with discharge)

---

accurate, correct, and appropriate information directed at providing essential information, correcting misinformation, and giving patients the opportunity to protect themselves from a devastating illness.

Wellness

A universal definition for wellness probably does not exist. The term has been used by different groups to define aspects of physical, social, and mental well-being. For some, the concept includes care providers; and for some, the individuals. For purposes of this discussion the following definition will be used:

> Wellness is a concept of personal health and well-being through personal improvement and effort coupled with appropriate health promotion and disease prevention strategies that lead to the minimizing of health risk factors and the use of appropriate health screenings. The goal is to achieve the highest level of physical, social, and mental well-being.

The care provider must be able to provide patient education concerning diet, exercise, behavior modification, risk factors,

identification of risk factors, and other patient concerns. Coupled with this education is the appropriate use of history, physical examination, and appropriate screening tests. The timing and use of screening tests can be controversial and open to debate. An excellent resource for information on screening tests is the *Guide to Clinical Preventive Services*.[1] Screening tests should be used when they are most effective, sensitive, specific, and reliable for detecting disease states and reducing morbidity and mortality. For every patient a plan should be developed that outlines personal contribution to wellness (diet, exercise, etc) and the care provider's contribution (appropriate education, screenings, etc). Both should adhere to their plans. Failure by the patient does not eliminate the obligations of the provider to continue the effort to counsel and encourage further effort.

Wellness may be seen by some as an individual and personal effort that is not related to medicine and its high-powered technology. Alternative forms of therapy may be sought for health problems (see Appendix II). Many people who have this perception will still see a place for medicine, however. In a broader sense, it seems reasonable to accept wellness as a partnership between the individual and the care provider. This partnership does not necessarily exclude alternative pathways, provided no harm is being done. The care provider should try to be informed on alternative modalities and their benefits and risks. The relationship that will succeed is the one that is open, honest, and in the best interest of patient and provider. For the patient, the goal is the achievement of the best possible physical, social, and mental well-being. For the care provider, the accomplishment is being an important part of helping people to achieve the best that their life offers. As time goes by, it becomes more obvious that it is better to prevent and lessen morbidity and mortality than to treat disease.

Conclusion

Behavior modification can be accomplished by a partnership between the health care provider and the patient. It takes commitment by both. A number of references, patient education aides, and information sources exist. Some are available free of charge and others are commercially available (see Chapter 3). Each provider should identify those materials he or she wants to use and share with patients. It is important to review these materials and update them regularly. If a patient succeeds in behavior modification and becomes healthier, the health care provider has achieved the goal of his or her profession.

Reference

1. *Clinician's Handbook of Preventive Services.* U.S. Government Printing Office, 1994.

5

Managing Medication Nonadherence

John Fuchs, Jr

Introduction

The National Council on Patient Information and Education describes nonadherence as "America's other drug problem."[1] It is a medical problem that should be identified and treated in a similar manner to hypertension, congestive heart failure, or diabetes mellitus. Nonadherence occurs when a patient fails to have an initial prescription filled or fails to take a medication correctly, as prescribed by the clinician. Unfortunately, it is difficult for health care workers to determine when it is occurring. This is a problem that may result in therapeutic failure and needless cost to the patient and the health care system. When medications are taken correctly, however, the result in most circumstances is cost-effective medical management. Nonadherence is a continuing medical problem and it is vital that health care workers continue to look for new and better ways of preventing, detecting, and correcting it.

A Major Health Problem

There have been many studies completed in the past four decades that have examined medication nonadherence or noncompliance. The majority of these studies do not support the assumption that patients will follow instructions on taking their medications. In fact, failure to achieve desired results from noncompliance ranges from 0% to 50% (average 40%) depending on the condition being treated (Table 5–1) and medication dose frequency (Table 5–2).[2,3] About 10% of all hospitalizations and 23% of all nursing home admissions are attributed to nonadherence.[4] The cost of nonadherence in the United States has been estimated at more than 100 billion dollars per year. This estimate is based on outcomes that include: (1) hospitalizations, (2) nursing home admissions, (3) lost productivity, (4) premature deaths, and (5) treatment costs in ambulatory patients. Improvement of nonadherence is likely to save billions of dollars per year in a health care system that is struggling.

Forms of Nonadherence

Table 5–3 lists the common forms of nonadherence. The forms or manifestations of nonadherence are easier to identify than the causes. Not having the initial prescription filled occurs at an estimated rate of 14% to 20%.[5–7] The reasons for not filling the initial prescription include: (1) patient didn't want the medication (or thought it wouldn't help), (2) patient didn't need the medication (rejected the diagnosis), (3) patient had a concern about adverse reactions, (4) cost, and (5) poor understanding of instructions or of importance of taking the medication. Nonadherence resulting from not having an initial prescription filled can largely be addressed by improving communications between the patient and practitioner. Other forms of nonadherence include: (1) taking an incorrect dose, (2) taking the medication at the wrong time, (3) forgetting to take one or more doses, and (4) stopping the medication too soon.

Reasons for Nonadherence

The reasons for nonadherence are listed in Table 5–4.[8] These include poor communication, drug regimen complexity, and patient behavior or unresolved concerns.

Poor Communication. Several studies have indicated that poor communication can be associated with nonadherence. Published reports indicate that only 82% of patients recall their health care provider telling them how long to take a medication and only 66% recall being told about re-

TABLE 5–1. RATE OF NONCOMPLIANCE BY DISEASE STATE

Condition	Rate of Noncompliance (%)
Asthma	20
Arthritis	55–71
Contraception	8
Diabetes	40–50
Epilepsy	30–50
Hypertension	40

TABLE 5–3. FORMS OF NONCOMPLIANCE

1. Not having the prescription filled
2. Taking an incorrect dose
3. Taking medication at the wrong time
4. Forgetting to take one or more doses

fill instructions.[7] Burgess reported that only 50% of patients received detailed instructions on how to take their medications.[9] In addition, it has been estimated that patients forget about half of the instructions they are given the minute they leave a health care provider's office.[10] It is advisable that patients be given verbal and written information about their condition and medications.

Drug Regimen Complexity. Complex drug regimens may also be associated with nonadherence. Patients receiving multiple medications and at a dosage frequency greater than twice daily are at increased risk for nonadherence. Reducing drug regimen complexity can be beneficial in promoting compliant behavior but only when the other reasons for nonadherence have also been addressed.

Patient Behavior. Table 5–4 lists examples of several concerns that can have a negative influence on patient compliance if left unresolved.

Management of Nonadherence

The management of nonadherence requires that it be recognized as one of the patient's medical problems. After it has been identified as a problem, an individual treatment plan can be developed. A treatment plan can then be implemented and assessed at follow-up clinic appointments.

Education is the cornerstone in the management of nonadherence. The goal is to present medication information

that is understood by the patient so that the patient is willing and capable of complying with the drug regimen. This may require providing information to the patient's caregiver. In general, the information should (1) be presented verbally and written (see Table 5–5 for specific information that should be provided on each medication); (2) be easy to understand, not too comprehensive, and allow patients to ask questions; (3) include detailed instructions for use on the medication container (avoid instructions such as "as directed"); and (4) be reinforced at each visit to the clinic or pharmacy.

Figure 5–1 depicts the management of nonadherence from two standpoints: prevention and treatment.

Nonadherence Prevention. Medication nonadherence is best avoided by educating the patient about a new drug or drug regimen. Drug regimens should be chosen that have the fewest number of medications and that permit the lowest daily dose frequency (once or twice daily if possible). Every attempt should be made to individualize the drug regimen to the patient's schedule and use reminder devices when appropriate. Patients should be allowed to participate in their treatment plan and feel as though they are involved with the decisions of their drug regimen. The patient should have no unresolved

TABLE 5–2. NONCOMPLIANCE BY DOSE FREQUENCY

Dose Frequency	Rate of Noncompliance (%)
Once daily	27
Twice daily	30
Three times daily	48
Four times daily	58

TABLE 5–4. REASONS FOR NONCOMPLIANCE

1. Poor communication (from health care provider to patient about disease and therapy)
2. Drug regimen complexity (increased number of medications or increased daily dose frequency)
3. Patient behavior (unresolved concerns)
   1. Poor perception of health: asymptomatic condition or long treatment duration (hypertension)
   2. High drug cost
   3. Rejection or denial of diagnosis; unwilling patient
   4. Fear or misunderstanding of adverse drug reactions
   5. Early abatement of symptoms (antibiotic therapy)
   6. Delayed onset (antidepressant therapy)
   7. Mental disorder (reduced ability to cooperate)
   8. Physical disorder (visual impairment, manual dexterity limitation)

TABLE 5–5. MEDICATION INFORMATION PROVIDED TO PATIENTS

1. Drug name (trade and generic) and the intended therapeutic effect
2. Dosage regimen (specify times) and integration with meals and other medications
3. Common adverse effects, including the significance and action to be taken if encountered
4. Action to be taken in event of missing dose
5. Storage and refill instructions

concerns about the drug or regimen. Caregivers should be notified when patients are incapable of compliant behavior.

Nonadherence Treatment. An approach to the treatment of nonadherence in a patient chronically receiving medication consists of four steps: (1) detection, (2) determination of the reason, (3) development and implementation of a plan, and (4) assessment.

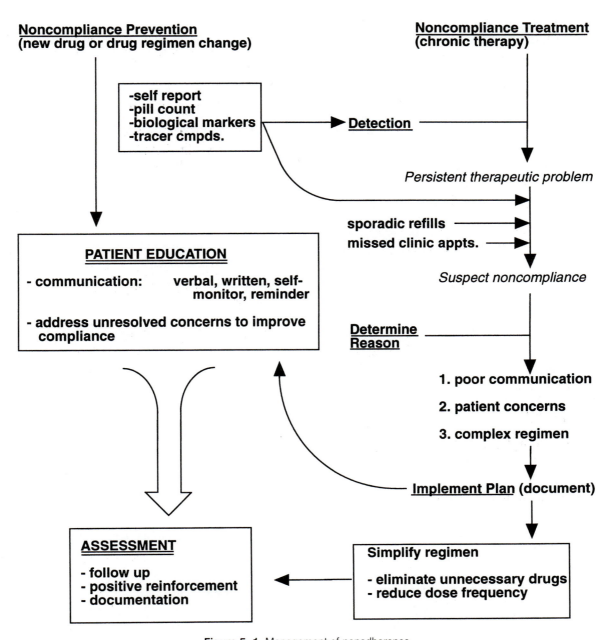

Figure 5–1. Management of nonadherence

Step I: Detection of Nonadherence. For nonadherence to be successfully treated, it must first be identified. Nonadherence should be suspected whenever a patient has a *persistent therapeutic problem*. Sporadic refill patterns or missed clinic appointments in the setting of a persistent problem can be useful to distinguish nonadherence from disease progression or an untreated illness. Subtherapeutic serum drug assays, pill counts,[11] biological markers, tracer compounds,[12,13] and interviews can also be used to identify nonadherence. These methods and their limitations are listed in Table 5–6.

Step II: Determine the Reason. Once nonadherence has been suspected, determining the reason (if possible) is helpful in developing an individual treatment plan. This may be accomplished by interviewing the patient or the patient's caregiver and reviewing the medication regimen. Table 5–4 lists the reasons for nonadherent behavior. They include poor communications, complex drug regimens, and patient behavior or unresolved concerns.

Step III: Develop and Implement a Plan. A plan should be developed according to the reasons identified. Patients receiving chronic medications may have barriers to adherence that can be addressed with the use of reminder devices such as drug calendars, medication organizers, blister packaging of unit-of-use doses, and electronic pill boxes (an alarm will sound when a dose is due). Phone calls or postcard reminders can be useful to remind a patient when refills are due. Some pharmaceutical companies (Table 5–7) have established adherence programs in which patients directly receive benefits from the company. These benefits include phone call reminders for refills, educational newsletters and videotapes, and cash rebates.[7,14] Self-monitoring should be recommended whenever possible. For example, home monitoring of

TABLE 5–6. LIMITATIONS OF NONCOMPLIANCE DETECTION METHODS

Method	Limitation
Self report; interview	subjective (overestimation)
Pill count	pill dumping (overestimation)
Serum drug assay	drugs with short half-lives reflect what patient ingested in previous 24 hours (overestimate)
Biological markers	objective (better estimate)
Tracer compounds	objective (better estimate)

TABLE 5–7. PHARMACEUTICAL COMPANIES AND COMPLIANCE PROGRAMS

Pharmaceutical Company	Medication
1. Zeneca	Tenormin, Tenoretic
2. Stuart	Zestril, Zestoretic
3. Marion Merrell Dow	Cardizem CD and SR
4. Lederle Labs	Prostep
5. Wyeth-Ayerst	Premarin
6. Merck & Co.	Proscar
7. Sandoz	Miacalcin
8. Becton-Dickinson	Insulin syringes
9. Schering-Plough	Nitro-Dur
10. Glaxo	Ventolin, Beclovent, Beconase

blood pressure, blood glucose, proteinuria, and many other disease indicators allow a patient to participate in the management of his or her own condition. Regardless of the method suggested to improve adherence, the treatment plan should be documented in the medical chart so an assessment can be made on subsequent visits.

Step IV: Assessment. The treatment plan should be assessed at the next follow-up visit. All objective information regarding adherent behavior should be reviewed. This includes the status of the therapeutic problem. Assessment is an important aspect of the treatment of nonadherence, not only from the standpoint of improving therapeutic outcome, but also as a continual reminder to the patient of the importance of correctly taking medications.

Conclusion

Medication nonadherence is a common occurrence that may be avoided or corrected through education and reminder programs. Some patients, however, have concerns about medications that represent resistant barriers. Some are either unwilling or incapable of adhering to the prescribed regimen. Nonadherence is a continuing issue; it is costly and it is a health problem. Health care providers must find new ways in preventing, detecting, and correcting medication nonadherence.

REFERENCES

1. Eraker SA, Kirscht JP, Becker MD. Understanding and improving patient compliance. *Ann Int Med*. 1984;100:258–268.

2. Emerging issues in pharmaceutical cost containment. Reston, VA: National Pharmaceutical Council. 1992;2(2):1–16.

3. Greenberg RN. Overview of patient compliance with medication dosing: a literature review. *Clin Ther*. 1984;6:592–599.

4. McKenney JM, Harrison TL. Drug-related hospital admissions. *Am J Hosp Pharm*. 1976;33:792–795.

5. Survey by Applied Research Techniques conducted for the American Association of Retired Persons. Washington DC: AARP; 1984.

6. National Prescription Buyers Survey. Kalamazoo, Mich: The Upjohn Co; 1985.

7. Debrovner D. Did you take your pill today? *Am Druggist*. 1992;(November):60–66.

8. Berg JS, Dischler J, Wagner DJ, et al. Medication compliance: a health care problem. *Ann Pharm*. 1993;27:S3–S22.

9. Burgess MM. Ethical and economic aspects of noncompliance and overtreatment. *Can Med Assoc J*. 1989;141:777–780.

10. Clepper I. Noncompliance. The invisible epidemic. *Drug Topics*. 1992;136(16):44–65.

11. Pullar T, Kumar S, Tindall H, et al. Time to stop counting the tablets? *Clin Pharmacol Ther*. 1989;46:163–168.

12. Feely M, Cooke J, Price D, et al. Low-dose phenobarbitone as an indicator of compliance with drug therapy. *Br J Clin Pharmacol*. 1987;24:77–84.

13. Maenpaa H, Javala K, Pikraraine NJ. Minimal dose of digoxin: a new marker for compliance to medication. *Eur Heart J*. 1987;8 (suppl 1):31–37.

14. Bond WS, Hussar DA. Detection methods and strategies for improving medication compliance. *Am J Hosp Pharm*. 1991;48:1978–1988.

6

Incorporating Patient Education into Clinical Practice

Albert F. Simon

Introduction

Over the years, issues relative to patient education have been relegated to a special status in medical education. This status has allowed patient education to have mention in various aspects of health professions' curricula and perhaps cursory attention on clinical rounds on the wards. What real importance does patient education have in our system of health care? With the shift in emphasis to focus more on primary care, many have called for an increase in patient education services as a means of achieving efficiency and cost containment. Some professional groups are highlighting patient education as part of their policy agenda for health care reform. In 1994, the American Academy of Family Practice issued a white paper calling for family physicians to assume a leadership role in patient education.[1] But how well do health care providers put patient education into practice? A recent study demonstrated that family practice and internal medicine residents seldom identified patient risk behaviors in their patients. Few attempted to provide patient education and counseling and those who tried did not possess adequate skills to perform the education effectively.[2]

*In outpatient private practice, patient education is often the first casualty to concerns of time and productivity. For the student or new practitioner, the emphasis to be placed on patient education can be confusing. In the case of the more seasoned practitioner, the issues of patient education are caught in a wrestle between an increasing schedule of patient commitments and less time in which to accomplish them. This chapter discusses a rationale for un-*dertaking patient education, suggests adjuncts to enhance one-to-one education, and looks ahead to patient education in the future.*

A Rationale for Patient Education

Should I undertake patient education at all? Even on an item as basic as this, there seems to be no universal agreement. Indeed, some argue that patient education is time-consuming, expensive, and ineffective. Research suggests that personal health behaviors are often unaffected by counseling.[3] The American health care system currently offers practitioners little incentive through reimbursement of preventive services or health promotion to perform patient education activities. Even with appropriate incentives, some practitioners may not be adequately prepared to provide health promotion strategies.[4] Others contend that significant reductions can be achieved in US mortality rates by the institution of appropriate life-style changes.[5,6] This promise of gain in the health of patients provides sufficient rationale to many providers to incorporate patient education into their everyday practice. However, there are other compelling reasons to undertake patient education.

The latter part of the 1990s promises to create tremendous change in the provision of medical care. Health care reform legislation, the move to system based primary care, and an emphasis on prevention signal changes that providers and patients will experience. Policy makers and legislators now expect that providers will provide comprehensive patient education in the day-to-day provision of their medical care. The seriousness of this expectation is reflected in a Dutch law that requires that a doctor always inform the patient about the treatment being given.[7] Patients are now more optimistic about the potential of preventive strategies. They are demanding more information from their health care provider and are more interested in the range of treatment options than in previous times. Many patients now expect their health care provider to be their partner in empowering them to attain health. Given these changes in the health care system and the characteristics of patient behaviors, providing ample information in a digestible fashion will help to meet the needs of a wide range of patients.

Making Patient Education More Effective

The time-honored method of providing patient education is through the one-to-one interaction between patient and practitioner. Even with the advent of technologic innovations, this interaction, established on the therapeutic relationship, will continue to be the predominant method of providing patient education. By approaching patient education in an organized fashion, the clinician has the potential to affect positive change in patient behavior. Each patient education encounter utilizes the same basic skills. A list of these skills is outlined in Chapter 1.

Adjunctive Strategies for Patient Education

Many additional strategies for enhancing patient education can be added to the basic techniques discussed in Chapter 1. The following discussion highlights several methods. Of course, not all of these methods may fit with each individual's practice style; each option may be modified or used as is to embellish patient education.

In any given practice setting, a pattern of common problems soon emerges. These constitute a list that the provider has to deal with over and over again. To help improve the process of patient education and to facilitate a uniform approach in any given practice, many practitioners develop patient information sheets (see Chapter 20). These sheets offer a written set of instructions for the patient to follow and engender consistency for the provider by offering an outline of talking points to use in each encounter. In some practices, clinicians have taken the time to construct "home-grown" versions of patient information sheets. In other practices, they have adopted educational pamphlets that are available from a variety of sources, including pharmaceutical companies, voluntary health agencies, and companies that exist just to publish

patient education materials (see Chapter 3). For the many practices that use prepublished educational materials, at least one problem exists; namely, how does one choose from the overwhelming numbers of materials that are available?

To address this issue, the Huffington Library of the American Academy of Family Physicians Foundation has created a health and patient education database for family practice. The database does not contain a comprehensive review of all patient education materials and does not warehouse any particular literature. However, it does serve to direct the user to the source of the information. Information on the ordering, cost, and contents of the referenced material is listed on the database report that one obtains from a search using a key word.[8] This database contains useful information for those in primary care who wish to use preprinted materials for patient education.

Another approach to providing adjuncts to patient education is the establishment of a patients' library. Collings et al, created a patients' library associated with a general practice that consisted of 200 books covering 107 medical topics.[9] The books were chosen by a general practitioner, in consultation with a medical librarian. At first the library was available to the patients only on the recommendation of one of the six general practitioners who staffed the practice. Later in the study, the library was moved into the patients' waiting room to allow the patients unlimited access to any of the collection. Analysis of the usage of the library over the 15 months of the study was based on responses to questionnaires returned by those who checked out books. Of the 163 respondents to the survey, only 12% were men. The respondents were asked to rate the information gained by their reading as of great usefulness, of some usefulness, of little use, or no use. Forty-seven percent of the respondents said that the reading was of great use and 50% indicated the reading was of some use. Only 2% found the reading to be of no use. These patients indicated that the books lacked specific relevance to their situation and thus were of no benefit. But would this access to information by the patients raise their level of anxiety? In the information from the respondents to the survey, only 6% said that their level of anxiety was raised by information from the reading in the patients' library. A full 44% of the patients reported that their anxiety level actually decreased after reviewing the information about their condition.

Adding another dimension to patient education are strategies designed to educate individuals in situations larger than the traditional one-to-one interaction. One approach to providing this type of experience is through patient education classes (see Chapter 3). The classroom setting allows for an in-depth coverage of a topic that would be impossible with patients seen in the office setting. In such sessions, instruction may also be tailored to meet the individual needs of the patient audience. Educational theory postulates that long-term knowledge benefit is likely from such sessions.[9,10] While there is potential for gain, some argue that the number of participants per session would tend to be low, thus making the venture a rather expensive proposition in terms of personnel investment. One alternative to help distribute the cost is to have health educators or others conduct the sessions instead of subtracting providers' time from seeing patients in the office. Schattner piloted the concept of conducting patient education classes in a general practice outside of Melbourne, Australia.[10] Ten educational sessions were conducted, each on a different topic over a period of about 2 months. The attendees were all patients recruited from his group's practice. Of the 113 invited, 55 actually attended at least one of the sessions. This resulted in an average of about 5 people per session. When surveyed, 96% of the attendees responded that they had learned something worthwhile and 90% indicated that they felt that, from the knowledge gained, they would be able to better control their condition. Each participant was pre-and posttested on information that was covered in each session. The participants' strong positive feelings about the learning gained in the sessions was not borne out by the results of the pre-and posttesting, which showed an improvement of only about 10% in base knowledge.

An effective method of sharing ideas about health and providing education may be the production of a newsletter for your practice. There are many successful health newsletters that have been produced around the country including the *Mayo Clinic News, The Harvard Health Letter*, and *The Help Newsletter*. While most practices would not attempt to produce a publication as ambitious as these, others have learned that a short, simple newsletter distributed to the patients in the practice may be an effective patient education tool. Dr. Glen Aukerman produces *Total Health*, a nationally circulated newsletter that started as a typed letter to the patients in his practice. The impetus for the newsletter developed as Dr. Aukerman noticed that he was spending significant time in educating patients about health concerns and that many of these concerns were similar from patient to patient. He envisioned producing a let-

ter to address these common health concerns that would be distributed to his patients. The common issues generated during discussions with patients would serve as the basis for topics in the next newsletter. After initial publication of the newsletter, Aukerman discovered a tremendous demand for copies of his publication, which is now distributed to over 6000 subscribers. Even with this success, Aukerman still bases many of the selections for articles from issues generated by discussions with the patients seen daily in his practice.

Any practice could use the newsletter concept as a forum to address issues that are topical for the patients whom it serves. Some suggestions to help make the newsletter effective that have worked in other publications include keeping the focus topical and germane to the patients in the practice and trying to "catch the reader's eye" with shorter news items as well as longer feature items. The newsletter can also serve as a vehicle to list upcoming classes, highlight services offered by the practice, or introduce new staff members.

The ideas discussed above allow one to add to one's basic skills and to provide one-on-one patient education as most providers typically do each day as they see patients. It is important to remember that these ideas are adjuncts to but do not replace the basic methods of providing patient education, as discussed in Chapter 1.

The Future of Patient Education

The line between the future and the present is a rather narrow one. How will technology influence the methods that providers use to provide education? Already many projects using computer systems to provide information to patients are being piloted (see Chapter 3). Computers offer the promise of being able to allow patients to choose between a menu of topics and locate the information of interest to them. It also allows the monitoring of the pattern of usage so that topics of concern that are not addressed currently by the system can be added. Stanley and Tongue found that use of a computer data system in the waiting area of a general practice office to provide patient education was well-accepted and well-utilized. Evidence in the literature supports the use of computer terminals over printed material as a source of information and indicates that they are well received by patients.[11–13]

Using the computer in the waiting area to provide patient education is only the beginning of how technology will alter the approach to patient education. With community access channels in most American communities, health care providers have access to, literally, every patient's home. Health programming can be conducted and made interactive by using a phone-in format or keypad access from the home. Although there are a few commercial programs broadcast (eg, Dr. Edell), the market is wide open in most communities to take advantage of cable access channels.

With the advent of the Internet and the number of personal computers, other possible avenues of interaction become available. The Internet provides a means to communicate with all of the patients that are "on line." Using this technology, it is possible to communicate with patients via electronic mail, a venue not commonly utilized at this point. The patient can also access any one of several worldwide databases. Perhaps soon a patient-oriented database service will be on line. The Internet also offers the ability to send still images, audio, and video. The advanced capabilities for interactivity created by the Internet set the foundation for a patient education network that would allow for patients and experts worldwide to converge and exchange information. The patient education library of the future may be access to a national network of interactive programs.

It is difficult to look ahead and predict all the changes that technology will bring. As we watch Star Trek, we see the holographic image that is the ship's doctor. This hologram is activated whenever health advice is needed and then stored electronically between consultations. It is doubtful that any of us seriously need to be worried about being reduced to bits on a CD. However, the emerging technology will challenge all of us who provide health care to think about patient education in new ways. Coming technologies should be viewed as an opportunity to complement our methods of patient education rather than as competition with them. If anything is certain,

it is that the bonds that develop between patient and practitioner, established through basic patient communication and education skills, will continue to be necessary for effective medical practice.

References

1. American Family Physicians. AAFP issues on patient education. *Special Med Rep*. 1994;15:673.
2. Hoppe RB, Farquhar LJ, Henry R, et al. Residents' attitudes towards and skills in counseling: using undetected standardized patients. *J Gen Intern Med*. 1990;5:415–420.
3. McMillin CL. Health promotion: strategies for family physicians. *Can Fam Physician*. 1993;39:1079–1085.
4. Cummings KM, Giovina G, Sciandra R, et al. Physician advice to quit smoking: who gets it and who doesn't? *Am J Med*. 1987;3:69–75.
5. What is wellness? *Hospitals*. 1991;3:14. Editorial.
6. Lawrence RS. The role of physicians in promoting health. *Health Aff (Millwood)*. 1990;Summer:122–132.
7. Donabedian A. *Explorations in Quality Assessment and Monitoring*. Ann Arbor: Health Administration Press; 1980.
8. Gibson PA, Ruby C, Craig MD. A health/patient education database for family practice. *Bull Med Libr Assoc*. 1991;79:357–369.
9. Collins LH, Pike LC, Binder AI, et al. Value of written health information in the general practice setting. *Br J Gen Pract*. 1991;41:466–467.
10. Schattner P. Patient education classes in general practice. *Aust Fam Physician*. 1993;7:1229–1238.
11. Fisher LA, Johnson TS, Porter D, et al. Collection of a clean voided urine sample: a comparison among spoken, written, and computer-based instructions. *Am J Public Health*. 1977;67:640–644.
12. Dove GAW, Wigg P, Clarke JHC, et al. The therapeutic effect of taking a patient's history by computer. *J R Coll Gen Pract*. 1977;27:477–481.
13. Deardorff WW. Computerized health education: a comparison with traditional formats. *Health Educ Q*. 1986;13:61–72.

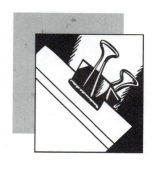

Part Two

Primary Care Disorders

Pulmonary Disorders

Doris J. Rosenow

■ CHRONIC OBSTRUCTIVE PULMONARY DISEASE

General Characteristics

Obstructive pulmonary disease includes a group of disease entities that are associated with chronic air flow limitation within the lung as a result of a decrease in the conducting air flow diameter or loss of the lung's integrity.[1,2] These conditions are characterized by difficult expiration, which is manifested by: (1) a more forcible use of accessory muscles of expiration to expel a given volume of air; (2) a reduction in expiratory air flow, as measured by the forced expiratory volume in 1 second (FEV_1); (3) varying degrees of dyspnea; and (4) chronic cough and sputum production.[3,4] The clinical term chronic obstructive pulmonary disease (COPD) is used to describe patients with at least two of the following diagnoses: chronic bronchitis, emphysema, and asthma. Although asthma is more often acute and intermittent, it can be chronic.

It is estimated that over 15 million Americans suffer from COPD.[1] It is the fifth leading cause of mortality in the United States, and second only to heart disease as a cause of disability in adults under 65 years of age.[3] The incidence of COPD increases with age, occurs more frequently in men over the age of 45 years, and is higher in whites than nonwhites. However, the incidence of COPD in women has been steadily increasing. Several factors have been implicated in the pathogenesis of COPD. The primary cause is cigarette smoking, accounting for 80% to 90% of all cases.[5] Other contributing factors are environmental and occupational dusts and gases, infection, and genetics.

Although chronic bronchitis, emphysema, and asthma are classified under a common clinical term (COPD), the pathophysiologic bases for the air-flow limitation is different in the different diseases (Figures 7–1 to 7–4). Because the clinical management of chronic bronchitis and emphysema is similar, the care for patients with either of these diseases is presented together.

■ *Chronic Bronchitis*

Bronchitis is defined as a chronic or recurrent excess mucus secretion into the bronchial tree for at least 3 consecutive months a year for 2 successive years.[6] It is an inflammation of the bronchi that is caused by a variety of environmental and occupational irritants or infection.[3] Although the inflammation can result from a variety of causes, the primary etiologic factor is cigarette smoke. While the primary action of cigarette smoke is to paralyze mucociliary activity, it also has some adverse effect on the inflammatory cell response in the pulmonary parenchyma.[7]

Bronchitis is characterized by an increased mucus production related to: (1) an increased number of goblet cells in the epithelial lining; (2) hypertrophy and hyperplasia of bronchial glands; and (3) impaired ciliary function. In the early development of bronchitis, the pathophysiologic changes affect the larger bronchi. As the disease progresses over several years, all airways are involved, whereby mucus plugging and inflammation in the peripheral airways contribute most to obstruction and airway trapping.[3,8] Consequently, these changes in the small airways begin to cause a ventilation-perfusion deficit, leading to hypoxemia and hypercapnia. The hypoxemia contributes to pulmonary hypertension, with subsequent right ventricular failure (cor pulmonale). Hypoxemia also

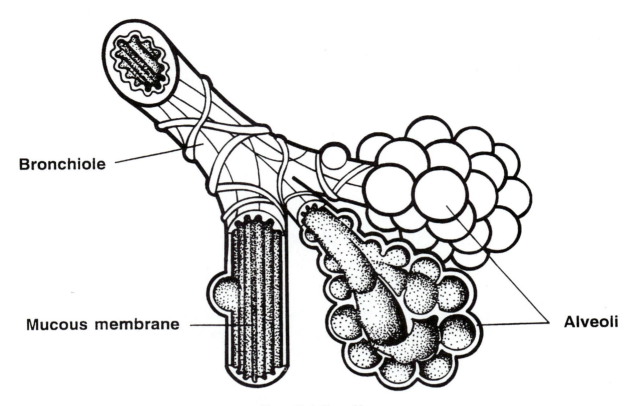

Bronchiole

Mucous membrane

Alveoli

Figure 7–1. Normal lung

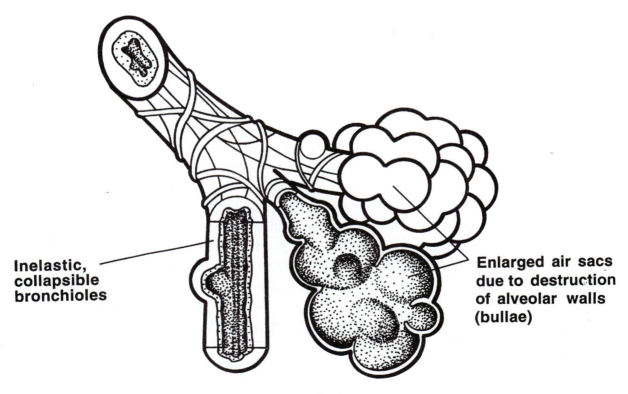

Inelastic, collapsible bronchioles

Enlarged air sacs due to destruction of alveolar walls (bullae)

Figure 7–2. Emphysema

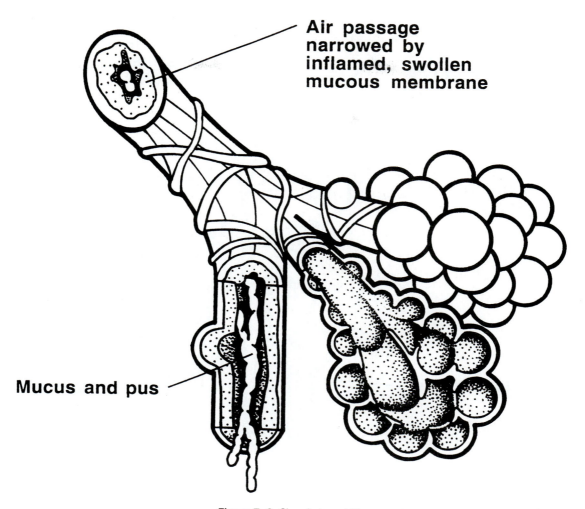

Air passage narrowed by inflamed, swollen mucous membrane

Mucus and pus

Figure 7–3. Chronic bronchitis

stimulates erythropoiesis, resulting in polycythemia, increased blood viscosity, and complications of confusion and stroke.[9]

Infectious organisms are the primary causative agent for exacerbations of chronic bronchitis. These exacerbations are mostly induced by viruses, primarily influenza, parainfluenza, adenovirus, and some strains of rhinovirus, followed by secondary bacterial invasion. The primary bacterial organisms that contribute to the exacerbations are aerobes, such as *Haemophilus influenzae* and *Streptococcus pneumoniae*.[7] Repeated respiratory infections lead to varying degrees of dyspnea and a decline in pulmonary function tests as the airways narrow as a result of inflammation-induced fibrosis of the bronchial wall.

In some patients, exacerbations may be due to an allergic response from an allergen causing eosinophilic inflammation in the bronchial airways. The patients with this condition are referred to as having asthmatic bronchitis, which is characterized by wheezing and airway obstruction that is partially reversible with pharmacologic agents. The irritation from chronic smoking of many years' standing and a person's genetic susceptibility to asthma form asthmatic bronchitis.

Signs, Symptoms, and Diagnosis

The symptoms in the early stages of chronic bronchitis are insidious, with infections causing acute exacerbations. As the disease progresses, a productive cough that is considered the hallmark of chronic bronchitis usually occurs on awakening and often produces substernal discomfort.[10] Mucopurulent sputum production may indicate a secondary bacterial infection, although this is not clearly supported.[11] For example, the traditional view is that yellow sputum represents pus, yet it may be due to inflammation related to asthma. While green

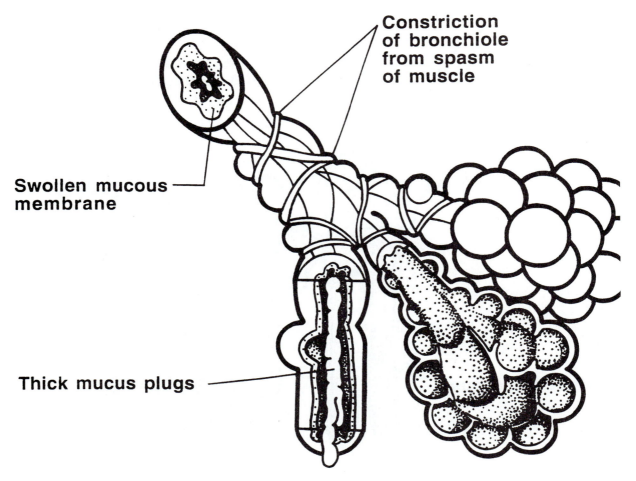

Figure 7–4. Asthma

sputum is a more likely sign of infection, it can also be due to noninfectious inflammation.[12] A fever of 38°C (101°F) usually is an indicator of a bacterial infection. In contrast, a low-grade fever often represents a viral infection.[7]

Other symptoms that lead individuals to seek medical care include decreased exercise tolerance and varying degrees of dyspnea. Individuals have to use accessory muscles more frequently to breathe. Although the expiration phase is prolonged, the anteroposterior (AP) diameter measurement of the thorax is normal. Auscultation of the lungs often discovers localized or diffuse inspiratory and expiratory wheezes and rhonchi. Airway obstruction results in hypoxemia and hypercapnia. If hypoxemia is not reversed, jugular venous distention, peripheral edema, hepatomegaly, and cyanosis are present as a result of pulmonary hypertension that eventually results in cor pulmonale and congestive heart failure. However, clubbing of the fingers is usually not present.

Patients with chronic bronchitis are often stocky or obese. The slang term "blue bloaters" is used frequently to describe these individuals because of the cyanosis, peripheral edema, and hypercapnia reflecting the severity of the disease process.

Diagnosis is made on the basis of physical examination, chest roentgenogram, pulmonary function tests, and arterial blood gas analysis.

The chest radiographic changes may include increased bronchovascular markings in the lower lung field and increased cardiac silhouette if right ventricular failure is present.[8] Pulmonary function test findings will indicate: (1) a decrease in vital capacity; (2) an increase in residual volume; (3) a decrease expiratory flow rate; and (4) the total lung capacity is usually within normal limits. Arterial blood gas findings will indicate: (1) low resting PO_2 (45 to 65 mm Hg); (2) elevated Pco_2 (50 to 60 mm Hg); and (3) an increase in Pco_2 and Po_2 during exercise.

In uncomplicated chronic bronchitis, electrocardiographic findings are within normal limits. However, when pulmonary hypertension and cor pulmonale are present, the findings are: (1) tall P waves in lead II, III, and aVF; (2) right axis deviation; and (3) atrial or ventricular dysrhythmias (often resulting from hypoxemia, acid-base imbalance, and electrolyte abnormalities).[4,8]

■ *Pulmonary Emphysema*

Pulmonary emphysema is defined as an abnormal enlargement of gas-exchange airways (acini) accompanied by destructive changes in the alveolar walls and enlarged air spaces distal to the terminal nonrespiratory bronchioles. The pulmonary obstruction results from changes in lung tissues, rather than mucus production and inflammation as seen in chronic bronchitis.[3,13]

Although the precise etiologic factors for the development of pulmonary emphysema are unknown, recent evidence has suggested that a genetic predisposing factor and cigarette smoking are strongly linked to the pathogenesis of emphysema. This genetic factor is a deficiency in a serum protein called alpha$_1$-antiprotease (antitrypsin). The purpose of the alpha$_1$-antiprotease is to block the enzymatic effect of protease on elastin and collagen, the major protein components of the lung parenchyma. When there is a breakdown in this factor or a deficiency, protease and elastase enzymes attack and destroy the lung connective tissue. Recent studies have shown that cigarette smoke increases elastase secreted by the alveolar macrophages and neutrophils. In addition, it oxidizes a critical amino acid residue of alpha$_1$-protease inhibitor, which then interferes with the activity of this protein.[14]

When elastin in the connective tissue is lost, the lungs become distended, without their normal elastic recoil ability, resulting in decreased lung compliance. Loss of elastin also causes the small airways to collapse or narrow, which allows air to become trapped in the distal spaces, causing increased airway resistance, leading to pressure on the diaphragm. In an effort to breath effectively, a person will use accessory muscles to move trapped air out of the lungs. This process not only increases intrapleural pressure, but it exacerbates airway collapse.[14]

There are two types of emphysema, depending on the site of pulmonary involvement: (1) centrilobular (centriacinar) and (2) panlobular (panacinar). In *centrilobular* emphysema, the respiratory bronchioles at the central lobules are affected: however, the alveoli are not involved. This form of emphysema usually occurs in the upper lobes of the lung. Individuals who smoke and have chronic bronchitis tend to have this type of emphysema. In *panlobular* emphysema, the destruction involves the entire distal acinus, alveolar ducts, and alveoli, resulting in air trappings in the alveoli. This type of emphysema often occurs in the elderly and individuals with a deficiency of alpha$_1$-antiprotease.[1,3,14]

Signs, Symptoms, and Diagnosis

Signs and symptoms associated with emphysema usually appear in the fourth decade, and disability from the disease usually occurs in the fifth or sixth decade of life. The chief complaint is dyspnea, with minimal cough. There is muscle wasting as a result of the poor nutritional intake from shortness of breath and activity intolerance; sexual function is also limited. Therefore, these patients are thin in physical appearance.

The breathing pattern of emphysematous individuals includes: (1) the use of accessory muscles; (2) an increased respiratory rate; (3) a prolonged expiratory phase resulting from the airway narrowing or collapse on expiration; and (4) decreased diaphragmatic excursion. Because of the reduced diaphragmatic excursion, these individuals present with "pursed-lips" breathing. Auscultation presents diminished breath sounds. The AP diameter of the thorax is increased (barrel chest) and there is hyperresonance to percussion and decreased fremitus on palpation.

The diagnosis is based on subjective and objective data. Subjective data should include the following: (1) history of character and onset of dyspnea, cough, sputum, smoking history, family history, exposure to irritants, medications, and self-care modalities.

Pulmonary function objective data include: (1) increased residual volume, residual capacity, and total lung volume; (2) decreased forced expiratory volume; and (3) vital capacity may be normal or only slightly reduced until late in the disease process. Chest x-rays usually show a flattened diaphragm and bullae. Arterial blood gas values may be near normal; however, many individuals develop respiratory alkalosis from hyperventilation to compensate for hypoxemia. Because the pink color they develop from this process, they are often referred to as "pink puffers."

Management

Chronic bronchitis and emphysema are usually irreversible. Therefore, the goals for both these diseases are the same: (1) smoking cessation; (2) bronchial hygiene; (3) prevention of infection; (4) reduction of the rate of progression of the disease process; and (5) health maintenance and compliance with treatment.

The most effective preventive measure against COPD is smoking cessation. In addition, other respiratory irritants should be avoided. Patients should be educated about how to perform bronchial hygiene, which includes postural drainage, adequate hydration, and breathing exercises. To avoid infection, prophylactic vaccination against influenza and pneumococcal pneumonia is recommended by the Centers for Disease Control and Prevention (CDC). To meet the increased metabolic needs related to the high calorie expenditure from increased work in breathing, a high-fat, reduced-carbohydrate diet is recommended. Patients should avoid carbohydrate intake because it requires more ventilation because of a high carbon dioxide production.

Antibiotic therapy is recommended for bacterial respiratory infections. The choice of antibiotic is based on the sputum strain of such patients. Oral ampicillin and amoxicillin are considered the drugs of choice in patients not allergic to penicillin. Other alternatives include tetracycline with sulfamethoxazole (Septra or Bactrim) and oral cephalosporins.

Life-style Changes

Concerns may be expressed about the progression of the disease and the patient's state of well-being. The major life-style change is smoking cessation, which is vital to prevent the progress of COPD. Clonidine transdermal patches (Catapres-TTS) and nicotine replacement therapy (Nicorette gum and transdermal nicotine) have enabled some persons to stop smoking (see Chapter 4). In addition, pulmonary rehabilitation programs are organized to include instruction on the disease process and medication, exercise activities, breathing parameters, and psychosocial support.

■ ASTHMA

Asthma is the most common chronic disease in the United States, afflicting more than 5% of the population; two thirds of asthma sufferers are adults. From the mid-1980s to the mid-1990s, the prevalence increased 60%.[15] The estimated economic cost of asthma in the United States in 1990 was $1.6 billion for inpatient hospital care and another $295 million for emergency care.[15] Despite recent advances in the treatment for asthma, the morbidity and mortality rates are increasing. It has been estimated that 80% to 90% of the deaths are preventable.[16] Most deaths occur outside the hospital as a result of inadequate assessment of the severity of airway constriction or obstruction by the patient or provider and inadequate therapy. Thus, the key to prevention of morbidity and mortality associated with asthma is health education and health promotion.

Asthma is defined as a reversible obstructive airway disorder characterized by a hyperreactivity (increased responsiveness of the airways to a wide variety of stimuli) of the airways.[1] While the stimuli triggering the episode of asthma may vary from one person to another, the end result is usually bronchial constriction, inflammation, edema, and mucus plugs producing variable dyspnea, wheezing, and a harsh cough. Prior to the late 1980s, it was believed that the obstruction of the bronchi and bronchioles was due to bronchospasm. However, new technologies have added substantially to our understanding that asthma is a chronic inflammatory disease with complex "interrelationships of immunology, biochemistry, and physiology contributing to the clinical presentation of asthma."[16]

Although asthma can affect all age groups, in the majority of the cases it begins before the age of 10. There appears to be a genetic predisposition, with the occurrence significantly higher for blacks than whites, and with it affecting males twice as often as females. Although asthma remains a common cause of admission to hospitals and emergency rooms, it affects different age groups at different times of the year. For asthmatic children and young adults, hospitalization usually peaks from September through November; among the middle-aged and older groups, it peaks in the winter.[17] These seasonal peaks are due to inflammatory mediators that initiate the asthma response, such as viral respiratory infections (colds, flu), sudden changes in weather, pollens, mold, and emotional stress.[17]

The etiology of asthma is usually classified according to precipitating factors and individual patterns of response to these factors. Some of the stimuli that can produce an attack of asthma include the following:

Allergens. Immunologic asthma is the result of an antigen-antibody reaction that results in the IgE-mediated allergic response. Allergens produce steric changes in a mast cell, leading to the production of chemical mediators. Some of the chemical mediators are histamine, slow-releasing substance of anaphylaxis (SRS-A), eosinophilic chemotactic factor, and bradykinin. The combined effects of all these factors cause two main reactions: (1) localized edema in the walls of the small bronchioles as well as secretion of thick mucus into the bronchiolar lumens and (2) spasm of the bronchiolar smooth muscle. As a result, the person with an asthmatic attack will have inflamed airways, bronchial hyperreactivity, variable dyspnea, labored breathing, and wheezing.

Some of the common precipitating factors for immunologic asthma include pollens, pollutants, smoke, irritating fumes and odors, change in humidity and air temperature, and dust.

Infections. Nonimmunologic or nonallergic asthma is frequently associated with a history of recurrent respiratory tract infections. Research studies have demonstrated that viral infections are responsible for the asthma response. Often the symptoms from the viral infection may resolve before the bronchial hyperresponsiveness, which may last for days or weeks.

Exercise. Exercise-induced asthma is defined as a decrease in forced expiratory volume in 1 second (FEV_1) of greater than 15% to 20% of baseline value. Although the etiology is unclear, it is thought to be due to heat or water loss from the central airways. Vigorous exercise in cold, dry air is more likely to cause an attack than exercise in warm, humid air. Symptoms of wheezing and coughing usually develop after 5 to 10 minutes of strenuous efforts or shortly after exercise ends.

Emotions. Psychological factors, such as emotional stress, usually do not precipitate asthmatic attacks but can often make the attack worse. Bronchoconstriction appears to be mediated through the parasympathetic nervous system. In addition, smooth muscles of the airways can become constricted as a result of hypocapnia from hyperventilation.

Other Factors. Aspirin sensitivity, sinusitis, rhinitis, and recurrent nasal polyps have been linked to asthma for many years. Inflammatory mediators from the nasal passages into the lung may precipitate bronchial hyperresponsiveness.

Signs, Symptoms, and Diagnosis

Signs and symptoms vary on a continuum from chronic, acute, to life-threatening status asthmaticus. An asthmatic attack is characterized by restlessness, anxiety, altered mental status, dyspnea with use of accessory muscles of respiration, a prolonged expiratory phase, wheezing on auscultation, cough productive of characteristic thick, sticky sputum with mucus plugs, and abnormal blood gas values. These clinical manifestations may occur immediately (early-phase reaction), appearing seconds after exposure to the antigen and can last about 1 hour. However, many individuals may experience a delayed (late-phase) reaction, which can occur 4 to 8 hours after exposure to the antigen and may last for days.

Status asthmaticus, a life-threatening syndrome, occurs when the bronchospasm can no longer be relieved by bronchodilators and corticosteroids, resulting in impaired gas exchange by the obstruction of distal airways. Symptoms include extreme dyspnea, cyanosis, wheezing, rapid and thready pulse, nausea or vomiting, and a harsh cough. The chest is hyperresonant, with diminished breath sounds. In severe attacks, both pulsus paradoxus and sensorium changes are present as a result of decreased cardiac output. Repeated attacks may cause irreversible emphysema, resulting in a permanent decrease in total breathing capacity.

The diagnosis of asthma should include a comprehensive clinical history of any prior episodes of cough, dyspnea, and wheezing. While wheezing is often one of the symptoms in asthma, it does not always indicate a diagnosis of asthma because all asthmatics do not wheeze. When the pulmonary air flow is severely impaired, the conducting airways may not be able to generate an audible wheeze. The medical history should also be elicited to determine evidence of: (1) common allergic triggers such as pets, pollens, dust mites, mold, and feathers; (2) environmental irritants such as cigarette smoke,

household cleaning products; (3) viral respiratory infections; (4) emotional stress; and (5) medication history.

Other data of importance to the diagnosis of asthma include pulmonary function tests, sputum examination, and chest x-rays. Pulmonary function tests vary greatly depending on the stage of the disease existing at the time of the test. The common findings during an asthma attack include: (1) marked decrease in flow rates; (2) reduced forced vital capacity (FVC); (3) increased residual volume (RV) and functional residual volume (FRV); and (4) ventilation-perfusion abnormalities. As a result, the patient can become hypoxemic, with blood gases varying from respiratory alkalosis to respiratory acidosis.[15]

Sputum examination provides information about the infectious process by an increase in neutrophils and eosinophils. Asthma with infection produces sputum that is purulent green or yellow and tenacious.

Chest x-rays are a mechanism by which to ascertain pulmonary complications. For example, hyperinflation, which is caused by increased lung volumes, is evidenced by a lower-than-usual placement of the diaphragm. If an infectious process is present, x-rays may reveal areas of atelectasis, infiltration, and other densities.

Management

The goals of medical management of asthma are to promote normal functioning of the individual and to prevent future attacks. The management of asthma is twofold: (1) pharmacologic therapy and (2) nonpharmacologic therapy. Some medications are principally used to eliminate acute exacerbations, while others are primarily used for prophylaxis to prevent exacerbations (Table 7–1).

Pharmacologic Therapy

Beta₂-Adrenergic Agonists. The $beta_2$-adrenergic agonists such as albuterol (Proventil, Ventolin) and metaproterenol (Alupent) are the most effective bronchodilators, which result in smooth muscle relaxation, mast-cell membrane stabilization, and skeletal muscle stimulation. The mode of delivery directly to the lungs via aerosol allows a reduced dosage, with a subsequent reduction of side effects.[16]

Corticosteroids. Because inflammation is the predominant feature in asthma, the National Heart, Lung, and Blood

TABLE 7–1. SELECTED ASTHMA DRUGS

Medication	Dosage	Side Effects
Proventil (albuterol)	Tablets — ≥12 years, 2–4 mg tid, 6–12 yrs, 2 mg tid-qid. Aerosol — ≥12 years, 2 inhalations q 4–6 h.	Tachycardia, palpitations, nervousness, tremors, nausea, and dyspepsia.
Alupent (metaproterenol sulfate)	Adult: 20 mg or 10 ml (2 tsp) tid or qid. Child (6–9 yr): 10 mg or 5 ml (1 tsp) tid or qid. Child > 9 yr: 20 mg or 10 ml (2 tsp) tid or qid.	Tachycardia, palpitations, nervousness, tremors, and nausea.
Ventolin (albuterol)	Adult and Child (≥ 4 yr): 2 inhalations q 4–6 h, as needed.	Tachycardia, palpitations, nervousness, tremors, nausea, and dyspepsia.
Theo-dur (theophylline anhydrous)	Adult and Child (≥6 yr): 200 mg q 12 h to, followed, if needed and tolerated, by an approximately 25% increase in dosage every 3 days.	Palpitations, tachycardia, extrasystoles, headache, irritability, restlessness, nausea, and vomiting.
Beclovent (beclomethasone dipropionate)	Adult and Child (≥12 yr): 2 inhalations tid or qid, or 4 inhalations bid, up to 20 inhalations/24 h, if needed. Child (6–12 yr): 1–2 inhalations tid or qid or 4 inhalations bid, up to 10 inhalations/24 h, if needed.	Suppression of hypothalamic-pituitary-adrenal function, immediate and delayed immune reactions, hoarseness, and dry mouth.
Deltasone (prednisone)	Adult: 5–60 mg/day to start, then gradually reduce dosage to lowest level consistent with maintaining an adequate clinical response.	Suppression of hypothalamic-pituitary-adrenal function, masks infection, glaucoma, cataracts, peptic ulcer, dermal atrophy.
Solu-Cortef (hydrocortisone sodium succinate)	Adult: 100–500 mg IV, repeated at intervals of 2, 4, or 6 h, as determined by patient's response and clinical condition. Infant and child: adult dosage may be reduced according to severity of disease and clinical response; minimum dose: 25 mg/day.	Suppression of hypothalamic-pituitary-adrenal function, masks infection, glaucoma, cataracts, peptic ulcer, dermal atrophy.
Intal (Cromolyn sodium)	Aerosol—adults and children over 5 yr: 2 inhalations 4 times daily. Solution—adults and children over 2 yrs: 20 mg administered by nebulizer 4 times a day.	Bronchospasms, throat irritation, bad taste, cough, wheezing, nasal congestion, and anaphylaxis.

Institute in 1991 recommended the use of anti-inflammatory agents (beclomethasone, prednisone, and others) to reduce and prevent recurrence of the asthma attack. Oral steroids are used for patients who do not respond to inhaled steroid therapy or for short courses during an acute attack. Dosages and choice of steroid vary; for unstable patients, higher dosages are required.[16]

Methylxanthines. Theophylline (Theo-Dur, Theo-24, and others) is the primary methylxanthine used to produce bronchodilation. Methylxanthines are ineffective by aerosol and therefore must be taken systemically. Because of the availability of slow-release oral preparations, theophylline preparations are often used for preventive therapy.[16]

Cromolyn Sodium. Cromolyn (Intal) is often used as a prophylactic agent. It inhibits the release of chemicals involved in air-flow obstruction. It is considered one of the safest asthma drugs and therefore it is often the first choice for children as well as adults who need medication. The majority of adults and children with mild to moderate chronic asthma will be adequately controlled with cromolyn. Cromolyn is only effective by inhalation and is available as a metered-dose inhaler, dry powder inhaler, and a nebulized solution.[16]

Anticholinergics. These drugs produce bronchodilation by blocking parasympathetic innervation at the cholinergic receptors on the larger airways. Ipratropium bromide (Atrovent) and atropine sulfate are two drugs that are used in aerosol form in patients with intractable asthma when cholinergic stimulation is thought to precipitate the attack.[16]

Oxygen. Oxygen therapy is given for hypoxemia. Low flow rates (1 to 3L/min) are used via nasal cannula with humidity.

Nonpharmacologic Therapy. Because bronchial secretions in asthma are characteristically thick and tenacious, with numerous mucus plugs, an important therapy is hydrating the patient through administration of fluids to thin secretions for mobilization and to improve the productive cough reflex. However, body fluid balance needs to be carefully monitored to prevent overhydration, especially in those individuals with compromised cardiac function.

Chest physiotherapy, including postural drainage with percussion and vibration, deep breathing, and coughing also facilitate removal of tracheobronchial secretions. The frequency and duration of these treatments should be scheduled according to the person's responses and tolerance. Effective pulmonary hygiene may preclude a life-threatening asthmatic attack. Therefore, patient education and teaching patients self-management is the cornerstone of management. Ensuring that the patient understands the pathogenesis of asthma and the appropriate use of his or her medications is important, but focusing on what allergens trigger the asthmatic attack is even more important. For example, the patient should control environmental factors, consider allergy shots for allergic rhinitis, and practice relaxation techniques to facilitate slow breathing pattern and to reduce emotional stress.

Life-style Changes

Most patients with childhood asthma will recover spontaneously. However, when the development of asthma occurs in later life, spontaneous recovery is less likely and patients will suffer with asthma all their lives.[15] Therefore, concerns may be expressed about achieving the best quality of life possible.

Quality of life for patients with asthma can be achieved through rehabilitation. The American Thoracic Society defines rehabilitation as a process to "return the patient to the highest possible functional capacity allowed by his or her pulmonary handicap and overall life situation."[18] Because a satisfying quality of life is a fundamental desire of all human beings, clinicians are in a unique position to assist asthmatic patients to higher levels of life quality through health education and health promotion. Thus the clinician's role is to have an individualized self-care plan for each patient. These plans can then be altered to fit in with any changes in the disease or the patient's life-style. The more aware asthmatic patients are about their self-care, the more likely they are able to control the disease process.

■ PNEUMONIA

General Characteristics

Pneumonia is an acute infection of the lower respiratory tract that causes an inflammatory process of the lung parenchyma involving interstitial tissues, distal airways, and acini.[19–24] As a result of the inflammation, the involved lung tissues become edematous with accumulation of exudate in the bronchioles and alveoli. Mode of transmission and clinical manifestations vary, depending on the etiologic agent. Most often, gas exchange cannot occur and nonoxygenated blood is shunted into the vascular system, causing hypoxemia.[25]

The pneumonias generally are classified into two groups: (1) community-acquired and (2) hospital-acquired (nosocomial). By definition, community-acquired pneumonias are contracted outside the hospital environment and usually begin as common respiratory illnesses that progress to fulminant pulmonary infections. Hospital-acquired, or nosocomial, pneumonias are contracted during hospitalization and are most commonly caused by bacteria.[26,27]

Pneumonia is the most serious respiratory infection and major cause of death in the United States. Overall, it is the fifth leading cause of mortality.[28] Pneumonia occurs throughout the year, with a higher rate during the winter months. More than 1 million cases of pneumonia are diagnosed each year,[28] affecting persons of all ages. It has been recognized that the mortality rate associated with pneumonia is the highest with the elderly, the very young, and the chronically ill person.[29]

Pneumonia can be caused by numerous etiologic agents, such as viruses, bacteria, mycoplasma, fungi, and parasites; however, the majority of pneumonias are caused by either bacteria or a virus. Although fungi are uncommon causes of pneumonia, they can be seen in immunosuppressed individuals. Examples include candidiasis, histoplasmosis, cryptococcosis, and aspergillosis.[29]

■ *Bacterial Pneumonia*

The most common cause of community-acquired bacterial pneumonia is *Streptococcus pneumoniae* (gram-positive diplococcus). It is estimated that *S. pneumoniae* accounts for 40% to 80% of all community-acquired pneumo-

nias.[21] This type of pneumonia is lobar pneumonia and is commonly referred to as pneumococcal pneumonia.[1] The onset begins acutely, with rapidly rising fever and shaking chills. The sputum is mucopurulent or rust-colored. Pneumococcal pneumonia is often seen in the following clinical situations:[1,30]

- COPD
- sickle cell disease
- congestive heart failure
- alcoholism
- diabetes mellitus

Haemophilus influenzae (gram-negative bacillus) infection often occurs following an episode of influenza A or B. It also causes a lobar type of pneumonia; therefore, *Haemophilus influenzae* may mimic pneumococcal pneumonia. This type of pneumonia has become more difficult to treat because the bacteria frequently produce beta-lactamase and become ampicillin- and amoxicillin-resistant.[29,31]

Staphylococcus aureus (gram-positive bacillus) pneumonia occurs most often as a secondary complication after an episode of influenza A or B and recent antibiotic therapy, which are predisposing factors to oropharyngeal bacterial colonization. *S. aureus* pneumonia is often seen in children under the age of 3, the chronically ill person, and the elderly in nursing homes.[29,31]

The most common causes of nosocomial pneumonia are the gram-negative microorganisms such as *Escherichia coli, Pseudomonas aeruginosa, Proteus* species, *Klebsiella pneumoniae, Bacteroides* species, and *Haemophilus influenzae*. However, alcoholics, nursing home residents, and diabetics are especially susceptible to *Klebsiella pneumoniae*. Clinically, the pneumonia developed in patients in the hospital can be overshadowed by an underlying disease. Nevertheless, pneumonia is usually suspected when there is fever or an increase in fever, pleuritic chest pain, and purulent sputum production.[28–31]

■ *Atypical Pneumonia*

Viral pneumonia usually develops after an episode of influenza, chickenpox (varicella), or adenovirus.[32] The risk groups include elderly persons with chronic diseases such as diabetes mellitus and congestive heart failure or pregnant women. The patient presents with severe dyspnea, cyanosis, scant sputum, fever, and persistent dry cough. The severity of the illness carries a high mortality rate because it progresses rapidly to acute respiratory failure.[33]

Mycoplasma pneumoniae infection is known as "walking pneumonia," which is frequently seen in school-aged children and young adults. The patient presents with chills, malaise, anorexia, sore throat, fever, and cough. The clinical course is usually benign and self-limiting.[34,35]

Pneumocystis carinii pneumonia occurs most frequently in immunocompromised persons with acquired immunodeficiency syndrome (AIDS) or those who have received organ transplants.[29] The organism occupies the surface of the alveolar epithelial lining and multiplies rapidly by going through continual cycles of trophozoite stage and cyst formation. Clinical manifestations usually begin insidiously and the patient presents with fever, nonproductive cough, night sweats, dyspnea, and hypoxemia. Examination of the lungs may be normal despite significant abnormalities on a chest x-ray.[29]

The major mechanisms by which the microorganisms gain access to the lower respiratory tract are:

- inhalation of microbes that are present in the air;
- aspiration of organisms from the oropharyngeal flora; and
- hematogenous spread to the lung from an extrapulmonary site of infection.

The infectious agents may reach the lung when there is significant impairment of the lung defense mechanisms or impairment of the blood supply, such as lack of phagocytic cells, antibodies, and other elements of the immunologic system, which deprive the lungs of their second line of defense.[10] Predominantly, there is a ventilation: perfusion mismatch ($\dot{V}:\dot{Q}$) and right to left shunting occurs when the alveoli are completely filled with inflammatory exudate.[21,29,33]

Signs, Symptoms, and Diagnosis

The clinical manifestations in the patient with pneumonia are varied because the interaction between the individual and the microorganism determines the manifestation. Some patients experience few symptoms, whereas others become critically ill. A history of exposure to tuberculosis must be sought, as well as the possibility of immunocompromising disease or therapies, since the signs and symptoms of pneumonia may be absent in the immunocompromised patient.

Pneumonias caused by anaerobic organisms are usually associated with aspiration and occur in patients with altered level of consciousness or impaired protective reflexes. A characteristic of this type of pneumonia is a cough productive of sputum with a foul odor.[36]

Pneumonias caused by bacteria, such as *Streptococcus pneumoniae* and *Haemophilus influenzae,* have an abrupt onset and are characterized by high fever, pleuritic chest pain, and shaking chills accompanied by a cough that becomes productive with mucopurulent sputum that is often rust-colored. Physical examination of the lungs reveals evidence of consolidations, including dullness to percussion over the affected area of the lungs with increased vocal fremitus, bronchophony, egophony, inspiratory rhonchi, decreased breath sounds, and rales. Chest x-ray findings include patchy infiltrates or consolidation over the affected area and occasionally pleural effusion. Arterial blood gas analysis shows evidence of hypoxemia. The white blood cell count is elevated, with an increase in the immature polymorphonuclear leukocytes.[29–30,33]

Atypical pneumonias, such as *Mycoplasma pneumoniae* and viral pneumonias, have a gradual, insidious onset of symptoms that include a sore throat, muscle soreness, fatigue, and headache, usually accompanied by a dry cough. Physical examination reveals a few scattered wheezes and crackles with minimal or no evidence of consolidation. Chest x-ray findings range from minimal infiltrates to substantial bilateral infiltrates. The white blood cell count can be slightly elevated but is usually less than 10,000/mL.[37]

The diagnosis of pneumonia is suspected after an adequate history and physical examination have been obtained. Chest x-ray confirms the presence of pneumonia in the affected lung fields. Examination of expectorated sputum for gram stain, culture, and sensitivity is done to identify the causative microorganism. Studies of the white blood cell (WBC) count will typically show an increase ($>$10,000) in bacterial pneumonias and may be normal or low in viral or mycoplasmal pneumonias. Acid-fast stains and cultures are done to rule out tuberculosis. Serologic studies that include acute and convalescent titers are done to diagnose viral pneumonia. A relative rise in antibody titers is suggestive of a viral infection. Arterial blood gases are routinely analyzed to determine respiratory status.

Management

Bacterial pneumonias are treated with antimicrobial drugs (Table 7–2) and supportive therapy. The choice of antibiotics will be determined by the information from bacteriologic studies. Usually pneumococcal pneumonia and anaerobic aspiration pneumonia are treated with penicillin. For penicillin-allergic patients, erythromycin is an alternative in pneumococcal pneumonia and clindamycin is the preferred alternative in anaerobic pneumonia. Ciprofloxacin is active against gram-positive cocci and gram-negative bacilli as well as *S. aureus* and *H. influenzae.*[1,30–31]

Viral pneumonias, unless complicated by bacterial superinfection, will not respond to antibiotics; however, some of the antiviral agents have been very effective. For example, acyclovir has been effective in the treatment of varicella zoster pneumonia and aerosolized ribavirin for respiratory syncytial virus. Supportive therapy is directed toward relief of symptoms; it generally includes bed rest, adequate hydration, proper nutritional intake, supplemental oxygen, antitussives, and mild analgesics to relieve muscle pain and fever.[1,30–31]

TABLE 7–2. SELECTED ANTIBIOTICS FOR PNEUMONIA

Medication	Dosage	Side Effects
Amoxicillin (Amoxil)	Adults: 500 mg q 8 h. Children: 40 mg/kg/day in 3 divided doses q 8 h.	Superinfection, anaphylaxis, urticaria, GI upset, blood dyscrasias, and hyperactivity.
EES (erythromycin ethylsuccinate)	Adults: 400 mg tid-qid. Children: 30–50 mg/kg/day in divided doses every 6 hours.	Hepatotoxicity, superinfection, GI upset, rash, reversible hearing loss, and arrhythmias.
Ceclor (cefaclor)	Adults: 500 mg q 8 h. Children: >1 month, 40 mg/kg/day in divided doses, max 1 g/day.	GI upset, diarrhea, rash, blood dyscrasias, hepatotoxicity, CNS stimulation, serum sickness-like reactions, superinfection.
Cipro (ciprofloxacin)	Adults: 500–750 mg q 12h. Children: <18 yrs not recommended.	CNS stimulation, superinfection, GI upset, headache, restlessness, rash, eosinophilia, elevated liver enzymes, and photosensitivity.
Biaxin (clarithromycin)	Adults: 500 mg q 12 h. Children: not recommended.	GI upset, abnormal taste, headache.
Bicillin (penicillin G benzathine and penicillin G procaine)	Adults: 1.2 million Im every 2–3 days until temperature normal Children: 60,000 units Im every 2–3 days until temperature normal.	Rash, drug fever, serum sickness, anaphylaxis, superinfection, blood dyscrasias, neuropathy, nephropathy.

■ TUBERCULOSIS

General Characteristics

Tuberculosis refers to infection caused by two microorganisms, *Mycobacterium tuberculosis* and *Mycobacterium bovis.*[28] However, the rod-shaped *Mycobacterium tuberculosis* bacillus is responsible for tuberculosis in humans.[38] *Tuberculosis infection* refers to a state in which the tuberculosis organism is established in a person; however, the person is asymptomatic, chest x-ray results are normal, and bacteriologic studies are negative. Consequently, there is no active disease process in these persons. In contrast, the term *tuberculosis* refers to the disease process involving one or more organs of the body. It is primarily a disease of the lungs, although extrapulmonary involvement is common in richly oxygenated sites such as the kidneys, heart, and growing bone tissues.[29,39]

Tuberculosis is an ancient infection that has plagued humans throughout recorded history. Although improved working conditions, housing, nutrition, and modern treatment has resulted in a decline in the mortality rate, tuberculosis remains a worldwide pathogen that causes approximately 3 million deaths annually. Since 1984, the number of US tuberculosis cases reported to the CDC has increased 20%. These increases are largely due to the susceptibility of persons with human immunodeficiency virus (HIV) to tuberculosis, people living in crowded living conditions that favor airborne spread of the bacilli, individuals who are debilitated (alcoholics or malnourished individuals), and those who report nonadherence to recommended drug regimens for the disease.[38,40]

M. tuberculosis is an acid-fast aerobic bacterium. It is most commonly found in particles known as nuclei. These droplet nuclei become airborne when a person with tuberculosis has coughed or exhaled into the air. The bacilli are then inhaled and most often lodge in the upper portion of the lung. However, extrapulmonary sites can be involved because blood and lymph can carry the *M. tuberculosis* to other tissues that are richly oxygenated such as the kidneys, heart, meninges, and growing bone tissues.[29,38,41,42]

Once the bacilli are lodged in the lung, they multiply and cause a nonspecific inflammation. This inflammation triggers the immune system to respond, causing neutrophils and macrophages to migrate to the area. If these cells are successful in engulfing and destroying the bacilli, a granulomatous lesion called a tubercle is formed. Within this fibrotic tubercle lesion, the bacilli may remain dormant for life. However, if the immune system becomes impaired, active disease can occur and the bacilli may spread through the blood and lymphatics to other tissues and organs.[1,41–42]

The *M. tuberculosis* organism is a robust bacillus that is capable of surviving for long periods under adverse circumstances. Because the tubercle bacilli generally must be inhaled for infection to occur, environmental surfaces are rarely associated with transmission of infection. Items such as food trays, utensils, or items that touch only intact skin do not transmit tubercle bacilli. Therefore, normal disinfection is required as for other patients. The focus is on the air exchanges in rooms or buildings, since the airborne droplets are carried on air currents and remain infectious until they die, are vented to the outdoors, or are killed by exposure to ultraviolet light. To lower the risk of transmission from infected persons, the indoor environment must have a large dilution of air, proper flow, and ventilation of air with ultraviolet irradiation (natural or artificial).[43–44]

Signs, Symptoms, and Diagnosis

Primary infection with *M. tuberculosis* bacilli may occur shortly after exposure to the bacilli or most often occurs within 1 to 2 years of exposure. However, all infected persons will not necessarily develop tuberculosis. For individuals who develop tuberculosis, the symptoms will vary from person to person depending on the extent of the disease. During the early stages, a person with a small inflammatory lesion will be asymptomatic. As the disease progresses, the most common symptom is a nonproductive cough that eventually becomes productive with mucopurulent sputum. Hemoptysis may develop when there is extensive cavitary disease. A sharp pleuritic type of chest pain will develop when the lung tissue adjacent to the pleura is involved. Other symptoms include fever, night sweats, malaise, weight loss, anorexia, and fatigue that develop insidiously after infection. For persons with HIV infection, the interval between infection and the development of symptoms usually is shorter than with HIV-negative persons with the infection.[29,41–42,44]

The diagnosis of tuberculosis begins with a history of the person's past or recent exposure to the bacilli. Chest x-ray findings are often nonspecific. However, the classic presentation shows upper lobe abnormalities, often with cavitation.[1,29]

The tuberculin purified protein derivative (PPD) skin test remains the most specific and sensitive diagnostic method for the detection of *M. tuberculosis* infection. Two types of tuberculin preparations are available in the United States: old tuberculin (OT), which is a filtrate of sterile, killed concentrates from cultures of tubercle bacilli and is available in multiple-puncture devices (rarely used), and PPD, a filtrate of OT, is available for both the Mantoux intradermal injection method and the percutaneous injection by multiple puncture (tine test). PPD is available in three strengths: 1,5, and 250 tuberculin units (TU). However, the 5 TU PPD preparation is the most widely used for the Mantoux test.[45–48]

Once the PPD is injected intradermally into the anterior surface of the forearm, a wheal of 6 to 10 mm is usually produced. The outer margin of the wheal is marked and the test is read 48 to 72 hours after injection. The diameter of induration is measured (Fig. 7–5). The reaction to injected tuberculin is a cellular hypersensitivity reaction characterized by a delayed response and induration secondary to cell infiltration. An induration of 5 mm is considered positive for high-risk persons such as persons with HIV disease and persons with chest x-ray findings consistent with healed tuberculosis.[45–48]

An induration of 10 mm is considered positive for high-risk persons who are exposed to active cases of tuberculosis (eg, health care workers), born in areas where the prevalence of tuberculosis is high (Asia, Central America, South Texas), or have certain diseases (diabetes mellitus, silicosis, malabsorption syndrome). An induration of 15 mm is considered positive for persons without any risk factors.[45–48]

Because of the current increase in tuberculosis, any person who has a positive tuberculin reaction, even one who has received the BCG vaccine (may produce a false positive), is considered to be infected with *M. tuberculosis*. Individuals who have a negative result and are highly suspected of having tuberculosis should have a repeated Mantoux test with another 5 TU or a 250 TU dose. In addition, it is highly recommended that if an anergic condition is suspected, as in HIV-infected persons, skin testing with mumps, tetanus, and candidal antigens is recommended by some to evaluate delayed hypersensitivity. A negative reaction to these antigens suggests an anergic state.[45–48]

When tuberculosis disease is active, the tubercle bacillus can be cultured from the sputum or body fluids and may be

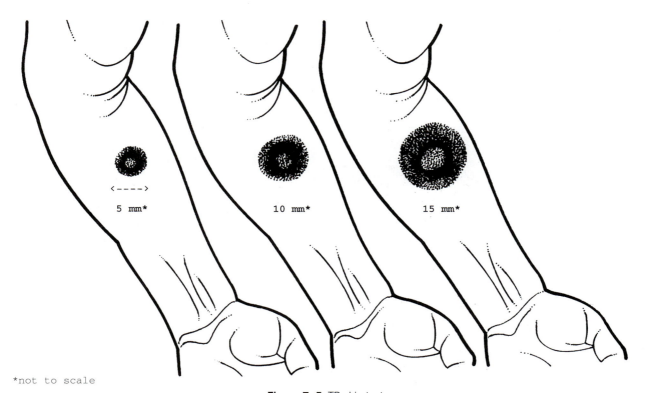

5 mm*   10 mm*   15 mm*

*not to scale

Figure 7–5. TB skin test

seen with an acid-fast stain. Often multiple specimens will be required to confirm the organism.

Management

Persons with active tuberculosis ideally will remain at home or, rarely, in the hospital until sputum cultures show that the active bacilli have been eliminated. If the person is adherant to the medication therapy, this usually takes a few weeks to 2 months. Treatment for both pulmonary and extrapulmonary active disease lasts 6 to 9 months. The recommended drugs are isoniazid (INH), rifampin, pyrazinamide, and ethambutol (Table 7–3). Although isoniazid is the most effective antituberculosis drug, it is recommended that three or more drugs be given to make sure that resistant organisms are covered. Because of the increased numbers of immunosuppressed and susceptible individuals and drug-resistant bacilli, it is recommended that a combination of these four drugs be given to these individuals.[38,41,42,47]

Serious side effects from these drugs such as peripheral neuritis, hyperuricemia leading to joint swelling and pain, liver toxicity, flulike syndrome, and gastrointestinal irritation can cause patients not to adhere to their medicine therapy. Nonadherence is a serious problem, which can cause treatment failure, drug resistance, continuing transmission of infection, and increase in morbidity and mortality. Vitamin B_6 (50 mg/d) is administered to prevent peripheral neuropathy from isoniazid. In addition, liver enzymes should be evaluated before drug therapy begins and then evaluated every month thereafter. To control drug resistant strains, some health departments require that persons with tuberculosis receive their medication under health supervision.[41,42,49]

Life-style Changes

Tuberculosis remains a challenging, deadly disease. To deter the rise of this disease, the American Thoracic Society and the CDC have provided preventive therapy guidelines. Treatment regimens are aimed at killing the rapidly growing mycobacteria. Consequently, a person's adherence to the drug therapy is critical to prevent the resurgence of the disease and drug-resistant tuberculosis. Patient education about the side effects of the medication and how to take the medication provides the gold standard of adherence. With early diagnosis and proper treatment, respiratory functional impairment will be unusual and a majority of people will be able to return to their occupation and live a normal life.

TABLE 7–3. ANTI-TUBERCULAR MEDICATION

Medication	Dosage	Side Effects
Nydrazid (Isoniazid)	Adults: 300 mg q day. Children: 10–20 kg q day. Usually given concurrently with pyridoxine (Vit B6).	Hepatitis, peripheral neuropathy, hepatic injury, GI distress, blood dyscrasias, pyridoxine deficiency, hyperglycemia, rheumatic and SLE-like syndrome.
Rifadin (Rifampin)	Adults: 600 mg q day. 10–20 mg/kg/day; max 600 mg/day.	Hepatitis, jaundice, GI upset, headache, drowsiness, ataxia, dizziness, confusion, visual disturbances, muscular weakness, fever, urticaria, blood dyscrasia.
Myambutol (ethambutol HCL)	Adults: Give in one daily dose. 15 mg/kg/day. Children: under 13 yrs not recommended.	Reduced visual acuity, optic neuritis, anaphylaxis, dermatitis, pruritus, joint pain, GI upset, fever, malaise, headache, dizziness, confusion, peripheral neuritis, gout.
Pyrazinamide	Adults and Children: 15–30 mg/kg once daily; max 2 g daily.	Hepatitis, liver dysfunction, gout, GI disturbances, arthralgia, myalgia, blood dyscrasia (rare).

Note: Combination preparations include Rifamate (Rifampin 300 mg and isoniazid 150 mg) and Rifater (Rifampin 120 mg, isoniazid 50 mg, and pyrazinamide 300 mg).

PULMONARY EMBOLISM

General Characteristics

Pulmonary embolus (PE) is an undissolved mass such as a thrombus (blood clot), lipids (fat), air bubble, tissue fragments, amniotic fluid, or foreign bodies (catheter tips) that travels in the systemic circulation to the pulmonary circulation and results in a partial or complete occlusion of the pulmonary artery (PA) or one of its branches[50–52] A thrombus becomes an embolus when it becomes detached from the inner lining of the vein and is carried by the bloodstream. Often these small emboli lodge in the distal branches of the pulmonary artery.[50] When vessels are too small for the emboli to pass through, destruction of the lung tissues occurs distal to the occlusion as a result of disruption of blood supply.[52,53]

Incidence. In the United States, it is estimated that pulmonary emboli contributes to 100,000 deaths per year and that approximately one half of the deaths occur within 2 hours after embolization.[51,53,54] Because a PE can mimic right heart failure, cardiogenic shock, pulmonary edema, or coronary insufficiency, these estimations may be low as a result of misdiagnoses, both in terms of overdiagnosis when not present, and underdiagnosis when present. Many of the instances have been diagnosed after death.[55–57] Pulmonary embolism can affect individuals of all ages; however, it rarely occurs in children.[51,58] Although a PE is a common occurrence in adult patients, it is one of the most difficult diagnoses to make because it is not a distinct disease entity but rather a serious complication of many medical and surgical disorders.[50,52,53]

Etiology. More than 95% of emboli are from a thrombus that begins in a deep vein of the leg (DVT) or pelvis, which can occur any time that blood pools in a vein.[51,59–61] The larger leg veins above the knee are the most common source of pulmonary embolism as compared to the small calf veins, which only pose a small risk of developing a PE.[62]

Virchow (1858) identified the following classic triad of risk factors that predispose individuals to venous thrombosis: (1) venous stasis; (2) injury to the vascular endothelium; and (3) blood hypercoagulable state.[51,53,54,57,61]

Venous stasis may result from a number of conditions such as immobility, obesity, congestive heart failure, prolonged bed rest, sitting for long periods of time, pregnancy, or atrial fibrillation, which causes blood stasis in myocardial chambers. Venous stasis remains the leading cause of DVT.[53,57] Vascular endothelium injury may result from mechanical injury to the intima of vessel walls from direct trauma as with surgery (especially hip, knee, and tibial), bone fractures, varicose veins, or chemical irritation from the infusion or injection of agents such as potassium or hypertonic glucose.[63] A hypercoagulable blood state can result from clotting disorders, polycythemia vera, sickle cell anemia, fever, as well of use of oral contraceptives, especially in women who smoke.[50–52,57,64]

Nonthrombotic risk factors include: catheter embolus that results when a piece of a catheter breaks off and lodges in a pulmonary vessel, foreign bodies that are injected into the vascular system by intravenous routes, amniotic fluid that is introduced into the venous circulation during pregnancy, an air embolus that enters into the bloodstream during an invasive procedure, and gas emboli, which may result from any condition that exposes people to increased atmospheric pressure.[58,64]

Pathophysiology. Most pulmonary emboli originate as thrombi in the deep venous system, and approximately 15% to 20% of these thrombi that embolize to the lungs occur when the proximal veins of the legs are involved.[51,63] The degree of hemodynamic compromise that occurs with a pulmonary embolus correlates with the degree of the pulmonary vascular obstruction. That is, the size of the pulmonary vessel and the number of emboli determine the respiratory and hemodynamic responses that lead to the severity of symptoms.[57,61–63]

As a result of the pulmonary blood flow obstruction, platelets aggregate and adhere to the embolus. It is presumed that these platelets release vasoactive substances such as histamine, serotonin, and prostaglandins, causing bronchoconstriction. These factors act together to produce a ventilation-perfusion ($\dot{V}/\dot{Q}$) mismatch.[57] There is adequate ventilation, but inadequate perfusion. Consequently, arterial hypoxemia results from any sustained V/Q mismatch. To compensate, the respiratory rate increases, resulting in a decreased Pco_2. Hypocapnia further increases the bronchoconstriction and vasoconstriction.[61] As the condition worsens, there is a decrease in surfactant production and surface-tension–reducing activity in the affected areas of the lung. Consequently, atelectasis develops with intrapulmonary shunting.[51,53,54,57,61,64–66]

Because of the decrease in arterial blood flow through the lungs, there is an increase in PA pressures and right ventricular afterload. The major hemodynamic consequence is pulmonary arterial hypertension. As the pulmonary vascular resistance increases, there is an increased work load of the right ventricle. When the right ventricle is unable to sustain the increase in work load, right heart failure develops. Cardiac output decreases because of the right ventricular dilatation and a decreased left ventricular preload. The sequela of these factors is systemic hypotension.[51,61,62,67–70]

Signs, Symptoms, and Diagnosis

The signs and symptoms of PE may be sudden and abrupt in onset, may be insidious, or may range from no symptoms to sudden death.[56,59–61] The extent and degree of clinical manifestations relate to the degree of vascular occlusion caused by the emboli. The most common symptom is a sharp, pleuritic pain (usually unilateral) accompanied by dyspnea and a cough. Tachypnea is the most common clinical sign as the body attempts to restore homeostasis initiated by the baroreceptors.[56,64] Other classic physical findings include: (1) apprehension, restlessness, and anxiety as a result of hypoxemia; (2) hemoptysis, which is an infrequent finding and usually an indicator of pulmonary infarction; however, absence of hemoptysis does not rule out a PE; (3) diaphoresis, nausea or vomiting, fever, and leukocytosis; (4) syncope episodes, which may be due to a decreased cardiac output; (5) nonspecific rales or wheezing; and (6) a gallop rhythm or murmur located in the pulmonic valve area and an increased S_2 heart sound as a result of pulmonary hypertension. A pulmonary infarction that extends to the pleura may produce a friction rub and a pleural effusion finding on chest x-ray. Massive blood vessel occlusion causes profound shock, hypotension, narrowing pulse pressure, tachycardia, and tachypnea.[50–56,61,69]

The diagnosis of PE should be suspected in any person who presents with suggestive clinical signs and symptoms. The evaluation of predisposing risk factors is an important aspect of diagnosis because the signs and symptoms of PE are nonspecific. In addition, objective testing methods are necessary in confirming the diagnosis.[52,56,63]

Pulmonary angiography is the "gold standard" for PE diagnosis.[56] It has the greatest diagnostic certainty in diagnos-

ing a PE. However, it is expensive and an invasive procedure that requires right heart catheterization and injection of dye into the pulmonary artery to visualize the pulmonary vessels. Consequently, this procedure exposes the patient to more radiation than a $\dot{V}/\dot{Q}$ scan.[57,60,64]

The $\dot{V}/\dot{Q}$ scan is the most frequently used objective testing method to diagnosis PE because it demonstrates a 90% accuracy rate.[7] A scan showing a $\dot{V}/\dot{Q}$ mismatch (normal ventilation and decreased perfusion) suggests a PE, as compared to a normal $\dot{V}/\dot{Q}$ scan, which excludes the diagnosis of PE.[71,72]

Arterial blood gas (ABG) levels may be normal, but often the ABG values will demonstrate hypoxemia (Pa_{O_2} <80 mm Hg), hypocarbia (P_{CO_2} <35 mm Hg), and respiratory alkalosis (pH > 7.45). However, a normal Pa_{O_2} does not rule out PE.[64,68]

More than 50% of patients with a PE will have electrocardiographic (ECG) changes.[68] The specific ECG changes for PE are S wave in lead I and a Q wave in lead III.[64,68] Other changes include a right axis deviation and inverted T waves in the right precordial leads. A new onset or incomplete right bundle branch block are indicative of pulmonary emboli.[50,64,68]

Laboratory studies such as coagulation studies, serum enzyme studies, and blood cell counts are generally nonspecific and have little value in the diagnosis of PE.[69] However, these studies are useful in differentiating a PE from other diagnosis such as myocardial infarction.[64,69]

Management

The main objective of PE management is directed toward maintaining adequate ABG exchange for cardiovascular and pulmonary functions. Because pulmonary embolism is a life-threatening condition, management is also directed toward prevention. General management of PE includes supplemental oxygen, either by nasal cannula, nonrebreathing mask, or mechanical ventilation, to correct the impaired gas exchange and to increase tissue perfusion. A high Fowler's position will also facilitate breathing and lung expansion.[61,68]

Before medication therapy is initiated (Table 7–4), a person's activated partial thromboplastin time (APTT) is obtained for a baseline measure and then at regular intervals for drug therapeutic maintenance. During the first 24 to 72 hours, thrombolytic therapy, such as streptokinase and urokinase, is administered for a more rapid restoration of hemodynamic properties. Patients receiving thrombolytic therapy need to be monitored closely because hemorrhagic complications often

TABLE 7–4. PULMONARY EMBOLISM MEDICATIONS

Medication	Dosage	Side Effects
Coumadin (warfarin sodium, crystalline)	Adult: 2–5 mg/day.	Tissue or organ hemorrhage, skin or tissue necrosis, alopecia, urticaria, dermatitis, fever, nausea, diarrhea, urine discoloration, abdominal cramping, purple toes syndrome, hepatic injury, priapism.
Heparin sodium	Adults: IV administration, 10,000 units to start, followed by 5–10,000 units q 4–6 h. Child: 50 units/kg by IV drip to start, followed by either 100 units/kg by IV drip q 4 h or 20,000 units/m^2/24 h by continuous IV infusion.	Bleeding, thrombocytopenia, local reactions.
Abbokinase (urokinase)	Adult: 4,400 IU/kg (15 ml) by infusion at a rate of 90 ml/h over a period of 10 min, followed by 4,400 IU/kg/h (15 ml/h) by continuous IV infusion for 12 h; total dose 195 ml.	Bleeding, fever, GI upset, transient changes in blood pressure, tachycardia, dyspnea, cyanosis, back pain, hypoxemia, acidosis, allergic bronchospasm, rash.
Activase (alteplase, recombinant)	Adult: 100 mg via IV infusion over 2 h.	Bleeding, reperfusion arrhythmias, urticaria.
Kabikinase and Streptase (streptokinase)	Adults: 250,000 IU by IV infusion over 30 min to start, followed by 100,000 IU/h by continuous IV infusion for 24 h.	Bleeding, hypotension, fever, urticaria, pruritus, flushing, nausea, headache, musculoskeletal pain, vasculitis, interstitial nephritis, anaphylactoid reactions, polyneuropathy, and noncardiogenic pulmonary edema.

occur. If hemorrhagic complications do occur, the drug is discontinued and fresh frozen plasma is given because it contains all the clotting factors. If no complications occur, heparin therapy is administered after the 24 to 72 hour time period.[73–76]

Continuous intravenous heparin remains the drug of choice because it slows the clotting by inactivating thrombin and preventing the conversion of fibrinogen to fibrin. Heparin therapy is titrated to maintain APTT between 60 and 80 seconds.[69] Heparin therapy is continued for 7 to 10 days, followed by warfarin therapy for several months. Warfarin is administered at any time during the heparin therapy to prevent a break in the level of anticoagulation when heparin is discontinued.[63,69]

Surgical interventions are options for patients for whom anticoagulation or thrombolysis is contraindicated. A percutaneous transvenous filter (Kimray-Greenfield filter) or an umbrella (Mobin-Uddin) is surgically inserted into the jugular vein and then advanced into the inferior vena cava. The purpose of these devices is to impede the flow of emboli by entrapping them, thus preventing emboli from becoming lodged in the pulmonary vascular system.[50,77]

Other interventions include cardiovascular support with inotropic drugs, vasopressors, and volume expander agents.

Narcotic medication should be administered to relieve pleuritic chest pain, to relieve anxiety symptoms by decreasing excessive sympathetic activity, and to prevent splinting and guarding, which can contribute to hypoventilation.

Life-style Changes

Concerns may be expressed by the patient about home anticoagulant therapy, activity, and diet. Anticoagulant therapy involves knowledge about the drug name, purpose, dose, schedule, and side effects, such as bruising, prolonged bleeding from cuts, spontaneous nosebleeds, black and tarry stools, and blood in urine and sputum. These findings should be immediately reported to the the health care provider.

Another concern is how to store the anticoagulant medications. Anticoagulant drugs taken by mouth are stored in a tight, moisture-resistant container because they can lose their potency when exposed to air. Also, medications should not be stopped without the clinician's approval. Other health care providers, such as the dentist, need to be informed that anticoagulants are being taken before any treatments are started.

Travel life-style changes include consulting with the physician before traveling to any area where a change in climate is expected. For example, when traveling to a hot climate from a cold one, the dose of the drug may need to be reduced. An identification card or a piece of jewelry that states the name of the drug and the physician's name and phone number should be on the person in case of an emergency.[63]

Dietary life-style changes include avoidance of foods rich in vitamin K, such as green leafy vegetables, cauliflower, tomatoes, fish, liver, cheese, egg yolks, and fats from red meats because they can interfere with anticoagulation. In addition, excessive alcohol intake should be avoided because of its effect on the liver and an increased tendency to bleed.[63,78]

Medication self-care life-style changes to be avoided are over-the-counter drugs such as salicylates and anti-inflammatory drugs (eg, aspirin and ibuprofen) because they increase the chance of bleeding. All prescribed and over-the-counter drug therapy should be evaluated by a clinician.[63]

Sedentary life-style changes to be avoided are prolonged sitting, crossing legs, and constrictive clothing in order to prevent venous stasis.[61,68,79] Elastic antiembolism stockings should be applied smoothly and evenly. They should be removed briefly every 8 hours for skin care and to inspect for redness, warmth, or tenderness.

■ UPPER RESPIRATORY INFECTIONS

General Characteristics

The upper respiratory tract consists of the nasal cavity, the pharynx, and the larynx. The purpose of the nasal cavity is to precondition atmospheric air before the air moves into the lungs. The nasal cavity is divided by the septum and has several projections called turbinates that provide the following functions: (1) warming the incoming air; (2) humidifying the incoming air; and (3) cleansing the incoming air.[80] The surfaces of the nasal passageways are lined with ciliated epithelial cells containing many mucous and serous glands. This mucous membrane of the nasal cavity protects the lower airway by acting as a second filter, entrapping foreign particles from the air. The entrapped foreign particles are moved by the ciliated epithelial cells into the throat to be swallowed or be removed when the nose is blown.[81] These physiologic processes of removing foreign particles from the air are very efficient, and rarely do any particles greater than 3 to 5 microns pass through the nose into the lower respiratory bronchial system.[80]

The pharynx, commonly called the throat, separates posteriorly into the trachea and esophagus (laryngopharynx). Food is separated from the air at this point; air passes through the larynx (voice box) into the trachea while the food passes into the esophagus to the stomach. Contained within the larynx are the vocal cords; they function to vibrate and generate sound. During swallowing, the vocal cords assist in preventing the aspiration of food into the lungs.

The sinuses are four paired air-containing spaces (maxillary, ethmoid, sphenoid, frontal), which are situated around the nasal cavity and adjoin the orbits and anterior cranial fossa[82] The sinuses are continuous with the ciliated epithelial mucous membrane of the upper respiratory tract. These ciliated cells facilitate drainage of the sinuses through small openings into the nasal cavity.[82,83] Approximately 0.5% of common colds are complicated by sinus infection, making it one of the most common medical problems seen in clinical practice.[84]

■ *Sinusitis*

Sinusitis is an acute or chronic inflammation of the mucous membranes of the paranasal sinuses.[85] The paranasal sinuses have small tubular openings called ostia that connect the sinus cavities together and facilitate drainage into the nose.[82,85]

When a sinus ostium becomes obstructed by inflammation from bacterial or viral infections of the respiratory tract, it results in stasis of the sinus secretions, which become a rich bacteriologic growth medium.[85] The maxillary sinus is the most often involved, followed in frequency by the ethmoid, frontal, and sphenoid sinuses.[86] Pansinusitis refers to a condition involving all the sinuses.

Sinusitis may be acute and chronic, depending on the duration of the inflammatory response. Acute sinusitis is frequently associated with the bacteria *Streptococcus pneumoniae, Haemophilus influenzae*, and gram-positive and gram-negative anaerobic bacteria.[86,87] Chronic sinusitis develops when acute sinusitis goes untreated or is improperly treated, causing irreversible epithelial changes or damage from the retention of secretions.

Signs, Symptoms, and Diagnosis

Signs and symptoms of acute sinusitis will vary depending on the intensity of the inflammation and the sinus or sinuses involved.[85] Some of the general clinical manifestations are a constant aching or stabbing pain in the forehead, behind the eyes, base of the skull, and upper teeth area. The intensity is usually increased by bending over, coughing, or straining.[85] Palpation over the maxillary and ethmoid sinuses may produce tenderness and pain. Other symptoms may include: (1) fever; (2) malaise; (3) nasal congestion; (4) headache that is worse in the morning or when bending forward; (5) feeling of pressure inside the head; and (6) mucopurulent or purulent discharge. If complete blockage of the sinus ostia exist, nasal purulence is absent.[85]

Diagnosis is made on a thorough history and clinical evaluation that include sinus radiographs taken from different angles. The common findings of sinusitis include: (1) air-fluid level within a sinus; (2) mucosal thickening; and (3) opacity of the sinuses. Depending on the severity of infection and chronicity, computerized tomographic (CT) scan of the sinuses can be done for diagnostic measurement.

Management

The treatment modalities may vary depending on several factors, such as the severity of the infection, the duration of the infection, and age of the person.[85] The goal of treatment is to control the drainage of the sinuses and eradicate the pathogens because the sinuses are close to the central nervous system. Broad-spectrum antibiotics are the mainstay of therapy (Table 7–5), and the selection of the appropriate agent is directed against the most likely pathogens.[82] Drugs commonly used for acute sinusitis are ampicillin and trimethoprim-sulfamethoxazole.[87] Duration of antibiotic treatment of acute sinusitis usually last 10 to 14 days and may extend to 30 days.[82]

Supportive therapy includes: (1) application of moist heat to relieve pain in the sinuses and nose area; (2) a cool-mist ultrasonic humidifier to help thin the secretions in order for them to drain more easily; and (3) analgesics, such as acetaminophen to relieve minor pain and discomfort. For stronger pain relief, narcotics may be prescribed.[82]

If the sinusitis is not responding to treatment, sinus drainage, sinus irrigation, or surgery may be necessary to drain the blocked sinuses. Usually clinical symptoms improve within 7 to 15 days with appropriate antibiotics and drainage procedures.

Life-style Changes

Concerns may be expressed about the possibility of complications. Complications such as meningitis or brain abscess and infection of the bone are very rare. However, life-style changes recommended during this period are reducing normal activities until acute symptoms have subsided. Although there is no

dietary restriction, drinking extra fluids is recommended to help thin the secretions.

Irritants such as cigarette smoke, dusts, and pollution should be avoided, as should exposure to cold, damp weather outdoors, and dry heat indoors. Nonprescribed nose drops or sprays should be avoided because they can interfere with normal nasal and sinus function and become addictive, causing the condition to get worse. Therefore, only nasal drops or sprays that have been prescribed by the clinician should be used for treatment.

■ Pharyngitis

Pharyngitis is an inflammation of the pharynx that is caused by a variety of germs; the most common ones are viruses, bacteria, and fungi. Frequently, pharyngitis is classified as a "sore throat." Pharyngitis may be acute or chronic, and it ranks third among the most common clinical symptoms for which people seek health care.[88]

Viral Pharyngitis. Viral pharyngitis may be caused by many viruses such as the rhinovirus, coronavirus, adenovirus, paramyxovirus, and picornavirus.[85] Each classification of viruses contains large numbers of antigenic subgroups or different types. For example, influenza is an acute, usually self-limited febrile illness that occurs in outbreaks of different severity primarily during the winter months.[89]

TABLE 7–5. SELECTED ANTIBIOTICS FOR UPPER RESPIRATORY INFECTIONS

Medication	Dosage	Side Effects
Amoxil (Amoxicillin)	Adults: 500 mg q 8 h. Children: 40 mg/kg/day in 3 divided doses q 8 h.	Superinfection, anaphylaxis, urticaria, GI upset, blood dyscrasias, and hyperactivity.
EES (erythromycin ethylsuccinate)	Adults: 400 mg tid-qid. Children: 30–50 mg/kg/day in divided doses every 6 hours.	Hepatotoxicity, superinfection, GI upset, rash, reversible hearing loss, and arrhythmias.
Pen-Vee K (penicillinase-sensitive penicillin)	Adults: 125–500 mg q 6–8 h. Children: 15–56 mg/kg/day in 3–6 divided doses.	GI upset, superinfection, anaphylaxis, urticaria.
Bactrim DS, Septra DS (sulfamethoxazole and trimethoprim)	Adults: 1 tablet q 12 h. Children: 8 mg/kg/day of trimethoprim and 40 mg/kg/day in 2 divided doses at 12 hr intervals.	Blood dyscrasias, megaloblastic anemia, hepatic or renal toxicity, crystalluria, pancreatitis, pseudomembranous colitis, drug fever, Stevens-Johnson syndrome, lupus-like syndrome, GI distress, peripheral neuritis, depression, convulsions, ataxia.
Biaxin (clarithromycin)	Adults: 500 mg q 12 h. Children: not recommended.	GI upset, abnormal taste, headache.

Influenza A virus constitutes one genus, influenza B virus another, and influenza C still another. These viruses are transmitted by the respiratory route. When a virus enters the upper respiratory tract, it invades the epithelial lining of the nasal cavity, sinuses, pharynx, and bronchi.[81] Histamine is released from the mast cell as a result of the inflammatory immune response, resulting in pain, redness, and swelling of the pharyngeal membrane. Although the physical findings are similar to those of a common cold, pharyngitis is generally a prominent symptom with fever.[89] The body temperature rises rapidly to a peak of 38° to 40°C within 12 hours after onset. However, as the temperature returns to the normal baseline, the symptoms also diminish.[89] The drug amantadine is useful as a prophylactic agent against influenza during an outbreak and often can shorten the duration of illness in an affected person.

Viral pharyngitis is also associated with cytomegalovirus and Epstein-Barr virus infections. The clinical symptoms produced by the cytomegalovirus are similar to infectious mononucleosis (a disease caused by the Epstein-Barr virus) such as pharyngitis, fever, myalgia, and hepatitis.[88] The incidence of mononucleosis is highest in late childhood to adolescence, influenza is common among different age groups,[82] and herpes simplex virus is more common among young adults.[90]

The general clinical findings of viral pharyngitis include a mild "scratchy" sore throat, fever, malaise, and headache. Often there is pain during swallowing (odynophagia), small ulcers with localized tenderness over the palate, posterior pharyngeal wall, and tonsillar pillars. Sometimes these areas are covered with a whitish exudate or a grayish membrane.

The diagnosis of a viral pharyngitis can be based on a throat culture to determine whether the causative agent is bacterial. However, the use of a throat culture as a diagnostic aid is controversial because of the expense and time it takes to get back the results.[91]

The treatment for viral pharyngitis is supportive to relieve symptoms and may include anesthetic gargles, warm saline gargles, and over-the-counter lozenges to relieve discomfort and reduce inflammation. In addition, a soft, bland diet can minimize pharyngeal irritation and discomfort when swallowing. The total duration of illness is self-limiting and rarely exceeds 10 days. However, some individuals may experience 1 or 2 weeks of lassitude.[92]

Bacterial Pharyngitis. Bacterial pharyngitis is caused by *Staphylococcus*; group A, C, and G beta-hemolytic streptococci; *Corynebacterium diphtheriae* (diphtheria), *Neisseria gonorrhoeae, Mycoplasma pneumoniae,* and *Borrelia vincentii* (Vincent's angina). The most common bacterial cause of pharyngitis is the group A beta-hemolytic *Streptococcus pyogenes*[85] often called "strep throat."

Streptococcal pharyngitis is an acute illness that has its peak during the winter and spring months. Although it affects all ages, it is more common in school-aged children. The bacteria are transmitted by airborne droplets; therefore, outbreaks occur among persons in crowded conditions. The illness is characterized by: (1) fever greater than 101°F; (2) red pharynx with white patches of exudate; (3) enlarged cervical lymph nodes, and (4) malaise and headache.

Most of the clinical signs and symptoms are due to the inflammatory response triggered by cellular injury. Those streptococci that produce exotoxins often generate the rash of scarlet fever.[85] Other complications that can occur from streptococcal infections include rheumatic fever and glomerulonephritis.

The initial diagnosis is frequently based on a throat swab. The latex-agglutination tests offers rapid identification of streptococci in the throat swab material. The latex particles will agglutinate if group A beta-hemolytic streptococci are present in the exudate on the throat swab. This reaction can be seen with the naked eye in less than 1 hour, whereas a throat culture usually takes 2 to 3 days, resulting in a delay of treatment. Not only are the latex-agglutination tests inexpensive, but they have a high correlation with results from throat cultures.[85,91] Therefore, latex-agglutination tests demonstrate high reliability and validity of diagnostic accuracy.

The general treatment of bacterial pharyngitis includes: (1) home care unless hospitalization is recommended by the clinician; (2) penicillin, which is the standard drug treatment of streptococcal pharyngitis, or erythromycin if the person is allergic to penicillin, and both drugs are given for at least 10 days[82,85] (Table 7–5); (3) nonprescription drugs such as acetaminophen for minor discomfort; and (4) extra fluids to maintain body homeostasis, especially during high fevers.

Life-style Changes

Concerns may be expressed about the expected outcome and complications. Although the recurrence of the illness is common, life-style changes for people who have colds include avoiding crowded places, infants, young children, elderly, and the chronically ill persons during the 3 to 6 days the viruses are being shed. To reduce the spread of the causative virus, lifestyle changes include frequent hand washing, covering the mouth when coughing or sneezing, and careful disposal of waste tissues.[93]

Complications with antibiotic therapy are uncommon but can include sinusitis, otitis media, mastoiditis, peritonsillar abscess, and rarely, pneumonitis, endocarditis, or meningitis.[94] Acute glomerulonephritis may develop when the causative organism has a surface protein that is nephrotoxic. There is no evidence that antibiotic therapy reduces the risk of this disease.[95]

Another concern may be the development of chronic pharyngitis. Chronic pharyngitis results from frequently recurring inflammation of the oropharynx and is usually caused by direct irritation of the mucosa from cigarette smoke, alcohol, dust, postnasal discharge, or excessive dryness resulting from the use of antihistamines. Therefore, life-style changes involve avoiding irritants and identifying and controlling the underlying causative agents. Warm saline gargles; a cool-mist, ultrasonic humidifier to increase air moisture and relieve the dry, tight feeling in the throat; and increased fluid intake all may aid in reducing discomfort.

References

1. Farzan S. *A Concise Handbook of Respiratory Diseases*. Norwalk, Conn: Appleton & Lange; 1992.
2. Jenkinson S, Zamora C. Introduction to pulmonary function test. In: DiPiro JT Talbert RL, Hayes PE, et al, eds, *Pharmacotherapy: A Pathophysiologic Approach*. Norwalk, Conn: Appleton & Lange; 1993.
3. McCance KL, Huether SE. *Pathophysiology: The Biologic Basis for Disease in Adults and Children*. St Louis, Mo: CV Mosby Co; 1990.
4. Cooper D. Patients with chronic obstructive pulmonary disease. In: Clochesy JM, Breu C, Cardin S, et al, eds. *Critical Care Nursing*. Philadelphia, Pa: WB Saunders Co; 1993.
5. Johannsen JM. Chronic obstructive pulmonary disease: current comprehensive care for emphysema and bronchitis. *Nurse Pract*. 1994;19(1):59–67.
6. American Thoracic Society. Standards for the diagnosis and care of patients with chronic obstructive pulmonary disease (COPD) and asthma. *Am Rev Respir Dis*. 1987;136:225–244.
7. Petty T, Raff MJ. Controlling bronchitis flare-ups in COPD. *Patient Care*. 1991;10:81–100.
8. Stratton M. Chronic obstructive lung disease. In: DiPiro JT, Talbert RL, Hayes PE, et al, eds. *Pharmacotherapy: A Pathophysiologic Approach*. Norwalk, Conn: Appleton & Lange; 1993.
9. Snider GL. Chronic obstructive lung disease: risk factors, pathophysiology, and pathogenesis. *Ann Rev Med*. 1989; 40:411–429.
10. Stauffer JL, Carbone JE. Pulmonary disease. In: Krupp MA, ed. *Current Medical Diagnosis and Treatment*. Los Altos, Calif: Lange Medical Publications; 1986.
11. Biller PL. Diagnosis and management of acute bronchitis and pneumonia in the ambulatory setting. *Nurse Pract*. 1987; 12(10):12–28.
12. Petty TL. Future trends in the management of asthma and chronic obstructive pulmonary disease. *Am J Med*. 1985; 79(6A):38–42.
13. Robins AG. Pathophysiology of emphysema. *Clin Chest Med*. 1983;4:413–420.
14. Weinberger S. *Principles of Pulmonary Medicine*. 2nd ed. Philadelphia, Pa: WB Saunders Co; 1992.
15. Cooper D. Patients with chronic obstructive pulmonary disease. In: Clochesy JM, Breu C, Cardin S, et al, eds. *Critical Care Nursing*. Philadelphia, Pa: WB Saunders Co; 1993.
16. Kelly HW, Hill MR. Asthma. In: DiPiro JT, Talbert RL, Hayes PE, Yee GC, et al, eds. *Pharmacotherapy: A Pathophysiologic Approach*. Norwalk, Conn: Appleton & Lange; 1993.
17. Reinke LF, Hoffman LA. How to teach asthma co-management. *Am J Nurs*. 1992;92(10):40–46.
18. American Thoracic Society. Standards for the diagnosis and care of patients with COPD and asthma. *Am Rev Respir Dis*. 1987;136;225–244.
19. Garobado R. Epidemiology of community acquired respiratory tract infections in adults. *Am J Med*. 1985;78(suppl 6B):32.
20. Griggith D, Wallace R. Bacterial pneumonia in the adult: diagnosis and therapy. *Hosp Med*. 1988;24:188.
21. Stratton CW. Bacterial pneumonias—an overview with emphasis on pathogenesis, diagnosis, and treatment. *Heart Lung*. 1986;15:226–244.
22. Baum GL, Wolinsky E. *Textbook of Pulmonary Diseases*. Boston, Mass: Little Brown & Co. Inc; 1993.
23. Wimbush FB, Wright J. Acute respiratory infection. In: Wright J Shelton BK, eds. *Desk reference for Critical Care Nursing*. Boston Mass: Jones and Bartlett Publishers; 1993.
24. Holloway N. Nursing the critically ill adult. In: Brunner L, Suddarth D. *Lippincott Manual of Nursing Practice*. Menlo Park, Calif: Addison-Wesley; 1986:154.
25. Karetzky M. Pneumonia: treatment and prognosis. In: Karetzky M, Cunha B, Brandstetter R, eds. *The Pneumonias*. New York, NY: Springer-Verlag; 1993.
26. Blinkhorn R. Community-acquired pneumonia. In: Baum GL, Wolinsky E, eds. *Textbook of Pulmonary Diseases*. Boston, Mass: Little Brown & Co. Inc; 1993.
27. Blinkhorn R. Hospital-acquired pneumonia. In: Baum GL, Wolinsky E, eds. *Textbook of Pulmonary Diseases*. Boston, Mass: Little Brown & Co. Inc; 1993.

28. Schillinger D. Infections of the lower respiratory tract. In: Schillinger D, Harwood-Nuss A, eds. *Infections in Emergency Medicine*. New York, NY: Churchill Livingstone; 1989;1.

29. McCance K, Huether SE. *Pathophysiology: The Biologic Basis for Disease in Adults and Children*. St Louis, Mo: Mosby Year Book; 1994.

30. Biller PL. Diagnosis and management of acute bronchitis and pneumonia in the ambulatory setting. *Nurse Pract*. 1987;12(10):12–28.

31. Brown R. Community-acquired pneumonia: diagnosis and therapy of older adults. *Geriatrics*. 1993;48(2):43–50.

32. Raffin TA. Diagnosis: viral pneumonia. *Hosp Med*. 1986;3: 19–48.

33. Bjornson HS. Diagnosis and treatment of bacterial pneumonia in the intensive care unit: an overview. *Respir Care*. 1987;32: 773–780.

34. Luby JP. Pneumonia caused by *Mycoplasma pneumoniae* infection. *Clin Chest Med*. 1991;12:237–244.

35. Mansel JK, Rosenow EC, Smith TF, et al. *Mycoplasma pneumoniae* pneumonia. *Chest*. 1989;95:639–646.

36. Pierce AK, Sanford JP. Aerobic gram-negative bacillary pneumonias. *Am Rev Respir Dis*. 1974;110:647–658.

37. Murray HW, Tuazon CU. Atypical pneumonias. *Med Clin North Am*. 1980;64:507–527.

38. Hellman S, Gram M. The resurgence of tuberculosis. *AAOHN J*. 1993;41(2):66–72.

39. Nardell EA. Pathogenesis of tuberculosis. In: Reichman LB, Hershfield ES, eds. *Tuberculosis: A Comprehensive International Approach*. New York, NY: Marcel Dekker Inc; 1993.

40. Comstock GW, Cauthen GM. Epidemiology of Tuberculosis. In: Reichman LB, Hershfield ES, eds. *Tuberculosis: A Comprehensive International Approach*. New York, NY: Marcel Dekker Inc; 1993.

41. Jo HS. Assessment and management of persons coinfected with tuberculosis and human immunodeficiency virus. *Nurse Pract*. 1993;18(11):42–49.

42. Madsen LA. Tuberculosis today. RN. 1990;53(3):44–50.

43. Centers for Disease Control. Guidelines for preventing the transmission of tuberculosis in health-care settings with special focus on HIV-related issues. *MMWR*. 1990;39 (RR-17): 1–29.

44. Ravikrishnan KP. Tuberculosis. *Postgrad Med*. 1992;91: 333–338.

45. Amin NM. Tuberculin skin testing. *Postgrad Med*. 1994; 95(4):46–56.

46. Dowling PT. Return of tuberculosis: screening and preventive therapy. *AFP*. 1991;2:457–467.

47. Raju L. Current diagnostic and treatment strategies. *Emerg Med*. 1993;25(2):159–168.

48. Davidson P, Diferdinando G, Reichman L, et al. TB: coming soon to your town? *Patient Care*. 1992;26:40–66.

49. Centers for Disease Control and Prevention. Tuberculosis control laws—United States, 1993. *MMWR Morb Mortal Wkly Rep*. 1993;42(RR-15):1–28.

50. Currie DL. Pulmonary embolism: diagnosis and management. *Crit Care Nurse Q*. 1990;13(2):41–49.

51. McCance KL, Huether SE. (1994). *Pathophysiology: The Biologic Basis for Disease in Adults and Children*. St Louis, Mo: Mosby Year Book; 1994.

52. Handerhan B. Recognizing pulmonary embolism. *Nursing 91*, 1991;2:107–110.

53. Sherman S. Pulmonary embolism update. *Postgrad Med*. 1991;89:195–202.

54. Bone RC. Pulmonary embolism: new approaches to a complex problem. *Emerg Med*. 1992;(October 15) 24(14):144–152.

55. Kinasewitz GT. Thromboembolism in the elderly. In: Mahler DA, ed. *Pulmonary Disease in the Elderly*. New York, NY: Marcel Dekker Inc; 1993.

56. Wyngaarden JB, Smith LH, Bennett JC. *Cecil Textbook of Medicine*. Philadelphia, Pa: WB Saunders Co; 1992.

57. Carson S, Kelly M, Duff A, et al. The clinical course of pulmonary embolism. *N Engl J Med*. 1992;326:1240–1244.

58. Wright JE, Shelton BK. *Desk Reference for Critical Care Nursing*. Boston, Mass: Jones and Bartlett Publishers; 1993.

59. Easton KL. Early detection of pulmonary embolism. *Rehabil Nurs*. 1992;17(4):199–201.

60. Sherman S. Pulmonary embolism update. *Postgrad Med*. 1991;89(8):195–202.

61. Dobkin J, Reichel J. Pulmonary embolism: Diagnosis and treatment. *Cardiol Clin*. 1987;5:577–582.

62. Moser KM. Venous thromboembolism. *Am Rev Respir Dis*. 1990;141:235–249.

63. Erdman SM, Rodvold KA, Friedenberg WR. Thromboembolic disorders. In: Dipiro JT, Talbert RL, Hayes PE, et al, eds. *Pharmacotherapy: A Pathophysiologic Approach*. Norwalk, Conn: Appleton & Lange; 1993:312–332.

64. Davis LA, O'Rourke NC. Pulmonary embolism: early recognition and management in the postanesthesia care unit. *J Post Anesth Nurs*. 1993; 8:338–345.

65. Counselman FL. Best tests for pulmonary embolism. *Emerg Med*. 1990;(December 1, 15):66–86.

66. Kelly, M. Unmasking pulmonary embolism. *Diagnosis*. 1987; 9(12):46–60.

67. Stratton M. Ventilation-perfusion scintigraphy in diagnosis of pulmonary thrombo-embolism. *Focus Crit Care*. 1990; 17:287–293.

68. Whiter R. Pulmonary embolus. In: Shoemaker W, Ayers S, Grenuik A, et al, eds. *Textbook of Critical Care*. Philadelphia, Pa: JB Lippincott Co; 1984:666–668.

69. Bell WR, Simon TL. Current status of pulmonary thromboembolic disease: pathophysiology, diagnosis, prevention, and treatment. *Am Heart J*. 1982;103:239–261.

70. McFadden ER, Braunwald E. Cor pulmonale and pulmonary embolism. In: Braunwald E, ed. *Heart Disease*. Philadelphia, Pa: WB Saunders Co; 1984.

71. Hull RD, Raskob GE, Coates G, et al. Clinical validity of a normal perfusion lung scan in patients with suspected pulmonary embolism. *Chest*. 1990;97:23–26.

72. Hull RD, Hirsh J, Carter CJ, et al. Diagnostic value of ventilation-perfusion lung scanning in patients with suspected pulmonary embolism. *Chest*. 1985;88:819–828.

73. Loscalzo J. An overview of thrombolytic agents. *Chest*. 1990;97 (suppl):117S–123S.

74. Marder VJ, Sherry S. Thrombolytic therapy: current status. *N Engl J Med*. 1988;318(pt 1):1512–1520.

75. A Cooperative Study. Urokinase pulmonary embolism trial phase I results. *JAMA*. 1970;214:2163–2172.

76. Sherry S. Thrombolytic therapy for noncoronary diseases. *Ann Emerg Med*. 1991;20:396–404.

77. Addonizio VP. Thrombotic problems. In: Wilmore DW, Brenna MF, Harken AH, et al, eds. *Care of the Surgical Patient*. New York, NY: Scientific American, 1989;2,sect 8:1–12.

78. Rosenberg RD. Actions and interactions of heparin and antithrombin III. *N Engl J Med*. 1975;292:146–150.

79. Prevention of venous thrombosis and pulmonary embolism. *JAMA*. 1986;256:744–749. Consensus Conference.

80. Guyton A. *Physiology of the Human Body*. Philadelphia, Pa: WB Saunders Co; 1979.

81. Kuhn MM. *Pharmacotherapeutics: A Nursing Process Approach*. Philadelphia, Pa: FA Davis Co; 1991:914.

82. LeBel M, Massoomi F. Upper respiratory tract infections. In: Dipiro JT, Talbert RL, Hayes PE, et al, eds. *Pharmacotherapy: A Pathophysiologic Approach*. Norwalk, Conn: Appleton & Lange; 1993:1560–1576.

83. Wald ER. Rhinitis and acute chronic sinusitis. In: Bluestone DD, Stool SE, Scheetz MD, eds. *Pediatric Otolaryngology*. Philadelphia, Pa: WB Saunders Co; 1990:729–744.

84. McHenry MC, Weinstein AJ. Antimicrobial drugs and infections. *Med Clin North Am*. 1983;67:5–16.

85. Ladenheim S, Mahood CF, Lesser RW. Upper respiratory infections. In: Schillinger D, Harwood-Nuss A, eds. *Infections in Emergency Medicine*. New York, NY: Churchill Livingstone; 1989:2:29–66.

86. Tierno PM. Microbiology of the nose and paranasal sinuses. In: Goldman JL, ed. *The Principles and Practice of Rhinology*. New York, NY: Churchill Livingstone; 1987;79.

87. Levy ML, Ericsson CD, Pickering LK. Infection of the upper respiratory tract. *Med Clin North Am* 1983;67:153.

88. Lowe R, Hedges JR. Early treatment of streptococcal pharyngitis. *Ann Emerg Med*. 1984;13:440.

89. Douglas RG. (1992). Influenza. In: Wyngaarden JB, Smith LH, Bennett JC, eds. *Cecil Textbook of Medicine*. Philadelphia, Pa: WB Saunders Co; 1992:1815.

90. Anderson LJ, Patriarca PA, Hierholzer JC, et al. Viral respiratory illness. *Med Clin North Am*. 1983;67:1009.

91. Hedges JR, Lowe RA. Sore throat: to culture or not to culture? *Ann Emerg Med*. 1987;15:312.

92. Couch RB. Orthomyxoviruses: influenza. In: Stein JH, ed. *Internal Medicine*. Boston, Mass: Little Brown & Co. Inc; 1983.

93. Hall CB. Respiratory syncytial virus. In: Madell GL, Douglas RG, Bennett JE, eds. *Principles and Practices of Infectious Disease*. New York, NY: John Wiley & Sons Inc; 1979.

94. Brook I. Pharyngotonsillitis. In: Schlossberg E, ed. *Infections of the Head and Neck*. New York, NY: Springer-Verlag; 1987.

95. Gillette RD. Pharyngitis: reevaluating diagnosis and treatment. *Consultant*. 1985;25(7):59.

8

Cardiovascular Disorders

Teresa A. Newman
Stephen D. Newman

■ HYPERTENSION

General Characteristics

Hypertension, or high blood pressure, is often called the "silent killer" because there are often no early warning signs or symptoms until it reaches advanced stages. This is the most common cardiovascular disorder, affecting approximately one out of every four Americans.[1] With this many Americans developing hypertension, several factors have been noted to increase the risk of this development (Table 8–1). However, in most cases the exact cause of hypertension is unknown.[2] This form of hypertension is known as essential or primary hypertension. When there is an identifiable cause for the hypertension, such as kidney disease, the term secondary hypertension is used.

Hypertension, or high blood pressure, is a condition in which the blood flows through the arteries under pressure that is higher than normal. Blood pressure for an adult should be less than 140/90 millimeters of mercury (mm Hg). The first number is systolic pressure, the amount of pressure in the arteries while the heart is pumping blood out to the body. The second number is the diastolic pressure, the amount of pressure in the arteries when the heart is at rest between beats. Hypertension ranges from mild to severe, depending on the systolic and diastolic pressures.[1]

Signs, Symptoms, and Diagnosis

There may not be any presenting symptom or sign with hypertension. However, some patients may complain of headaches. Taking the blood pressure with a sphygmomanometer is the primary way to diagnose hypertension, although hypertension should not be diagnosed by one office visit. Elevated blood pressures should be confirmed, on at least two separate office visits.[2] A complete physical examination of the hypertensive patient needs to be performed to determine the cause and possible sequelae of this disease.

Several laboratory tests should be performed for all patients with hypertension to determine the cause and management for each individual (Table 8–2).[1,2] Other studies may be performed on patients who appear to have secondary hypertension (eg, renal scans and pyelograms).

Management

The most important goal in the treatment of hypertension is to keep the blood pressure under control and prevent further damage to end organs (Table 8–3). If the hypertension is secondary, the underlying cause needs to be treated or corrected. If the patient has primary or essential hypertension, life-style changes and medications may be indicated. If the life-style changes are not controlling the blood pressure, or if the patient has moderate to severe hypertension, the clinician may prescribe an antihypertensive medication or a drug combina-

TABLE 8–1. RISK FACTORS FOR HYPERTENSION

Male
African American
Increase in age
Family history of hypertension
Overweight
Smoker
Excessive alcohol consumption

TABLE 8–2. EVALUATION OF THE HYPERTENSIVE PATIENT

Complete blood count
Serum electrolyte levels
Urinalysis and serum creatinine determination
Total cholesterol and lipid profile
Fasting blood sugar test
Thyroxine level
Electrocardiogram
Chest x-ray
Echocardiogram (optional)

TABLE 8–3. COMPLICATIONS OF HYPERTENSION

Myocardial infarction
Stroke
Kidney failure
Congestive heart failure

tion until the blood pressure is under control with minimum side effects (Table 8–4).[1] Diuretics and beta-blockers are recommended initially. Some prefer angiotensin converting enzyme (ACE) inhibitors and calcium channel blockers. Increasing the dose, switching to another drug, or adding a second agent from another class may be necessary if blood pressure remains uncontrolled. It should be stressed to the patient that these medications may need to be continued for the rest of his or her life and should not be discontinued unless directed by her or his health care provider.

Life-style Changes

Several life-style changes for the hypertensive patient may help to control blood pressure (Table 8–5).[1] Exercise and weight

TABLE 8–4. SELECTED ANTI-HYPERTENSIVE MEDICATIONS

Medication	Dosage	Side Effects
Accupril (quinapril HCL)	Adult: Initially 10 mg once daily. Usual maintenance: 20–80 mg daily in 1–2 divided doses. Dosing may be different when on diuretic. Children: not recommended.	Headache, dizziness, fatigue, cough, GI upset, hyperkalemia, back pain, tachycardia, dry mouth, somnolence, sweating, sinusitis.
Zestril (lisinopril)	Adults: Initially and if not on diuretics: 10 mg daily. Usual: 20 mg–40 mg daily; max 80 mg daily. Dosing may be different when on diuretic. Children: not recommended.	Dizziness, headache, fatigue, diarrhea, upper respiratory symptoms, cough, nausea, orthostatic hypotension, hyperkalemia, renal impairment, angioedema. Liver dysfunction and blood dyscrasias (rare).
Inderal (propranolol HCl)	Adults: Initially 40 mg twice a day; max 640 mg daily. Children: Initially 1mg/kg daily in 2 divided doses; max 16 mg/kg/day.	Heart failure, hypotension, bronchospasm, bradycardia, heart block, fatigue, dizziness, depression, GI upset, pharyngitis, agranulocytosis.
Tenormin (atenolol)	Adults: Initially 50 mg daily; max 100 mg/day. Children: not recommended.	Heart failure, bronchospasm, bradycardia, angina, MI, heart block, dizziness, fatigue, GI upset, depression, orthostatic hypotension, cold extremities.
Cardizem CD (diltiazem)	Adults: Initially 180–240 mg once daily; adjust at 2 wk intervals; usual max dose 480 mg/day. Children: not recommended.	Edema, headache, dizziness, asthenia, 1st-degree AV block, bradycardia, flushing, nausea, rash. CHF and liver abnormalities (rare).
Procardia XL (nifedipine)	Adults: Initially 30–60 mg daily; max dose 120 mg/day. Children: not recommended.	Edema, headache, fatigue, dizziness, constipation, nausea, palpitations, muscle cramps. Increased angina, acute MI (rare).
Lozol (indapamide)	Adults: Initially 1.25 mg q am. May adjust at 4 week intervals to 2.5 mg then 5 mg q day. Children: not recommended.	Electrolyte disorders, hyperglycemia, hyperuricemia, gout, arrhythmias, headache, nervousness, blurred vision, muscle cramps, dizziness, fatigue, orthostatic hypotension, cough, GI disturbances.
Dyazide (triamterene and hydrochlorothiazide)	Adults: 1–2 caps once daily. Children: not recommended.	Drowsiness, muscle cramps, weakness, headache, GI disturbances, dizziness, impotence, arrhythmias, hypotension, dry mouth, urine discoloration.

TABLE 8–5. LIFE-STYLE CHANGES FOR THE
HYPERTENSIVE PATIENT

Exercise and weight loss program
Reduction of alcohol consumption
Reduction of salt and fat intake
Stopping smoking

loss should be addressed if indicated. Smoking cessation programs should be discussed with the hypertensive smoker (see Chapter 4). Decreasing the patient's alcohol consumption should also be addressed, since heavy alcohol use can increase arterial pressure. A low-salt and low-fat diet should be encouraged and dietary consultation obtained. These life-style changes are very difficult for most people to start and continue. It may be necessary to allow the patient to start with one life-style change and then make additional changes over several months. These patients need support and encouragement throughout their treatment.

■ PERICARDITIS

General Characteristics

Pericarditis is defined as inflammation of the pericardium, or pericardial sac. The pericardial sac surrounds the heart, as seen in Figure 8–1. It holds the heart in place in the chest and protects it from infections located in other areas of the chest.[3] The thin layer of pericardial fluid also helps to reduce the friction on the heart as it beats.

The etiology of acute pericarditis is usually unknown.[4] However, certain viruses, bacteria, fungi, tumors, and connective tissue diseases have been known to cause acute pericarditis (Table 8–6).[3,4]

Signs, Symptoms, and Diagnosis

The presenting symptom is usually chest pain.[3,4] It is typically described as a sharp, retrosternal pain on the left side of the chest that may radiate to the left shoulder and may worsen with deep inspiration or lying supine. It may be relieved by sitting up and leaning forward. In some patients the pain may

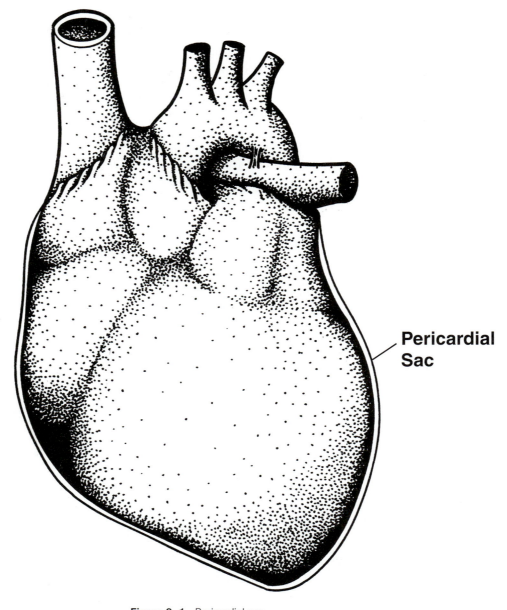

Pericardial Sac

Figure 8–1. Pericardial sac

TABLE 8–6. MOST COMMON ETIOLOGIES OF PERICARDITIS

Viruses	Coxsackie, echo, adenovirus
Bacteria	*Haemophilus, Staphylococcus, Pneumococcus, Nocardia*
Mycobacteria	*Mycobacterium tuberculosis*
Fungi	*Aspergillus, Candida, Histoplasmosis*
Tumors	Breast cancer, lung cancer, metastatic lymphoma
Connective tissue disease	Rheumatoid arthritis, scleroderma, systemic lupus erythematosus

also be described as dull. The pain may be accompanied by fever and myalgias.

The classic finding on physical examination is the pericardial friction rub, which may be described as scratchy, squeaky, leathery, or grinding and is heard best in the lower left sternal edge and cardiac apex but may be heard all over the precordium.[3,4] It is best heard with the diaphragm of the stethoscope firmly placed on the chest wall because movement of chest hair may simulate a pericardial friction rub.

A 12-lead electrocardiogram (ECG) is the most useful laboratory test.[3,4] There will be ST segment elevation but without reciprocal ST segment depression as in myocardial infarction. The ECG may also show PR segment depression and T wave inversion. A chest x-ray may be normal, show an enlarged heart with pericardial effusion, or show a pleural effusion. Blood tests such as erythrocyte sedimentation rate and complete blood count (CBC) may show an elevated rate and elevated white blood cell count. If cardiac enzymes are drawn to rule out myocardial infarction, they are usually normal in pericarditis. However, they may be elevated if there is extensive epicarditis.[3]

Management

If the etiology of the pericarditis is known, treatment of the underlying cause may help.[3] However, if the etiology is viral or unknown, management consists of analgesics and nonsteroidal anti-inflammatory drugs for pain relief.[3,4] Pericarditis may recur within a few months. In these cases, a longer course of anti-inflammatory drugs should be used. Corticosteroids should be reserved for patients who have multiple recurrences over 5 to 10 years. The only other complications, besides recurrences, is the development of a pleural effusion[3,4] and the accumulation of pericardial fluid. Rapid accumulation of pericardial fluid may lead to cardiac tamponade requiring pericardiocentesis.

Life-style Changes

If chest pain associated with pericarditis is severe, the patient may need to be put on bed rest. Otherwise, after 2 to 6 weeks, when the pericarditis has resolved, there should be no further problems unless it recurs.

■ MURMURS AND VALVULAR HEART DISEASE

General Characteristics

The four valves of the heart: tricuspid, pulmonic, mitral, and aortic allow blood to flow within the heart in one direction (Fig. 8–2). They act as gates to keep the blood in the four chambers of the heart. When one of the valves becomes damaged by a disease such as rheumatic fever, endocarditis, or a deformity in the heart, a murmur may develop.[5] When this happens, the valve may not open completely (stenosis) or may not close completely, allowing blood to flow backwards (regurgitation).[5,6]

Many people have a heart murmur sometime in their life, but it may not have occurred during the time they were examined by their clinician. There are three groups of murmurs that are based on the mechanism of production:

1. innocent murmurs,
2. physiologic murmurs, and
3. organic murmurs.[5]

Innocent murmurs, also called functional murmurs, are not caused by a problem with the heart or one of its valves and usually disappear by adulthood. Physiologic murmurs may be

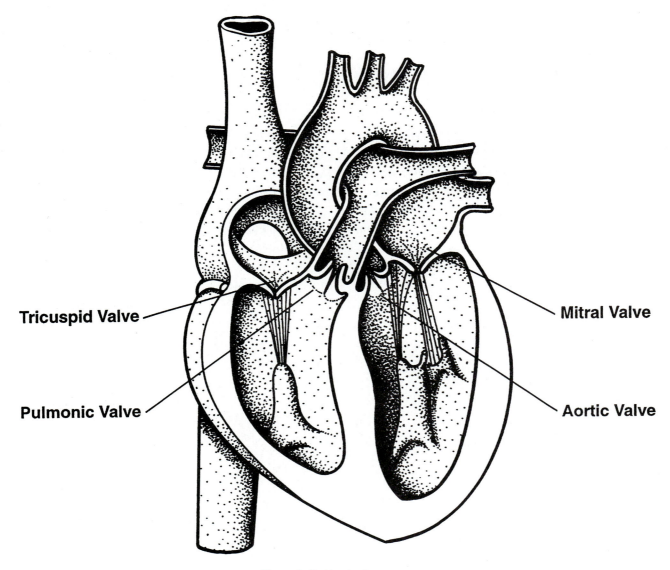

Tricuspid Valve

Pulmonic Valve

Mitral Valve

Aortic Valve

Figure 8–2. Heart valves

caused by a disorder in another area of the body that alters the function of the heart (eg, anemia, pregnancy, fever, and thyrotoxicosis). Organic murmurs are usually caused by a defect in the heart, the valves, or the central circulation (eg, congenital heart disease).

Signs, Symptoms, and Diagnosis. Although the patient may be asymptomatic with a heart murmur, some patients may present with the complaint of fatigue, shortness of breath, chest pain, syncope, or edema.[6] The patient may also present with a manifestation of valvular diseases such as congestive heart failure.

Careful listening through a stethoscope can narrow down the differential diagnosis, but special maneuvers, such as leaning forward or having the patient hold his or her breath, may help the clinician differentiate the etiology of the murmur.

There are several tests that can be performed to diagnose the defect of the valve and any manifestation of the valvular disorder (Table 8–7).[5,6] The chest x-ray can show enlargement of the heart resulting from a stiff valve not opening completely. This is referred to as cardiac hypertrophy. The echocardiogram shows the severity of the valvular disease and the possible etiology. It can also be used to follow the course of the disease and suggest possible need for valvular repair or replacement.[5,6] The transesophageal echocardiogram can be used to evaluate valvular abnormalities in patients with poor transthoracic echocardiographic images. It can also be used intraoperatively to follow valvular repair or replacement. The electrocardiogram can demonstrate associated cardiac abnormalities and associated arrhythmias. Cardiovascular laboratory tests include: right heart catheterization, left heart catheterization, contrast ventriculography, and aortography. Right heart catheterization will allow pulmonary pressures, left heart filling pressures, and pressure gradients to be measured. Left heart catheterization will allow pressure gradients, associated coronary artery disease, and left ventricular and aortic pres-

TABLE 8–7. DIAGNOSTIC TESTS FOR VALVULAR HEART DISEASE

Chest x-ray
Echocardiography
    Transthoracic echocardiography
    Transesophageal echocardiography
Electrocardiography
Cardiovascular laboratory tests
    Left heart catheterization
    Right heart catheterization
    Contrast ventriculography
    Aortography

sures to be measured. Contrast ventriculography will demonstrate left ventricular function, mitral valve regurgitation, and associated anatomical abnormality (eg, ventricular septal defect). Aortography will show aortic insufficiency if present.

Management

The management of valvular disorders is to prevent and treat any manifestations of the disorder.[5] For example, in a patient with mitral regurgitation, the patient should receive prophylactic antibiotics prior to dental and surgical procedures to prevent bacterial endocarditis. Medications such as diuretics and digitalis may be needed in patients with pulmonary congestion and arrhythmias.[5] The patient needs to be followed closely to decide if and when valvular repair and replacement may be indicated. The patient needs to be educated about his or her valvular disease and reassured that continuation of a normal, productive life is possible until symptoms or tests prove otherwise. Arrhythmias should be treated, since they can worsen symptoms for some valvular disorders.

Life-style Changes

Patients with valvular disease usually do not have any reduction in their physical activity as long as the valvular dysfunction is mild. It can worsen with time. Patients need to be informed to use antibiotics prophylactically if indicated and to watch for symptoms that might indicate worsening of their valvular disorder.

■ CONGESTIVE HEART FAILURE

General Characteristics

Congestive heart failure results when the heart can no longer pump an adequate amount of blood to meet the metabolic needs of the body.[7] The body attempts to compensate for this decrease in cardiac output by retaining sodium and water and dilating the ventricles, resulting in congestion of the systemic or pulmonary venous systems, once it exceeds the heart's reserve. This can occur acutely, after an extensive myocardial infarction, or insidiously, after chronic valvular disease.[7]

One of the most common causes of congestive heart failure in the United States is coronary artery disease.[8] Atherosclerosis leads to narrowing of the coronary arteries and deprives the heart muscle of needed oxygen and nutrients that are supplied by coronary vessels. There are many factors that may lead to congestive heart failure (Table 8–8).[8] Some of these factors may cause permanent damage to the heart muscle, while others, such as hyperthyroidism or acute valvular dysfunction, may make the heart work beyond its capacity, leading to transient congestive heart failure. However, once the abnormalities are corrected, the congestive heart failure may resolve.

The mechanisms of congestive heart failure can be divided into those affecting the systolic, or emptying function of the ventricle, and those affecting the diastolic, or accepting function of the ventricle. Systolic overload of the left ventricle can result from those conditions that cause increased resistance to emptying of the left ventricle.[8] Examples are aortic stenosis or hypertension, in which the ventricle must generate increased pressure to overcome the resistance to emptying. Systolic overload can also occur in right ventricular failure. Conditions that cause increased resistance to emptying of the right ventricle include acute pulmonary embolus, cor pulmonale in chronic obstructive pulmonary disease (COPD), and pulmonary hypertension. Diminished systolic function can also result from factors that directly affect the muscle of the heart.[8] These include coronary artery disease and cardiomyopathies. In addition, symptoms of congestive heart failure can be precipitated by tachyarrhythmias, hyperthyroidism, and severe anemias in patients with otherwise normal ventricular function. Congestive heart failure can also result from abnormalities in the relaxing, or diastolic, portion of the cardiac cycle.[8] During this diastolic period, the ventricles relax and accept blood from the corresponding atria. This blood normally fills the ventricles with minimal resistance, loading the ventricles for the next systolic cycle. In disorders in which an abnormal volume of blood enters the ventricles, the resistance to the normal ventricular filling is increased. This is seen with aortic regurgitation or congenital heart disease, such as a patent ductus arteriosus. The ventricles may not be able to relax for other reasons, such as a pericardium that becomes thickened and diseased and restricts the normal expansion or relaxing of the ventricle.

TABLE 8–8. FACTORS CAUSING CONGESTIVE HEART FAILURE

Coronary artery disease
Myocardial infarction
Hypertension
Congenital or acquired valvular heart disease
Anatomical heart defects
Myocarditis
Endocarditis
Pulmonary embolism
Hyperthyroidism (thyrotoxicosis)
Arrhythmias
Pericarditis
Cardiomyopathies
Anemia
Pregnancy

Signs, Symptoms, and Diagnosis

Patients with congestive heart failure usually present with fairly typical symptoms (Table 8–9). The major differences have to do with the primary ventricle affected.[7,8] Left heart failure usually causes symptoms relating to pulmonary congestion (Fig. 8–3). These include orthopnea, paroxysmal nocturnal dyspnea, shortness of breath, and cough. Right heart failure, which is commonly a result of left heart failure, results in symptoms associated with congestion of the systemic circulation (Fig. 8–4). Patients may note peripheral edema, ascites, or right upper quadrant pain. Patients may present with more subtle complaints of fatigue or decrease in their exertional capacity. They may also note a weight increase unrelated to an increase in their caloric intake.

TABLE 8–9. SIGNS AND SYMPTOMS OF CONGESTIVE HEART FAILURE

Left Heart Failure	Right Heart Failure	Both
Dyspnea	Peripheral edema	Fatigue
Orthopnea	Nocturia	Anorexia
Cough	Ascites	Cool extremities
Paroxysmal nocturnal dyspnea	Hepatomegaly	Tachycardia
Rales	Peripheral edema	Cardiomegaly
S_3 gallop	Jugular venous distention	Narrow pulse pressure
Tachypnea	Splenomegaly	Elevated blood pressure
		Confusion
		Cheyne-Stokes respirations

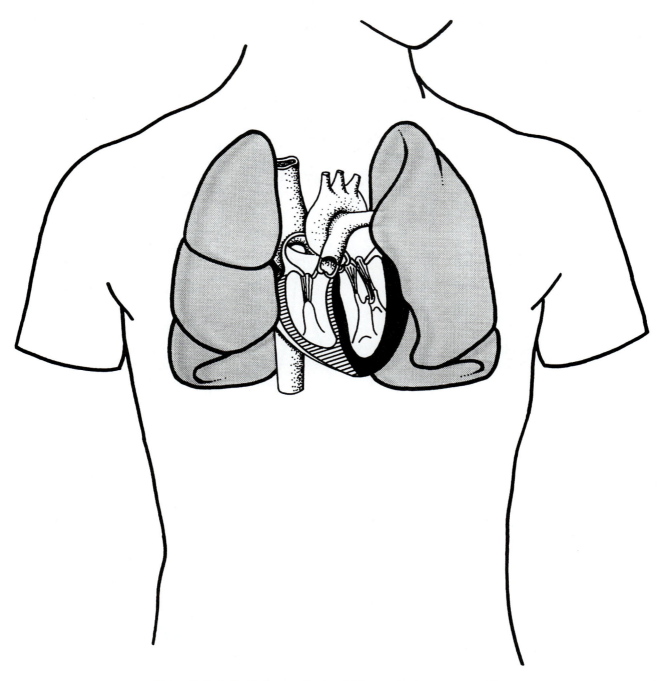

Figure 8–3. Left-sided congestive heart failure and pulmonary congestion

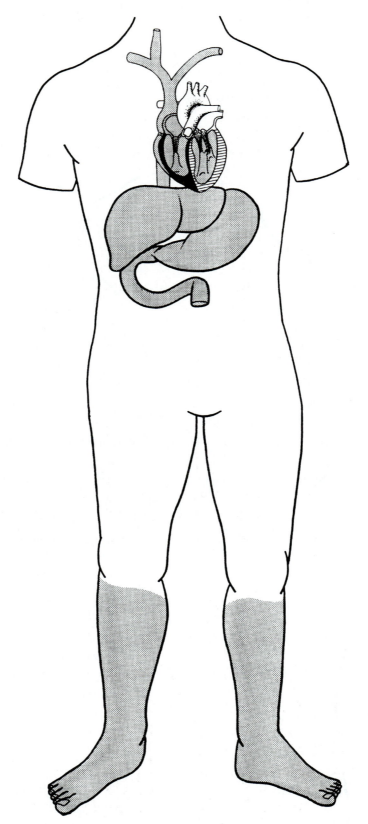

Figure 8–4. Right-sided congestive heart failure and systemic congestion

The physical findings depend on whether there is left or right ventricular dysfunction, or both. Left heart failure is usually associated with tachypnea, pulmonary rales, left ventricular S_3 gallop, and perhaps other physical findings that may suggest the etiology of the heart failure, such as hypertension or valvular stenosis.[7,8] Right heart failure is usually suggested by findings of systemic congestion. Findings of right ventricular failure include elevated jugular venous pressure, right sided S_3 gallop, pleural effusions, hepatomegaly, ascites, and peripheral edema in the ambulatory patient, and sacral edema in the bedridden patient.[7,8]

More advanced degrees of congestive heart failure may result in hypoperfusion of multiple organs. This may include confusion resulting from cerebral dysfunction, pulsus alternans, Cheyne-Stokes respirations, and frothy pink sputum of pulmonary edema and impending respiratory arrest.[7,8]

Diagnostic tests are performed to determine the presence, etiology, and severity of congestive heart failure. Once the diagnosis of congestive heart failure has been demonstrated by physical examination, one will employ various diagnostic tests and procedures to further assist with determining the diagnosis and appropriate therapy (Table 8–10).[7,8] It is important not only to perform those tests that determine the cardiac function, such as echocardiography, but to evaluate renal and hepatic function, since in advanced heart failure, perfusion to the renal and hepatic circulation can be significantly diminished. Chest radiographs may demonstrate signs of pulmonary congestion or effusions or cardiomegaly. Diagnostic tests should be used to enhance or clarify those findings on physical examination.

Management

The management goals of congestive heart failure are to reduce the cardiac work load, optimize cardiac performance, and control excess salt and water.[7,9] Bed rest can be instituted during more severe impairment. However, as symptoms improve, increased activity is encouraged. Assisting the patient to obtain ideal body weight and control those factors that may result in decreased cardiac performance, such as hypertension or ischemia, should be undertaken. Those factors that cannot be controlled by medications alone may require surgical intervention, such as heart valve surgery or coronary bypass.[7,9] Specially designed stockings to prevent the likelihood of embolic disease should be employed in those patients on bed rest or

TABLE 8–10. TESTS FOR CONGESTIVE HEART FAILURE

Chest x-ray
Electrocardiogram (ECG)
Echocardiogram
Exercise stress test
Holter monitor
Radionuclide ventriculography
Cardiac catheterization
Urinalysis for proteinuria
Blood urea nitrogen and creatinine levels
Liver transaminase levels
Arterial blood gas analysis
Serum electrolyte levels

with significant peripheral edema. Reducing the dietary sodium intake to approximately 2 grams per day and providing dietary teaching on the preparation and purchasing of foods should also be initiated.

Medical therapy (Table 8–11) includes the use of diuretics to control excess volume and ACE inhibitors to reduce the afterload, or resistance the ventricle must work against to empty.[7,9] Digoxin can be employed to improve the contractility of the dysfunctional ventricle. Thorough monitoring of the patient's symptoms for toxicity and careful use of digoxin in those patients with renal and hepatic disease should be employed.

More acute episodes of congestive heart failure require rapid assimilation of the historical and clinical data. For acute episodes of congestive heart failure, intravenous nitroprusside, nitroglycerine, or ACE inhibitors can be used as well as agents such as dopamine and dobutamine to optimize the acutely diminished ventricular function.[7,9] Patients with significantly reduced ventricular function may require the addition of oral anticoagulants, such as warfarin, to prevent embolic disease. These patients will require close monitoring of the medications used, electrolytes, and renal function. Patients should keep track of their body weight and notify their health care provider when significant change in weight occurs.

Life-style Changes

The most important life-style changes in congestive heart failure are the diet and fluid restrictions. The patient should have a clear understanding of the allowable amounts of salt and how to interpret labels before buying groceries. This can be accomplished through dietary education and assistance in selecting appropriate foods and substitutes. The patient will need

TABLE 8–11. SELECTED CONGESTIVE HEART FAILURE MEDICATIONS

Medications	Dosage	Side Effects
Lanoxin (digoxin)	Digitalization and maintenance varies in adults and children depending on the clinical situation: see literature.	Premature ventricular contractions, ventricular tachycardia, severe bradycardia, ECG changes, heart block, arrhythmias (especially in children), anorexia, nausea, vomiting, diarrhea, CNS effects, visual disturbances.
Lasix (furosemide)	Adults: initially: 20–80 mg q day. May repeat or increase after 6–8 h; max 600 mg daily. Children: Initially: 2 mg/kg after 6–8 h; max 6 mg/kg/day.	Excessive diuresis, fluid or electrolyte imbalance, GI upset, dizziness, vertigo, paresthesias, orthostatic hypotension, hyperglycemia, jaundice, hyperuricemia, rash, photosensitivity, tinnitus, hearing loss, blood dyscrasias, renal calcification in premature infants.
Nitro-bid IV (nitroglycerin)	Adults: 5 micrograms via IV infusion, to start; increase dosage in increments of 5 at 3–5 min intervals until response is noted. Children: not recommended.	Headache, crescendo angina, rebound hypertension, hypotension, anaphylactoid reactions, methemoglobinemia (rare).
Accupril (quinapril hydrochloride)	Adult: 5 mg bid to start, if needed increase weekly to 20–40 mg daily in 2 equally divided doses. Children: not recommended.	Headache, dizziness, fatigue, cough, GI upset, hyperkalemia, back pain, tachycardia, dry mouth, somnolence, sweating, sinusitis.
Capoten (captopril)	Adult: Take 1 h before meals, initially: 25 mg 3 times daily, max 450 mg day. Children: not recommended.	Headache, dysgeusia, rash, pruritus, dizziness, fatigue, cough, proteinuria, nephritis, GI upset, hyperkalemia, hyponatremia, back pain, tachycardia, excessive hypotension, dry mouth, jaundice, somnolence, sweating, sinusitis, impotence.
Vasotec (enalapril)	Adult: Initial: 2.5 mg 1–2 times daily, max 40 mg/day. Children: not recommended.	Cough, headache, dizziness, fatigue, diarrhea, rash, orthostatic hypotension, asthenia, hyperkalemia, renal impairment, nausea.

to be more aware of his or her weight and weigh at least three times a week. It is important to instruct the patient to keep a diary of weights and symptoms and, if possible, blood pressures. Negative habits such as smoking should be addressed and smoking cessation classes recommended. The patient should understand that he or she is to remain as active as symptoms will allow. This will vary with the etiology of heart failure and associated conditions. An exercise prescription should be determined by someone knowledgable about the patient's cardiovascular disorders. Patients with associated rhythm disturbances may require work limitations or driving restrictions. This can be determined on an individual basis, since many patients do well when heart failure is compensated for by medications and dietary measures.

■ ENDOCARDITIS

General Characteristics

Endocarditis is an inflammation of the endocardium, the endothelial lining of the heart (Fig. 8–5).[10] It can be infective or noninfective. Infective endocarditis is caused by a bacterium such as *Staphylococcus* or *Enterococcus*. These bacteria can enter the bloodstream during surgical and dental procedures or with injecting drug use. They can produce vegetations on heart valves, but these may occur anywhere on the endothelial lining. Noninfective endocarditis is a sterile vegetation, actually thrombotic rather than infective. Risk factors for endocarditis include a history of rheumatic fever, congenital or acquired defect in the heart or valves, intravenous drug use, and placement of an artificial heart valve.[10] Persons with any of these risk factors should be counseled on the prevention of endocarditis.

Signs, Symptoms, and Diagnosis

Symptoms of endocarditis include fatigue, fever, myalgia, weight loss, and anorexia.[11] The onset is often vague and insidious and only after treatment does the patient realize how long he or she has not felt well. The classic triad of endocarditis is fever, anemia, and the occurrence of a murmur, although murmurs may be absent initially when the patient complains primarily of flulike symptoms.[10] One or more murmurs are found in nearly every patient with endocarditis. The two most common murmurs are aortic and mitral regurgitation. Other signs that may be seen with endocarditis are: splinter hemorrhages in the nails, Osler's nodes in the extremities, Janeway lesions on the palms and soles of the feet, conjunctival petechiae, and clubbing of the fingers.[10] If pulses are decreased

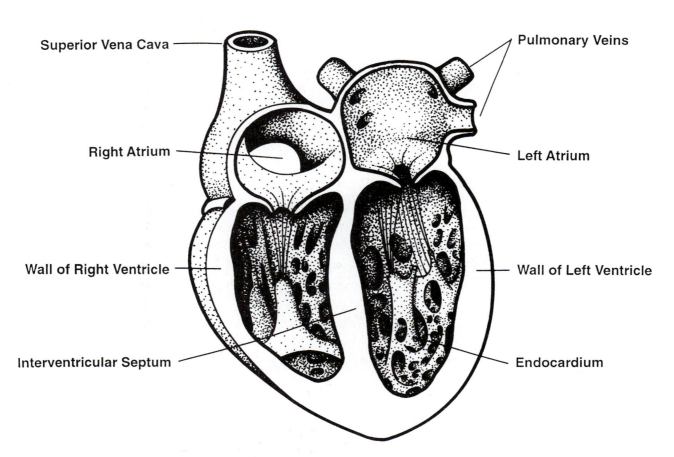

Figure 8–5. Heart anatomy

TABLE 8–12. DIAGNOSTIC TESTS FOR ENDOCARDITIS

Blood cultures
Complete blood count (CBC)
Urinalysis
Erythrocyte sedimentation rate (ESR)
Electrocardiogram (ECG)
Echocardiogram (transthoracic or transesophageal)
Chest x-ray

or absent, one should be suspicious of an embolism from a fragment of the vegetation. Splenomegaly can also occur with endocarditis.

There are several diagnostic tests in the evaluation of endocarditis (Table 8–12).[10,11] A CBC will usually show a normocytic, normochromic anemia. There will also be an elevation in the erythrocyte sedimentation rate. Urinalysis shows proteinuria and possibly hematuria. The most important test for endocarditis is the blood culture.[10,11] Four to six blood cultures should be obtained. Most blood cultures are positive in patients with endocarditis. If the blood cultures continue to be negative and there is a high suspicion for endocarditis, it may be necessary to do arterial blood cultures or even a bone marrow culture if an unusual pathogen is suspected.[11] An ECG should be performed during initial diagnosis and treatment to look for a silent myocardial infarction from embolized fragments of the vegetations or further infection into the myocardium.[10] Echocardiography can be helpful in seeing the vegetation but does not rule out endocarditis if a vegetation is not seen, since vegetations of less than 5 mm are not seen and require use of transesophageal echocardiography. Chest x-ray helps if there is suspicion of congestive heart failure, lung abscess, or pneumonia.

Management

Treatment with antibiotics should begin immediately when the diagnosis is made. These are usually intravenous antibiotics that are sensitive to the bacteria identified on blood cultures. Examples include cefazolin (Ancef, Kefzol) and penicillin G procaine (Wycillin) (Table 8-13). Endocarditis can be fatal if treatment is withheld or if it is undertreated.[11] Surgery is indicated in patients with prosthetic valve endocarditis, fungal endocarditis, persistent positive blood cultures while on therapy, recurrent emboli, heart failure, large vegetation, and possibly renal failure.[11]

Life-style Changes

Prophylaxis is the most important life-style change. Persons with the risk factors mentioned should be given antimicrobial drugs prior to any dental, upper respiratory, or genitourinary tract procedures, eg, amoxicillin 3 g orally 1 hour before the procedure and 1.5 g 6 hours after the procedure.[10]

TABLE 8–13. MEDICATIONS USED IN ENDOCARDITIS

Medication	Dosage	Side Effects
Kefzol, Ancef (cefazolin)	Adults: 1-1 5 g q 6 h IV or IM. Max 12 g/day. Children (≥1 month): 25–100 mg/kg/day in 3–4 equal divided doses.	Local reactions, drug fever, rash, pruritus, diarrhea, anaphylaxis, superinfection, blood dyscrasias, elevated liver enzymes.
Wycillin (penicillin G procaine)	Adult: 600,000–1,000,000 units/day IM. Child (≥12 yr): 600,000 units/day IM.	Rash, drug fever, serum sickness, anaphylaxis, superinfection, blood dyscrasias, neuropathy, nephropathy.

■ ANGINA

General Characteristics

Approximately 3 million Americans have angina, also known as angina pectoris.[12] Angina is a symptom of coronary artery disease. Coronary artery disease is the leading cause of death in United States and is caused by atherosclerosis (hardening of the arteries).[13] The arteries that carry oxygen-filled blood to the heart muscle become narrow as we age and the walls become irregular, which may allow for build up of fat, cholesterol, clot-forming platelets, and fibrous plaques.[13] When a coronary artery narrows, not allowing blood flow to a certain area of the heart, the heart develops ischemia and the patient develops angina (Fig. 8–6).

Risk factors for developing coronary artery disease and angina are not totally understood but should be discussed with all patients, no matter what their age, in hope of prevention of this problem (Table 8–14).

There are several types of angina: stable, unstable, and variant.[12] Patients with stable angina have pain that is predictable, ie, onset with exertion or stress, and can be relieved with rest and nitroglycerin in about 5 minutes. Heavy meals and emotional stress may also cause angina.

Patients with unstable angina may develop discomfort or pain at rest, with minimal exertion, or for prolonged periods

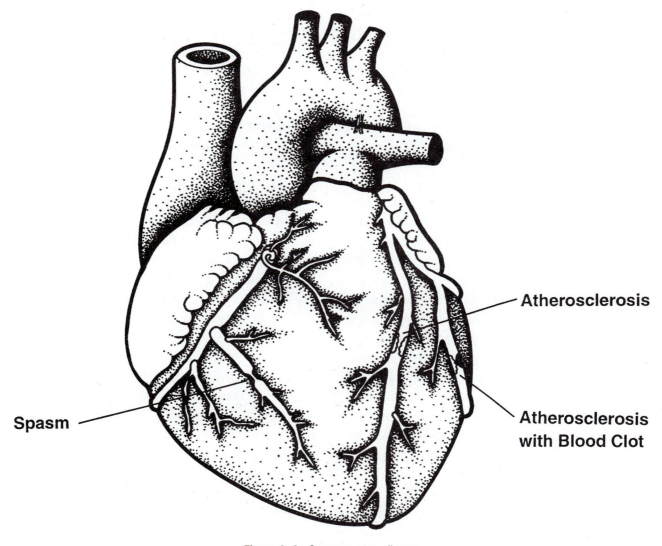

Atherosclerosis

Spasm

Atherosclerosis with Blood Clot

Figure 8–6. Coronary artery disease

TABLE 8–14. RISK FACTORS FOR CORONARY ARTERY DISEASE

Hypertension
Diabetes
Elevated cholesterol
Cigarette smoking

TABLE 8–15. TESTS FOR CORONARY ARTERY DISEASE AND ANGINA

Diagnostic Tests
Electrocardiogram (ECG)
Exercise stress testing (not performed in unstable angina)
Echocardiogram at rest or with exercise (stress echo)
Exercise perfusion imaging with thallium or technetium
Holter monitor (evaluate for ST segment elevation with variant angina)
Coronary angiography
Blood Tests
Cholesterol and fractions of low-density lipoprotein (LDL) and high-density lipoprotein (HDL) cholesterol
Complete blood count (CBC)

of time.[12] Unstable angina is considered the stage between stable angina and myocardial infarction.[12]

Variant (Prinzmetal's) angina is an unusual form of angina.[12] Patients with variant angina develop discomfort almost exclusively at rest, without physical exertion or emotional stress.[13] Variant angina is thought to be caused by coronary artery spasm. Variant angina may be associated with acute myocardial infarction, severe cardiac arrhythmias, and sudden death.[13]

Signs, Symptoms, and Diagnosis

People with angina may complain of chest discomfort, not necessarily chest pain. A thorough history of the anginal episode needs to be taken, with special attention paid to the onset, character, location, radiation, severity, length, and recurrence of the discomfort. The description of this chest discomfort may include heaviness, squeezing, constricting, bursting, strangling, or burning.[13] The onset may or may not occur with physical activity or emotional stress. With unstable angina or variant angina, the pain or discomfort may occur at night.[13] The location is usually in the substernal area with radiation to the shoulders, neck, jaw, and arms. The discomfort or pain of angina usually lasts from 5 to 15 minutes and may be relieved with rest or nitroglycerin. A history of pain or discomfort lasting longer than 15 minutes accompanied with profound fatigue may indicate a myocardial infarction.[13]

The physical examination may appear entirely normal or may show signs of coronary artery disease such as corneal arcus and xanthomas.[13] The blood pressure and arterial pulses should be evaluated. The physical examination may also indicate the etiology of the coronary artery disease such as diabetes, obesity, and hypertension.[13] A thorough cardiac examination should be performed.

Several tests can be performed to assist with the diagnosis of angina or infarction (Table 8–15).[12,13] Blood tests may be performed to evaluate cholesterol and lipid levels as well as to screen for diabetes. An ECG should be obtained when the pa-

tient is having pain.[12,14] If this is not possible, exercise stress testing may be helpful to reproduce the pain or discomfort during increased cardiac demand while an ECG is performed.[14] Other tests listed in Table 8–15 may be performed to evaluate presence and severity of coronary artery disease and if there has been any damage to the heart.[14]

Management

The goal of therapy (Table 8–16) is to improve the quality of life of the patient with angina.[12] Patients with stable angina may only need to take nitroglycerin sublingually as needed or prior to performing a task that brings on chest pain. The patient needs to be instructed to go for emergency evaluation if the chest pain is not relieved with two to three tablets in a 15-minute period. The patient also needs to learn the difference between chest pain caused by musculoskeletal factors or esophagitis.[12]

The patient needs to be informed about the use and care of nitroglycerin. Nitroglycerin should be stored in a cool, dark place. It usually causes a tingling sensation under the tongue and may cause side effects such as headaches and flushing.[12] If the tablets are losing their potency, the patient may not have the sensation or side effects when using tablets. Long-acting nitrates may be applied to the skin, where they are absorbed slowly and provide longer control of symptoms.[12] This is good for patients who have nocturnal angina. Other medications that may be given for angina are beta-blockers, calcium channel blockers, and aspirin.

Patients with unstable angina are usually admitted to the hospital and continuously monitored by electrocardiography,

TABLE 8–16. SELECTED ANTIANGINAL MEDICATIONS

Medications	Dosage	Side Effects
Corgard (nadolol)	Adult: 40 mg once daily to start, followed by increments of 40–80 mg/day q 3–7 days.	Bradycardia, dizziness, fatigue, cold extremities, heart failure, heart block, bronchospasm, GI upset, rash pruritus.
Adalat, Procardia (nifedipine)	Adult: 10 mg tid to start, followed by gradual increases in dosage. The usual effective dosage is 10–20 mg tid.	Peripheral edema, hypotension, headache, flushing, dizziness, fatigue, constipation, muscle cramps, rash, exacerbation of angina, heart failure.
Calan, Ispotin (verapamil hydrochloride)	Adult: 80–120 mg tid, followed by daily or weekly increases in dosage, up to 480 mg/day, as needed, until optimum clinical response is obtained.	Hypotension, impaired AV conduction, edema, bradycardia, CHF, constipation, dizziness, headache, fatigue, nausea, dyspnea, elevated hepatitis enzymes, rash, flushing, paralytic ileus.
Cardizem (diltiazem hydrochloride)	Adult: 30 mg qid, to start, followed, if necessary, by a gradual dosage increase q 1–2 days.	Edema, headache, dizziness, asthenia, first degree AV block, bradycardia, flushing, nausea, rash, CHF, hypotension, liver abnormalities.
Norvasc (amlodipine besylate)	Adult: 5–10 mg once daily.	Rash, headache, GI upset, orthostatic hypotension, flushing, dizziness.
Isordil (isosorbide dinitrate)	Adult: tablets, 5–10 mg to start, followed by 10–40 mg, q 6 h; Controlled release capsules, 40 mg to start, followed by 40–80 mg q 8–12h.	Headache, flushing, dizziness, weakness, orthostatic hypotension, paradoxical bradycardia, rash.
Nitrostat (nitroglycerin)	Adult: 1 tab dissolved sublingually or buccally at the first sign of an acute anginal attack and repeated about q 5 min until relief is obtained, up to 3 tabs in 15 min.	Headache, dizziness, flushing, orthostatic hypotension, tachycardia, palpitations, nausea, and rash.
Transderm-Nitro (nitroglycerin)	Adult: 0.2–0.4 mg/h.	Headache, dizziness, flushing, orthostatic hypotension, tachycardia, nausea, rash.

and often they are given intravenous anticoagulants if pain persists.[12,14] The medications used in unstable angina are similar. However, it may be necessary to administer nitroglycerin intravenously to reduce the chest pain. Patients with unstable angina need bed rest, sedation, and attention given to predisposing factors.[14] Patients with unstable angina usually do not undergo a stress test, but they may have coronary angiography to evaluate the coronary arteries. If significant obstruction not responsive to medical therapy is present, balloon angioplasty or a coronary bypass grafting should be performed.[12,14]

Patients with coronary artery disease without symptoms may have coronary angiography performed to see if angioplasty or bypass is required.[12,14] All of these patients can benefit from aspirin taken daily if there are no contraindications.

Life-style Changes

There are many life-style changes that need to be a part of the management of coronary artery disease and angina. There should be a good relationship between the clinician and the patient in order to work on these changes together. The risk factors discussed earlier should be modified. Ideal weight and blood pressure should be obtained and maintained.[12,14] Diet and exercise to achieve this will also lower lipid levels. A diet low in fat and salt should be discussed with the patient, using examples of cookbooks and recipes. A nutritionist or dietitian is extremely helpful to teach the patient the proper diet. If the patient has angina, moderate exercise can be started and as the patient's tolerance increases he or she can increase the exercise level. The patient needs to be informed on the hazards of cigarette smoking and its effect on coronary artery disease and angina. All patients should be encouraged to stop smoking. Stress is another risk factor that needs to be addressed. The patient needs to be informed on the different ways to reduce stress. All of these are major life-style changes. The patient should not be expected to do all of them at once. The patient and clinician should decide on one change to start with and then build up to the next change.

■ MYOCARDIAL INFARCTION

General Characteristics

Acute myocardial infarction (MI), also known as a heart attack, is the major cause of death in the United States.[15] An MI occurs when a coronary artery becomes obstructed, not allowing blood to reach an area of the heart (Fig. 8–7). This area becomes damaged or "infarcted." This can be caused by coronary artery disease (atherosclerosis), coronary artery spasm, thrombosis in the coronary artery, or a combination of them.[15,16]

Signs, Symptoms, and Diagnosis

The patient having an MI usually has angina-type pain but may not have any pain, as in a silent MI.[16] The angina-type pain may be described as a heavy pressure or squeezing sensation that radiates to the jaw and upper extremities. The longer the pains continue, the more the damage to the heart. The patient may also experience shortness of breath, anxiety, nausea, vomiting, fatigue, or a combination of these.[15,16]

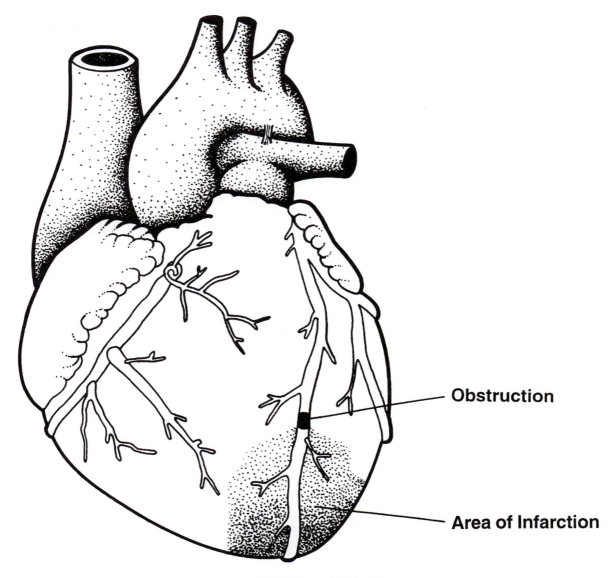

Obstruction

Area of Infarction

Figure 8–7. Myocardial infarction

TABLE 8–17. CARDIAC ENZYMES

Aspartate aminotransferase (AST) (also known as glutamic-
    oxaloacetic transaminase [SGOT])
Lactic dehydrogenase (LDH)
Creatine kinase (CK)
    CK-MB (an isoenzyme of CK)

On physical examination, the patient may appear diaphoretic and anxious, with mild shortness of breath. However, there are no specific physical findings for an MI.[15,16] The ECG is the most important diagnostic test for MI, but there may not be significant changes in the ECG in the early stage of an MI. Certain blood tests, known as cardiac enzymes, can help diagnose a MI (Table 8–17). The creatine kinase-MB (CK-MB) isoenzyme is currently the preferred enzyme to check.[15] Radionuclide imaging can be useful to see how much damage to the heart may have occurred.

Management

There are three important goals in the management of a patient with MI:

1. to alleviate any pain or discomfort the patient may have,
2. to preserve as much of the heart as possible by increasing blood flow to the damaged area, and
3. observe the patient continuously in a specialized unit for any complications that may occur and need to be treated.[16]

Oxygen, narcotics and intravenous nitroglycerin are often used to decrease the pain and discomfort the patient is having. There are several drugs that may be used to increase or preserve blood flow to the injured area of the heart (Table 8–18).[16] The patient's history and severity of MI should be taken into account when deciding which drug will benefit the heart the most. When the patient is stabilized or if possible in the first few hours, coronary angiography may be performed to evaluate for possible angioplasty or coronary artery bypass.

The patient should be monitored in a special care unit for any complications (Table 8–19).[16] If no complications develop, the patient should begin cardiac rehabilitation after the first 24 hours. In fact, the patient should be encouraged to progress through activity as quickly as tolerated. Several diagnostic tests may be performed on the post-MI patient before discharge to assess the risk of reinfarction. These include exercise stress test, exercise stress echocardiography or thallium imaging, and coronary angiography.[16] The patient may be continued on medications such as a beta-blockers, nitroglycerin, calcium channel blockers, ACE inhibitors, and aspirin after discharge from the hospital.

Life-style Changes

As part of cardiac rehabilitation, there are several life-style changes that need to be addressed with the post-MI patient

TABLE 8–19. COMPLICATIONS OF MYOCARDIAL INFARCTION

Cardiac arrhythmias
Congestive heart failure
Cardiogenic shock
Mitral regurgitation
Ventricular septal rupture
Free wall rupture
Pericarditis
Ventricular aneurysm
Recurrent angina

TABLE 8–18. MEDICATIONS FOR MYOCARDIAL INFARCTION

Medication	Dosage	Side Effects
Nitro-bid IV (nitroglycerin)	Adults: 5 micrograms via IV infusion, to start; increase dosage in increments of 5 at 3–5 min intervals until response is noted.	Headache, crescendo angina, rebound hypertension, hypotension, anaphylactoid reactions, methemoglobinemia (rare).
Streptase (streptokinase)	Adults: 1,500,000 IU by infusion within 60 min, alternatively, 20,000 IU as a bolus directly into thrombosed coronary artery, followed by 2,000 IU/min by intracoronary infusion for 60 min.	Bleeding, hypotension, fever, urticaria, pruritus, flushing, nausea, headache, musculoskeletal pain, vasculitis, interstitial nephritis, anaphylactoid reactions, polyneuropathy, and noncardiogenic pulmonary edema.
t-PA	Adults: 100 mg over 3 h: 10 mg as a bolus, followed by 50 mg over the first hour and 40 mg over the next 2 hours.	Bleeding.

TABLE 8–20. LIFE-STYLE CHANGES AFTER MYOCARDIAL INFARCTION

Low-fat, low-salt diet
Exercise in moderation
Decreased stress
Lowered blood pressure
Lowered cholesterol levels
Lowered lipid levels
Stopping smoking

(Table 8–20).[15,16] Although the patient cannot be expected to tackle all of these changes at once, the clinician needs to discuss each problem and help the patient decide on starting with one and then adding more as the patient becomes more confident. Patients who have had a uncomplicated MI may return to work as early as 4 to 6 weeks post MI.[16] The patient should be encouraged to try to resume life as it was before the MI. The patient may need to be reassured that he or she can still perform sexually. However, some patients may develop depression during their rehabilitation. Careful attention should be paid to each patient to prevent this and to refer the patient who develops depression.

References

1. Whelton PK, Goot VL. Systemic hypertension. In: Harvey AM, Johns RJ, McKusick VA, et al, eds. *The Principles and Practice of Medicine.* Norwalk, Conn: Appleton & Lange; 1988: 127–144.

2. Chobanian AV, Haralambos G. Hypertension. *Clin Symp.* 1990;42(5):2–32.

3. Shabetai R. Diseases of pericardium. In: Hurst JW, Schlant RC, Rackley CE, et al, eds. *The Heart: Arteries and Veins.* New York, NY: McGraw-Hill Inc;1990:1348–1353.

4. Achuff SC. Pericarditis. In: Harvey AM, Johns RJ, McKusick VA, et al, eds. *The Principles and Practice of Medicine.* Norwalk, Conn: Appleton & Lange; 1988:76–79.

5. Fortuin NJ, Achuff SC, Ross RS. Cardiac murmurs and other manifestations of valvular heart disease. In: Harvey AM, Johns RJ, McKusick VA, et al, eds. *The Principles and Practice of Medicine.* Norwalk, Conn: Appleton & Lange; 1988:63–75.

6. Rackley CE, Edwards JE, Wallace RB, et al, Valvular heart disease. In: Hurst JW, Schlant RC, Rackley CE, et al, eds. *The Heart: Arteries and Veins.* New York, NY: McGraw-Hill Inc; 1990:795–876.

7. Baughman KL. Congestive heart failure: pathophysiology, evaluation, and approach to management. In: Harvey AM, Johns RJ, McKusick VA, et al, eds. *The Principles and Practice of Medicine.* Norwalk, Conn: Appleton & Lange;1988: 50–63.

8. Braunwald E, Grossman W. Clinical aspects of heart failure. In: Braunwald E, ed. *Heart Disease: A Textbook of Cardiovascular Medicine.* 4th ed. Philadelphia, Pa: WB Saunders Co; 1992:444–463.

9. Smith TW, Braunwald E, Kelly RA. The management of heart failure. In Braunwald E, ed. *Heart Disease: A Textbook of Cardiovascular Medicine.* 4th ed. Philadelphia, Pa: WB Saunders Co;1992:464–509.

10. Durack DY. Infective and noninfective endocarditis. In: Hurst JW, Schlant RC, Rackley CE, et al, eds. *The Heart: Arteries and Veins.* New York, NY: McGraw-Hill Inc; 1990:1230–1255.

11. Mann JJ. Infective endocarditis. In: Harvey AM, Johns RJ, McKusick VA, et al, eds. *The Principles and Practice of Medicine.* Norwalk, Conn: Appleton & Lange;1988:613–618.

12. Fortuin NJ, Walford GD. Thoracic pain and angina pectoris. In: Harvey AM, Johns RJ, McKusick VA, et al, eds. *The Principles and Practice of Medicine.* Norwalk, Conn: Appleton & Lange; 1988:88–98.

13. Braunwald E. The history. In: Braunwald E, ed. *Heart Disease: A Textbook of Cardiovascular Medicine.* 4th ed. Philadelphia, Pa: WB Saunders Co; 1992:1–12.

14. Hurst JW. The recognition and treatment of four types of angina pectoris and angina equivalents. In: Hurst JW, Schlant RC, Rackley CE, et al, eds. *The Heart: Arteries and Veins.* New York, NY: McGraw-Hill Inc; 1990:1046–1052.

15. Guerci AD, Weisfeldt ML. Acute myocardial infarction. In: Harvey AM, Johns RJ, McKusick VA, et al, eds. *The Principles and Practice of Medicine.* Norwalk, Conn: Appleton & Lange; 1988:99–110.

16. Morris DC, Walter PF, Hurst JW. The recognition and treatment of myocardial infarction and its complications. In: Hurst JW, Schlant RC, Rackley CE, et al, eds. *The Heart: Arteries and Veins.* New York, NY: McGraw-Hill Inc; 1990:1054–1078.

9

Rheumatologic Disorders

Angela Wegmann

■ OSTEOARTHRITIS

General Characteristics

Arthritis is a disorder of joints that causes pain and loss of movement. The name literally means joint inflammation. There are over 100 kinds of arthritis, yet the most frequently encountered type is called osteoarthritis. Almost 16 million Americans suffer from this disease, which is characterized by deterioration of articular cartilage and bone proliferation. This disease is thought to be caused by simple "wear and tear" from normal everyday activity. Almost all persons over age 60 have developed osteoarthritis in one or more joints; however, degenerative changes of osteoarthritis will commonly exist in asymptomatic joints. Injury, obesity, and certain repeated stressful activities are factors that increase one's risk for developing symptomatic osteoarthritis. Osteoarthritis may develop in any joint but most commonly affects the hips, knees, feet, hands, and spine. It rarely affects the wrist, elbow, shoulder, or ankle unless the joint was previously injured. The disease affects men and women equally.

Signs, Symptoms, and Diagnosis

The most common symptom of osteoarthritis is pain in one or a few joints after overuse. Stiffness may occur in the morning or after rest, but it is usually brief (less than 30 minutes). Patients frequently notice that it requires more energy to move the affected joint and with advanced disease they may have limited range of motion. Nodular bony overgrowths called Heberden's or Bouchard's nodes may occur at interphalangeal joints, while small, cool effusions can be present in larger joints. Although osteoarthritis may develop in any joint the pattern of involvement is typically asymmetrical.

Diagnosis is based on the characteristics of joint involvement (Fig. 9–1, 9–2), radiographic features, and normal laboratory studies. Characteristic radiographic changes show narrow joint spaces, bony cysts, and osteophyte formation. If possible, joint fluid analysis should be included in the initial evaluation.

Management

Management consists of symptomatic relief combined with functional rehabilitation. Pain relief can be obtained with nonsteroidal anti-inflammatory drugs (NSAIDs) or aspirin (Table 9–1). Intermittent use is encouraged when possible to reduce gastrointestinal effects. Daily activities must be revised to avoid excessive strain on joints. Joint protection with splinting, walkers, or canes may be necessary. Physical therapy followed by a routine home exercise program is crucial to slow further joint deterioration. Corticosteroid injection may be used infrequently in refractory cases. For patients with advanced disease and loss of function or intractable pain, surgery is an option.

Life-style Changes

Patients should be encouraged to notice the relationship between pain and their activity. If possible, any activity that increases discomfort should be reduced or avoided. Gentle exercise to strengthen the joint-supporting structures can be recommended by a therapist and should be performed regu-

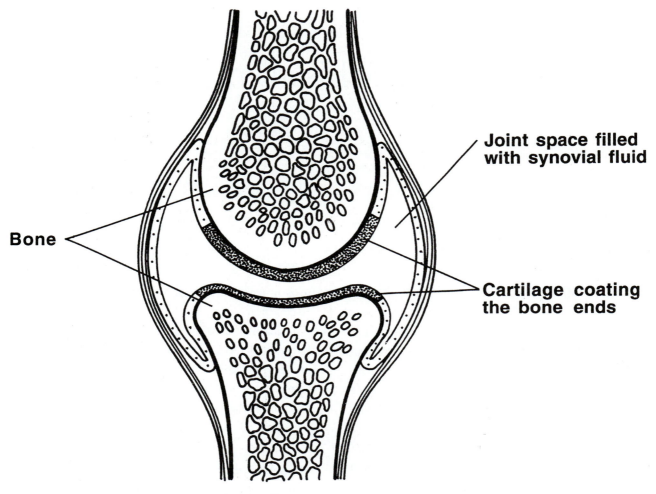

Figure 9–1. Normal joint

TABLE 9–1. COMMON OSTEOARTHRITIC MEDICATIONS

Medication	Dosage	Precautions
Anaprox (Naproxen sodium)	275–550 mg bid, up to 1650 mg/d	GI bleeding, ulceration, and perforation; renal toxicity; liver function abnormalities
Ansaid (Flurbiprofen)	200–300 mg/d in divided doses (50–100 mg bid to qid), up to 100 mg/dose or 300 mg/d	GI bleeding, ulceration, and perforation; renal toxicity; liver function abnormalities
Clinoril (Sulindac)	150 mg bid, followed by up to 400 mg/d	GI bleeding, ulceration, and perforation; visual disturbances; liver function abnormalities
Disalcid (Salsalate)	1 g tid or 1.5 g bid	Factors influencing plasma salicylic acid levels
Easprin (Aspirin)	975 mg tid or qid	Salicylate intoxication, GI bleeding
Feldene (Piroxicam)	20 mg/d in single or divided dose	GI bleeding, ulceration, and perforation; renal toxicity; visual impairment
Motrin (Ibuprofen)	300 mg qid or 400–800 mg tid or qid	GI bleeding, ulceration, and perforation; renal toxicity; ophthalmic changes

GI, gastrointestinal.

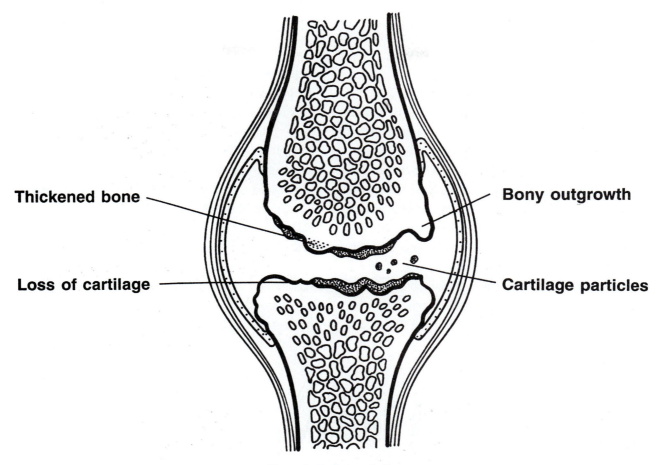

Thickened bone

Bony outgrowth

Loss of cartilage

Cartilage particles

Figure 9–2. Osteoarthritis

larly. Patients should be counseled on balancing rest and exercise. Resting a day or two after a joint has been strained is advisable. Overweight patients should be encouraged to lose weight. Maintaining good posture can help reduce strain on the lower back. Applying hot or cold packs can be used to reduce discomfort temporarily. In most cases, osteoarthritis is a manageable disease with few long-term complications.

■ RHEUMATOID ARTHRITIS

General Characteristics

More than 35 million Americans suffer from some form of arthritis. One of the more common forms is rheumatoid arthritis (RA), which is characterized by symmetrical inflammatory synovitis. Although the predominant symptom is polyarthritis, the disease is often extraarticular, affecting the eyes and cardiovascular, pulmonary, and neurologic systems. The prognosis is variable as the clinical course can range from intermittently symptomatic to rapidly progressive with deformity and disability. The etiology appears to be a normal but misdirected inflammatory response, which some experts believe is orchestrated by a virus. This autoimmune response causes inflammation of synovium and destruction of the joint space. The overall incidence is 1%, with females being affected more often than males.

Signs, Symptoms, and Diagnosis

The hallmark of RA is symmetrical polyarthritis. Most patients will complain of joint pain with motion and morning stiffness for longer than 1 hour after arising. Gelling commonly occurs during the day after periods of inactivity. Constitutional symptoms such as malaise, fatigue, and weight loss reflect the systemic nature of the disease. The joints most frequently involved include the proximal interphalangeal, metatarsalphalangeal, wrist, and knee joints (Fig. 9–3). Signs of inflammation such as swelling, heat, erythema, and limited range of motion secondary to pain are noted on examination. Occasionally rheumatoid nodules and atrophy of adjacent muscles will be seen. Joint deformities such as ulnar deviation and hammer toes may develop after persistent inflammation. The clinical course varies, but symptoms usually follow one of

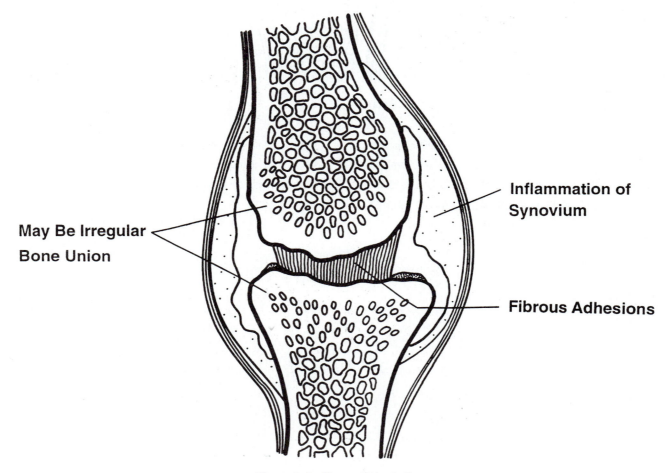

May Be Irregular Bone Union

Inflammation of Synovium

Fibrous Adhesions

Figure 9–3. Rheumatoid arthritis

three patterns: sporadic, insidious and progressive, or rapid and aggressive.

No laboratory test or set of symptoms is diagnostic for RA. Diagnosis is based on clinical manifestations, the presence of radiographic changes, and certain laboratory abnormalities. Helpful laboratory tests are synovial fluid analysis, erythrocyte sedimentation rate (ESR), complete blood count (CBC), and rheumatoid factor. An elevated ESR and a positive rheumatoid factor are suggestive of RA but can be present in other disease processes. Likewise, a negative rheumatoid factor does not rule out RA, as 20% of patients will have a seronegative form. Radiographs usually show some degree of joint space erosion but can also be negative in early stages of the disease.

Management

The primary goals of management are joint preservation and reconditioning. A combination of agents is usually required to obtain this goal. Treatment is commonly initiated with aspirin or NSAIDs (refer to osteoarthritis discussion for treatment options). Rest, gentle exercise, and judicious splinting are used in conjunction with NSAIDs as a conservative initial program. However, this will not significantly alter the course of disease in most patients. Disease-modifying agents such as hydroxychloroquine, gold compound, and methotrexate are now being used earlier in the course of the moderate-to-severe dis-

ease to combat inflammation and slow disease progression (Table 9–2). The toxicity of these drugs seems to be dose-related, and most RA patients tolerate them reasonably well. Pulse dosing with high-dose corticosteroids can be used for acute flares of RA. Long-term therapy with steroids is not recommended because of adverse effects.

All patients should undergo some physical or occupational therapy to recondition and protect joints and adjacent soft tissues. Physical therapy can increase range of motion and muscle strength. Cold or hot packs can be used prior to exercise to relieve pain. Occupational therapy teaches patients energy conservation and joint protection by providing special devices and techniques.

Life-style Changes

Numerous life-style changes are necessary to preserve or reestablish maximal joint function. A careful balance of rest and exercise is of primary importance. Regular gentle exercise and resting after activity or straining must be emphasized. Patients should avoid joint overuse and reduce the frequency of any activity that exacerbates symptoms. If pain continues more than 2 hours after exercise or is worse than baseline the following day, the patient should reduce the amount of exercise he or she is doing. A well-balanced, low-fat diet is recommended to maintain an optimal weight and reduce strain on knees and feet. Morning stiffness can be relieved by applying

TABLE 9–2. MEDICATIONS FOR RHEUMATOID ARTHRITIS

Medication	Dosage	Side Effects
Plaquenil (hydroxychloroquine sulfate)	Adults: 400–600 mg daily with food or milk.	Visual disturbances, hematologic disorders, muscle weakness.
Rheumatrex (methotrexate)	Adults: initially, 7.5 mg/wk in a single dose or three 2.5 mg doses at 12 hr intervals; max 20 mg/wk.	Elevated hepatic enzymes, bone marrow suppression, nausea, vomiting, diarrhea, stomatitis, rash, pruritus, alopecia, dizziness.
Ridaura (auranofin)	Adults: initially 6 mg daily in 1–2 divided doses. If response inadequate after 6 months, may increase to 3 mg tid.	Bone marrow suppression, proteinuria, hematuria, diarrhea, GI upset, ulcerative colitis, rash, pruritus, exfoliative dermatitis, stomatitis, conjunctivitis, nephrotic syndrome, cholestatic jaundice, gold bronchitis, pneumonitis, peripheral neuropathy.
Solganal (aurothioglucose)	Adults: Initially, 10 mg IM intragluteally. After 1 and 2 weeks: 25 mg.	Bone marrow depression, blood dyscrasias, dermatitis, skin pigmentation, proteinuria, nausea, diarrhea, hepatitis, ulcerative colitis, pruritus, stomatitis, conjunctivitis, nephrotic syndrome, anaphylaxis, gold bronchitis, pneumonitis, peripheral neuropathy.

heat with a hot shower or bath. Patients with RA that affects the hands are encouraged to avoid clothing with buttons or use a button hook. Wearing comfortable shoes and using a shoehorn will decrease strain on hands and feet. Various devices are available to enlarge or extend gripping surfaces and protect the joints of the hand. Lastly, patients taking NSAIDs should be advised to avoid alcohol in order to minimize the possibility of gastrointestinal side effects.

■ SYSTEMIC LUPUS ERYTHEMATOSUS

General Characteristics

Systemic lupus erythematosus is a multisystem autoimmune disorder with diverse clinical manifestations. The incidence in the United States is approximately 7 per 100,000, with a female preponderance of 9 to 1.[1] Certain racial groups also appear to be predisposed to the disease, with blacks and some asians being affected more than whites. Systemic lupus erythematosus (SLE) may occur at any age, but onset is typically between 15 to 25 years of age.

The etiology is not entirely clear but it is generally believed that unknown factors cause deregulation of suppressor T cell activity and overproduction of autoantibodies. These antibodies, which are directed against antigens like native DNA, platelets, and cell membrane constituents, form immune complexes that activate the complement system. These reactions in turn lead to widespread inflammatory damage to the vascular, nervous, musculoskeletal, and other systems (Fig. 9–4).

Signs, Symptoms, and Diagnosis

Presentation varies greatly depending on the organ systems involved and the severity of involvement. Cases range from mild and episodic to life-threatening. The most common complaint is constitutional symptoms such as fever, fatigue, and malaise. Photosensitive rashes and symmetrical joint pain occur in almost all patients. Pleuritis and pericarditis are fairly common

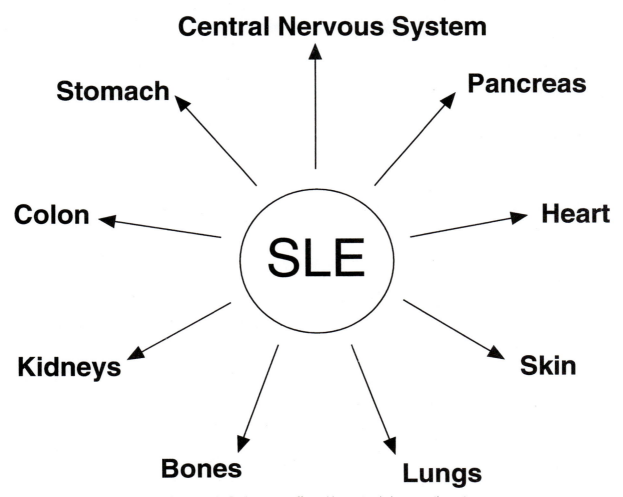

Figure 9–4. Body organs affected by systemic lupus erythematosus

and may present with dyspnea. Silent but potentially fatal kidney disease occurs in approximately half of patients. A variety of neurologic problems such as seizures, psychosis, hemiplegias, and peripheral neuropathies can be seen in varying degrees. Gastrointestinal symptoms, although common, are usually nonspecific. The course of the disease is punctuated by exacerbations (often triggered by infection, stress, or exposure to sunlight) and remissions. Overall survival rates are good and approximate 90% at 10 years.[2] The prognosis is even better for patients with milder disease.

Diagnosis is complicated, as no single test or laboratory study is confirmatory. Rather, SLE is considered probable if four or more specific criteria are present simultaneously or serially (Tables 9–3 through 9–5). A detailed history and physical examination as well as certain laboratory and diagnostic tests need to be performed to screen for these criteria. These may include hematologic and immunologic studies, urinalysis, 24-hour urine collection, chest x-ray, electrocardiogram, and echocardiogram.

Management

At present there is no cure for SLE. Treatment is determined by the systems involved and the severity of involvement. Patients with mild disease may require only supportive or preventive measures, such as wearing sunscreen or avoiding ultraviolet light. Lupus arthritis and fever can be managed with NSAIDs or salicylates (refer to osteoarthritis discussion for treatment options). Topical steroids can be used for milder skin lesions,

TABLE 9–3. CRITERIA FOR DIAGNOSIS OF SYSTEMIC LUPUS ERYTHEMATOSUS

Malar rash
Discoid rash
Photosensitivity
Oral ulcerations
Arthritis
Serositis
Renal disorder
Neurologic disorder
Hematologic abnormality
Immunologic abnormality
Positive antinuclear antibody test

TABLE 9–4. COMMON LABORATORY ABNORMALITIES FOUND IN SYSTEMIC LUPUS ERYTHEMATOSUS

Antinuclear antibodies
Anemia
Leukopenia
Thrombocytopenia
Proteinuria
False positive Venereal Disease Research Laboratories (VDRL) test
Anti-DNA antibodies
Low serum complement levels

whereas antimalarials such as hydroxychloroquine may be required for more severe skin or joint symptoms (Table 9–6). Major flares of SLE, particularly with cardiopulmonary, renal, or neurologic involvement, are usually treated with high-dose systemic corticosteroids for at least a month. Steroids may be slowly tapered after symptoms are controlled. Immunosuppressive agents such as cyclophosphamide and azathioprine are reserved for serious cases that are unresponsive to steroids.

Life-style Changes

Life-style changes may be numerous, depending on the severity of the disease, and may include:

- Wearing sunscreen or protective clothing in sunlight
- Avoiding fatigue by taking daily naps, pacing activity, and scheduling events by balancing rest and exercise
- Eating a balanced diet and taking a daily multivitamin
- Exercising regularly to build strength and increase mobility

TABLE 9–5. COMMON MANIFESTATIONS OF SYSTEMIC LUPUS ERYTHEMATOSUS

Malar rash
Arthritis
Cardiopulmonary disease
Renal disease
Nervous system disorders
Vasculitis/Raynaud's phenomenon

TABLE 9–6. MEDICATIONS FOR SYSTEMIC LUPUS ERYTHEMATOSUS

Medication	Dosage	Precautions
Hydroxychloroquine (Plaquenil)	Initial dose: 400 mg 1–2 times/d for several weeks or months, depending on response; prolonged maintenance, 200–400 mg/d	Visual disturbances; hematologic disorders; muscle weakness
Triamcinolone (Aristocort)	20–32 mg/d to start, followed by maintenance therapy; patients with severe symptoms may require ≥48 mg/d and higher daily maintenance doses	Infection; ocular damage; hypertension; salt and water retention
Triamcinolone acetonide (Kenalog-40)	60 mg IM to start; followed as needed by IM doses of 40–80 mg; in some cases, 20 mg or less	Infection; ocular damage; hypertension; salt and water retention

IM, intramuscular.

- Discussing birth control with physician, as pregnancy can exacerbate SLE
- Participating in support groups or professional counseling to control anger or depression
- Reducing stress with biofeedback or guided imagery techniques

References

1. Kamen B. Systemic lupus erythematosus and lupus-like syndromes. *Phys Assist.* 1991;15:10–26.
2. Stevens MB. Systemic lupus erythematosus: the latest in diagnosis and management. *J Am Acad Phys Assist.* 1993; 6:275–282.

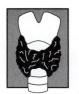

10

Endocrine Disorders

Roberto Canales
Bernadette M. Montgomerie

■ DIABETES MELLITUS

General Characteristics

Diabetes mellitus is perhaps one of the most common and least understood problems that exists in the world today. There are two main forms of the disease, non–insulin-dependent diabetes mellitus (NIDDM), formerly known as maturity-onset diabetes, and insulin-dependent diabetes mellitus (IDDM), once called juvenile-onset diabetes. An estimated 8 million people in the United States are known to have diabetes, of whom 680,000 have the IDDM type.[1]

Type II, or NIDDM, usually affects persons over the age of 40, who are most commonly overweight. As people gain weight, their individual fat cells grow, and sometimes these cells appear to lose their ability to receive and "hold on to" insulin. Such cells are then less efficient at taking up glucose and burning it or converting it to fat for storage.

The prevalence of diabetes is higher among blacks than whites, with black women showing a rate twice that of white women. Among Hispanics the rate is even higher. Black women over the age of 75 have the highest rate of type II diabetes mellitus, about one in four. The population of black and Hispanic elderly is increasing, and it is expected that these groups will constitute a larger proportion of older adults with diabetes in the future.[2] Heredity is an important factor also, in almost a third of all cases of NIDDM.

The type I form of the disease or IDDM occurs mainly in children and young adults because there is a defect in the pancreas that depletes, or completely destroys, the insulin-producing beta cells. Only 10% to 15% of all diabetics are type I. It is still not known exactly what causes the destruction of these beta cells; however, it is thought to be the result of some kind of autoimmune response. Many studies have shown that antibodies to the beta cells can be detected in the blood months and years before the symptoms of type I diabetes appear.[3]

Both forms of diabetes may be exacerbated by other diseases such as acromegaly, hyperthyroidism, Cushing's syndrome, and pancreatitis. This is known as secondary diabetes and in some instances, the condition continues even after the main disease has been successfully treated.

Signs, Symptoms, and Diagnosis

IDDM and NIDDM may present subtly with a common symptom being fatigue caused by energy deficiency or, in the case of IDDM, may begin dramatically with ketoacidosis.

Insulin deficiency causes hyperglycemia. The high blood glucose pulls fluid from body tissues, causing osmotic diuresis, polyuria, and ultimately dehydration. For both types, symptoms may include polydipsia, dry mucous membranes, and poor skin turgor. Edema and glucose deposits may cause visual changes. When diabetes causes ketoacidosis or hyperglycemic hyperosmolar nonketotic coma, dehydration may cause hypovolemia and shock. Wasting of glucose in the urine usually produces weight loss and hunger in IDDM, even if the patient eats voraciously.[4]

The diagnosis of diabetes is based on the criteria established by the National Diabetes Data Group in 1979. Unless there are unequivocal symptoms present when a random glucose level is over 200 mg/dL, two fasting blood glucose readings over 140 mg/dL are necessary to diagnose diabetes. Oral

101

glucose tolerance tests are generally not recommended for older adults.[1]

Ophthalmologic examination may reflect diabetic retinopathy. Random urinalysis should be performed to test for glucose and acetone.

Management

Management of the diabetic patient primarily consists of strict dietary controls, with the goal of controlling blood glucose levels, maintaining fasting levels of less than 200 mg/dL, and reaching and maintaining an appropriate body weight. Along with this, nutritional needs must be met to maintain the general health of the patient. For NIDDM, dietary management alone is sufficient to control the disease. Other patients may also require insulin injections and/or oral hypoglycemic agents (Table 10–1). For IDDM, the primary purpose is to prevent the long-term complications of diabetes through maintaining fasting blood glucose levels of less than 140 mg/dL. Insulin is recommended along with diet, exercise, and home blood glucose monitoring.

In general, multiple injections of regular insulin or regular insulin mixed with Neutral Protamine Hagedorn (NPH) or Lente insulin, controls blood glucose levels better than a single daily injection of long-acting insulin. The effects of diet and insulin may also be modified by the patient's activity level, which affects blood sugar and lipid metabolism.

The treatment for long-term diabetic complications, while still placing strong emphasis on careful blood sugar con-

trol, may also include vascular surgery for large vessel disease. It is currently believed that chronic hyperglycemia is causally related to the devastating chronic angiopathic and neuropathic complications of diabetes. Cerebrovascular disease is at least twice as frequent in diabetes, with the relative risk being highest for females. Hypertension is a major risk factor, as is being of African American or Asian American ethnic background. Coronary artery disease tends to be more severe, with more affected vessels, in patients with diabetes.

Diabetes is associated with more than 50% of the nontraumatic lower limb amputations in the United States, and interrelated factors, such as sensory and autonomic neuropathy and peripheral vascular disease can precipitate lower extremity morbidity.[5] Patients with type I diabetes often show evidence of nephropathy 15 to 20 years after diagnosis, and 30% to 40% of these patients will progress to end stage renal disease (ESRD). Patients with type II diabetes may show evidence of nephropathy 5 to 10 years after diagnosis, and approximately 3% to 5% of these patients will progress to ESRD. In attempting to prevent ESRD, it is of great importance that the health care professional ensure avoidance of nephrotoxic drugs in these patients. Nonsteroidal anti-inflammatory drugs, in particular, may cause tubular necrosis, interstitial nephritis, and glomerular impairment. When the diabetic is a child or adolescent, extra problems may arise. Here the health care professional's attention and availability could be crucial. For instance an adolescent girl with type I diabetes may feel "her life is over" when she discovers she has the disease. All diabet-

TABLE 10–1. ORAL HYPOGLYCEMIC AGENTS

Medication	Dosage	Precautions
Glyburide (DiaBeta)	2.5–5.0 mg/d to start maximum daily dosage: 20 mg/d	Cardiovascular risk; gastrointestinal reactions

Chlorpropamide (Diabinese)	250 mg/d to start; increase or decrease dosage as
	  needed by 50–125 mg/d, allowing 5–7 d to
	  elapse between start of therapy and first change
	  and 3–5 d to elapse between each adjustment
	Do not exceed 750 mg/d
		Cardiovascular risk; gastrointestinal disturbances

Glipizide (Glucotrol)	5 mg/d to start; increase dosage as needed by
	  2.5–5.0 mg/d, allowing several days between
	  each adjustment
	Do not exceed 40 mg/d
		Cardiovascular risk; gastrointestinal disturbances

Tolbutamide (Orinase)	1–2 g/d to start Maintenance: 0.25–2.0 g/d or up to 3 g/d in special cases	Cardiovascular risk; gastrointestinal disturbances
Tolazamide (Tolinase)	If glucose <200 mg/dL, 100 mg/d; if glucose >200 mg/dL, 250 mg/d. Do not exceed 1 g/d	Cardiovascular risk; gastrointestinal disturbances

ics can learn to be responsible for maintaining their own records of food exchanges and glucose levels and should be actively encouraged to take responsibility for their own health.[2]

Very little work has been done on the psychosocial impact of diabetes on older adults; however, their emotional response is similar to the response of younger people. Self-esteem, bodily integrity, self-worth, autonomy, independence, and control may all be challenged by a diagnosis of diabetes. The ability to deal with these feelings is affected by previous coping style, social support, and economic factors.[1]

Life-style Changes

Patients with diabetes mellitus must assume a major role in the medical management of the disorder. Since the goal of this management is to control blood glucose levels, patients may be required to test urine and blood glucose levels, take and adjust medications, make dietary decisions, and regulate their activity levels.

Acute complications of diabetes, such as hypoglycemia and acidosis, can be prevented or treated by a well-educated patient. The chronic or long-term complications of diabetes involving the cardiovascular system, renal function, visual impairment, and neurological dysfunction are believed to be slowed or eliminated when the patient maintains good glycemic control.[6]

Sexual function, particularly in men, may be impaired. The development of penile prosthesis implants has been a great help to such men.

■ HYPERTHYROIDISM

General Characteristics

Thyroid disease is one of the most common endocrine disorders, second only to diabetes mellitus. Hyperthyroidism accounts for most of the thyroid diseases occurring in both sexes and at virtually all ages. It is common in women and frequently occurs between the ages of 20 and 40.[7] Refer to Figure 10–1 to review the location of the thyroid and pituitary glands.

The thyroid gland is regulated by thyroid-stimulating hormone (TSH). TSH is produced by the pituitary gland. The thyroid gland in turn produces its own hormone, thyroxine (T_4). A portion of this T_4 is then broken down into triiodothyronine (T_3). Both T_4 and T_3 feed back negatively on the pituitary and inhibit the secretion of TSH (Fig. 10–2). Hyperthyroidism is usually characterized by an increased secretion rate of thyroid hormone causing in turn an increase in serum plasma levels.[8]

Hyperthyroidism is also known as thyrotoxicosis. There are many causes of this disorder (Table 10–2). Graves' disease is the most recognizable one because of the easily identifiable exophthalmos and pretibial myxedema associated with it. It is an autoimmune disorder with a familial tendency. The pathogenesis of Graves' disease involves the formation of autoantibodies that bind to the TSH receptor in the thyroid cell membranes and stimulate the gland to hyperfunction.[9] Toxic adenoma is not as common, and the signs of exophthalmos, pretibial myxedema, and thyroid antibodies are usually absent. Thyroiditis is thought to be caused by a viral infection and typically presents with an enlarged and tender thyroid gland.[9] Excess exogenous iodine can occur from intake of large amounts of iodine in the form of radiographic contrast materials or drugs, especially amiodarone. Contamination of ground beef with bovine thyroid gland can also be a cause. TSH-producing tumors are a rare cause of hyperthyroidism. Factitious hyperthyroidism can result from ingestion of synthetic T_4 or T_3. This condition can occur in dieters using thyroid hormones to lose weight. Trophoblastic tumor results in secretion of excess chorionic gonadotropin (beta hCG) from the tumor, which interacts with TSH receptors. Serum TSH is usually undetectable.[10] Struma ovarii is also a rare cause in which thyroidlike tissue rests within the ovary and can become hyperplastic.

Signs, Symptoms, and Diagnosis

Thyroid hormone receptors can be found in organ tissues throughout the body. As a result, thyroid dysfunction can have a profound effect. It can also make diagnosing hyperthyroidism confusing. Most clinicians think of a patient with hyperthyroidism as presenting with an obvious goiter, exophthalmos, and pretibial myxedema which is, in fact, the case for patients with Graves' disease. But there are several other causes of hyperthyroidism and many presenting signs and symptoms. The metabolic, cardiovascular, gastrointestinal, neuromuscular, and endocrine systems as well as skin, eyes, and behavior may all be notably affected (Table 10–3).

Patients can present with lethargy and somnolence in place of irritability, especially the elderly. Weight gain, as opposed to weight loss, can also occur and is often accompanied by osteoporosis. Elderly patients are also more likely to experience dry skin and pruritus. Graves' ophthalmopathy can occur acutely or several years after the onset of hyperthyroidism.[10] Abnormal liver function tests may also be seen. Muscle atrophy is a rare occurrence and usually indicates severe hyperthyroidism. Other autoimmune endocrine diseases such as IDDM or Addison's disease can occur with or before Graves' disease.

Diagnosis of hyperthyroidism is made by first excluding other causes of abnormal behavior or laboratory data. Diagnostic tests must include (1) radioimmunoassay measurement of serum T_4, T_3 and TSH, (2) determination of the percentage of radioactive iodine uptake (RAIU) by the thyroid gland, and (3) a thyroid scan. Serum T_4 and free T_4 concentrations are elevated and TSH level is low in most disorders listed in Table 10–2. The exception is a TSH-producing pituitary tumor.[10] Radioactive scanning is helpful in diagnosing toxic adenoma or a toxic multinodular goiter. RAIU can be reduced in thyroiditis, factitious hyperthyroidism, and in excessive exogenous iodine.[10] Trophoblastic tumor is associated with a near zero TSH level.

Management

Options in the treatment of hyperthyroidism include antithyroid drugs, radioiodine, and surgery (Table 10–4).[11]

Propranolol is a beta blocker normally used to treat hypertension, but it is also useful in controlling symptoms, as is

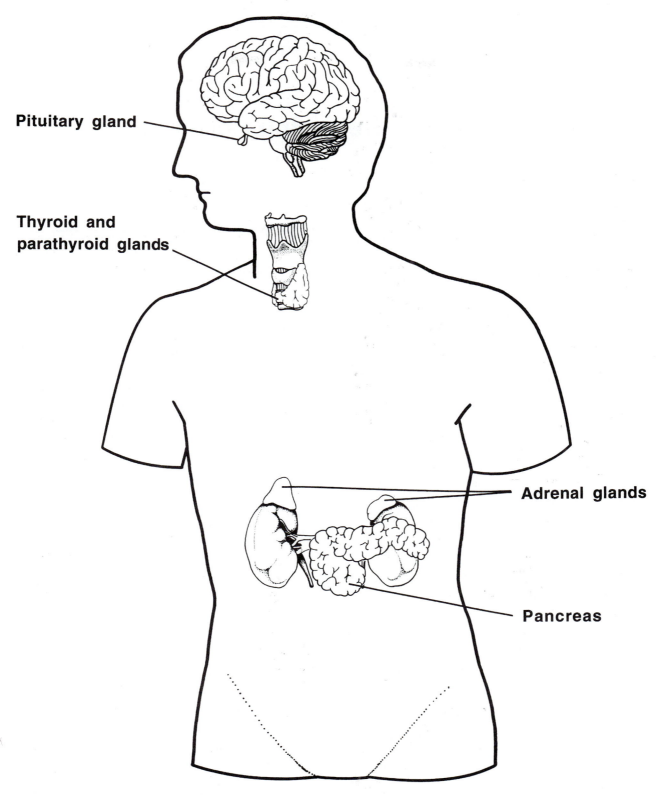

Pituitary gland

Thyroid and parathyroid glands

Adrenal glands

Pancreas

Figure 10–1. Anatomic Location of Endocrine Glands

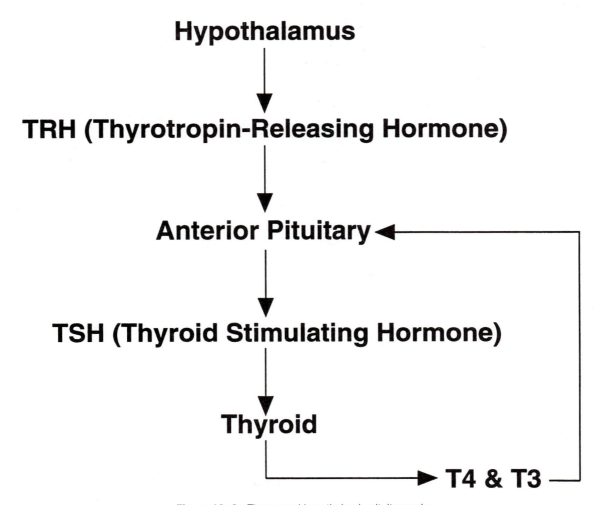

Figure 10–2. The normal hypothalamic pituitary axis

a class of drugs known as thioureas, which includes methimazole and propylthiouracil. These are usually reserved for children, young adults, pregnant women, and those awaiting surgery. Radioactive iodine (^{131}I) is used mainly for the destruction of overfunctioning thyroid tissue. This is to be

TABLE 10–2. CAUSES OF HYPERTHYROIDISM[10]

Graves' disease
Toxic adenoma
Toxic multinodal goiter
Hyperthyroidism with thyroiditis
Factitious hyperthyroidism
TSH-producing tumor
Trophoblastic tumor
Struma ovarii
Excess exogenous iodine

avoided in pregnant women. Thyroid surgery is used mainly for Graves' disease and toxic nodular goiter and can be used in children. Complications from surgery include damage to the laryngeal nerve and hypoparathyroidism.

Specific therapy is usually not recommended for hyperthyroidism associated with thyroiditis.[10] Hyperthyroidism caused by tumors or neoplasm is treated with excision and chemotherapy. Factitious hyperthyroidism is treated by removing excess exogenous T_4, T_3, or iodine.

Graves' disease may resolve spontaneously or may result in hypothyroidism, but more commonly it progresses. The ocular, cardiac, or psychologic complications may become irreversible despite adequate treatment.[9] Radioactive iodine therapy or subtotal thyroidectomy may result in posttreatment hypothyroidism. Radioactive iodine is not associated with an increased incidence of thyroid cancer, leukemia, or other cancers.[9]

TABLE 10–3. SYSTEMIC EFFECTS OF HYPERTHYROIDISM

Behavioral	Anxiety, irritability, insomnia, fatigue
Metabolic	Weight loss, heat intolerance, low-grade fevers
Cutaneous	Dry skin, pruritus, urticaria, thinning of hair
Ocular	Exophthalmos, conjunctivitis, periorbital edema, extraocular muscle dysfunction
Cardiovascular	Tachycardia, wide pulse pressure, systolic hypertension, atrial fibrillation
Gastrointestinal	Diarrhea, hepatomegaly
Neuromuscular	Tremor, weakness, periodic paralysis, delirium, stupor, coma
Endocrine	Irregular menses, impotence, gynecomastia, decreased libido, infertility

Management requires regular follow-up because of the potential for hypothyroidism to develop regardless of the treatment used. This is due in part to the fact that autoimmune thyroid disease may in itself be thyroid-destructive.

Life-style Changes

The physical signs, which may be persistent if not lifelong despite therapy, may result in emotional problems. The scar tissue associated with thyroidectomy may be cosmetically unacceptable for many patients but can easily be covered with makeup. Men who experience a decrease in libido may require alternatives to express sexuality with their partners. Special care should be taken with elderly patients because of their predisposition to experience cardiac abnormalities. Exercise modification and dietary changes are essential for this patient population. Finally, parents who are diagnosed with hyperthyroidism and have children should be aware of the possible familial tendency of this disease.

TABLE 10–4. HYPERTHYROID AGENTS

Medication	Dosage	Precautions
Methimazole (Tapazole)	15 mg/d (mild disease); 30–40 mg/d (moderately severe disease); 60 mg/d (severe disease) in 3 equally divided doses q 8 h Maintenance: 5–15 mg/d in 3 equally divided doses q 8 h	Blood dyscrasias, hepatotoxicity, rash
Propylthiouracil	Initially: 300 mg/d in 3 equally divided doses q 8 h Severe hypothyroidism or very large goiters: 400–900 mg/d in 3 equally divided doses Maintenance: 100–150 mg/d	Blood dyscrasias, hepatotoxicity, rash

■ HYPOTHYROIDISM

General Characteristics

Hypothyroidism affects people of all ages but is more common in the elderly and women. The onset of symptoms can take months to years to occur.

TSH is secreted by the pituitary gland. It stimulates the thyroid gland to release T_4 and a small amount of triiodothyronine T_3. T_4 is then absorbed by the tissues from the plasma. Once in the peripheral tissues, T_4 is converted to T_3. T_3 and T_4 in turn regulate TSH secretion via a negative feedback loop (see Fig. 10–2).[12] This mechanism becomes important when determining the underlying cause of hypothyroidism.

The most common cause of primary hypothyroidism is chronic autoimmune thyroiditis.[13] Other causes include treatment of hyperthyroidism with radioactive iodine, thyroidectomy, irradiation, certain medications, or iodine ingestion. (Table 10–5).

Severe hypothyroidism is called myxedema coma. This is a medical emergency and involves hypothermia, hypoventilation, hypoxia, hypercapnia, and hypotension. The term cretinism is used to describe congenital hypothyroidism. Juvenile hypothyroidism refers to children with this disorder, which leads to delayed growth and delayed skeletal maturation. Mental retardation can also occur if early symptoms are not properly identified and treated.

Signs, Symptoms, and Diagnosis

Before treatment can be initiated, a complete evaluation must be made to identify the etiology and to detect the presence of other, preexisting conditions. Every organ system is affected (Table 10–6).

TABLE 10–5. CAUSES OF HYPOTHYROIDISM

Autoimmune thyroiditis (Hashimoto's disease)
Idiopathic
Iatrogenic: Ablation
        Medication
        Contrast media
        Surgery
Diet (high levels of iodine)
Subacute thyroiditis secondary to infection
Postpartum thyroiditis

From Martinez et al.[12]

TABLE 10–6. SIGNS AND SYMPTOMS OF HYPOTHYROIDISM

System	Sign or Symptom
Cardiovascular	Bradycardia
	Cardiomegaly
	Arrhythmias
Respiratory	Hypoventilation
	Hypoxia
Nervous	Psychosis
	Dementia
	Slowed speech
	Hyperreflexia
Musculoskeletal	Arthralgia
Genitourinary	Irregular menses
Gastrointestinal	Constipation
	Nausea
	Vomiting
	Abdominal distention
Hematologic	Anemia
Integumentary	Xerosis

A TSH assay is essential for the diagnosis and treatment of hypothyroidism. Primary hypothyroidism is characterized by a high TSH level, which correlates with low T_3 and T_4 concentrations in the tissues.[12] An elevated TSH with a normal serum T_4 level represents "subclinical hypothyroidism," which does not necessarily require treatment.[14] Antimicrosomal and antithyroidal antibodies have been found circulating in some patients and appear to block the action of TSH. High antibody titers along with a high TSH level increase the chance of subsequent overt hypothyroidism.[14]

Management

Management with levothyroxine should be initiated once a diagnosis is made (Table 10–7). Treatment is usually 0.1 mg per day in young, healthy adults and titrated cautiously in the geriatric population, who are more at risk to experience side effects or who have underlying coronary artery disease, which

TABLE 10–7. HYPOTHYROID AGENT LEVOTHYROXINE SODIUM

Medication	Dosage	Precautions
Levothroid, Synthroid	Adults: 0.1 mg/d Children: doses vary with age (see package insert)	Monitor thyroidal symptoms and dosage closely

can be aggravated by the use of levothyroxine (Levothroid, Levoxine, Synthroid). The effects of hypothyroidism should improve within 2 weeks and resolve within 3 to 6 months.[12] TSH assay can take up to 6 months to return to normal. Thyroid function test should be assessed every 6 to 12 months in the patient who is not experiencing signs or symptoms and who is also on a therapeutic dosage.

Newborns should be identified immediately and aggressively treated. If a newborn is not treated during the first year of life, irreversible mental disturbances can occur. If therapy is started soon after birth, normal development occurs.[13]

There are many drugs that affect thyroid function tests, such as amiodarone, corticosteroids, some cough medications, dopamine, estrogens, lithium, phenytoin, and salicylates.

The prognosis is good when proper diagnosing, adequate treatment, and regular follow-up care is provided. Relapse will occur if treatment is interrupted. There is a return of abnormal appearance and mental functioning. Finally, chronic therapy with large doses can lead to bone demineralization.[15]

Life-style Changes

Because therapy is usually a lifelong commitment, the patient must learn to overcome his or her personal anxieties in dealing with this chronic disease. Chronic debilitating fatigue can result when the patient does not comply with self-administering daily oral medication. Once the patient resumes daily dosing, even after a very brief omission of therapy, the resulting signs and symptoms could take as long as 6 months to resolve. This can result in acute depression when this loss of control is realized by the patient with hypothyroidism. For this reason, psychosocial support is an essential part of the therapy for these patients.

■ ADDISON'S DISEASE

General Characteristics

Primary adrenocortical insufficiency is the term used to describe Addison's disease, which is commonly an autoimmune disease.[16] Refer to Figure 10–1 to review the location of the adrenal glands. Aldosterone is the major mineralocorticoid secreted by the adrenal glands and serves to promote sodium reabsorption and potassium excretion in the renal tubule.[17] Its secretion is stimulated by hypovolemia involving the renin-angiotensin cycle. Cortisol is the major glucocorticoid also secreted by the adrenal gland. Its purpose is to maintain vascular tone, counteract the effects of insulin, and to assist in the inhibition of protein synthesis in muscles.[17] Cortisol secretion is regulated by exercise levels, increasing with exercise.

Primary adrenocortical insufficiency, an uncommon disorder, is primarily due to autoimmune destruction of the adrenal glands, and accounts for approximately 80% of cases.[17]

Other causes of adrenal insufficiency include secondary adrenal insufficiency, caused by pituitary or hypothalamic hypofunction, and acute adrenal insufficiency, which may result from sudden withdrawal of chronic exogenous steroid therapy or from physical stress on the body.

Tuberculosis was previously a leading cause of Addison's disease, but this is no longer the case. However, it is still a problem in those countries where tuberculosis remains an epidemic.

Addison's disease can occur with hyperthyroidism, hypothyroidism or IDDM. Other associated endocrinopathies are listed in Table 10–8.

Signs, Symptoms, and Diagnosis

The signs and symptoms can mimic many other endocrine disorders related to specific organ systems or psychologic causes. It is because of this that the clinician must first confirm the diagnosis with supportive laboratory data before initiating a treatment plan. Most commonly the signs and symptoms will include weakness, fatigue, weight loss, anorexia, nausea, vomiting, gastrointestinal complaints, skin hyperpigmentation, hypotension, and diarrhea (Table 10–9).

Laboratory tests are not always able to indicate the cause of a patient's symptoms. Here is a typical presentation.

> A patient presents with a gradual increase in weakness, fatigue, nausea, and weight loss. On examination the patient is found to have a heart rate of 90, blood pressure of 110/60 lying, which falls to 60/40 when standing. A review of laboratory values reveals sodium of 122, potassium 5.5, and chloride 87.[18]

Refer to Table 10–10 to review the usual laboratory manifestations seen in a patient with Addison's disease.

The cosyntropin stimulation test is used to help diagnose Addison's disease. This involves administering cosyntropin and drawing a pre- and postadministration serum plasma cortisol level. A diagnostic test for Addison's disease must demonstrate a failure in the patient to increase plasma or urinary corticosteroid levels into the normal range.[16] A computed tomographic (CT) scan or magnetic resonance imaging (MRI) of the abdomen can be useful in assessing adrenal glands for calcification, cancer, or enlargement. A chest x-ray can be useful if problems such as tuberculosis, fungal infections, or cancer are suspected.

TABLE 10–8. ASSOCIATED ENDOCRINOPATHIES IN ADDISON'S DISEASE

Hyperthyroidism
Hypothyroidism
Diabetes mellitus
Gonadal dysfunction
Hypoparathyroidism

TABLE 10–9. SIGNS AND SYMPTOMS OF ADDISON'S DISEASE

Weakness and fatigue
Weight loss
Salt craving
Nausea and vomiting
Diarrhea
Lethargy
Disorientation
Skin hyperpigmentation
Hypotension
Buccal (tongue) discoloration
Vitiligo

TABLE 10–10. ADDISON'S DISEASE MANIFESTATIONS

Hyponatremia

Hyperkalemia

Antiadrenal antibodies

Azotemia

Fasting or reactive hypoglycemia

Eosinophilia

Hypercalcemia

Low white blood cell (WBC) count (neutropenia)

Management

Management should be initiated after diagnosis but also after reviewing a differential diagnosis. Weight loss can be caused by anorexia nervosa, skin changes may be a normal variant, cancer, diabetes mellitus, or hypoparathyroidism may also cause similar signs and symptoms. Treatment usually involves replacement therapy with glucocorticoids and mineralocorticoids. This usually involves hydrocortisone and fludrocortisone acetate (Table 10–11). The latter drug is used when there is in-

sufficient salt-retaining capability. Prednisone can also be used in place of hydrocortisone. Hyperkalemia or hyperpigmentation despite treatment may represent inadequate or inappropriate glucocorticoid therapy.

Without treatment, Addison's disease can be fatal. It is usually benign when under good control, and with continuous appropriate treatment, there is a near normal life expectancy.

Life-style Changes

Despite the mortality associated with untreated Addison's disease, it is a relatively benign disorder when treated appropriately. Because there is a lack of glucocorticoids, special attention should be paid to everyday infections such as colds and wounds to ensure that they heal properly. Women of child-bearing potential should be made aware that pregnancy can aggravate the disease. Also, as with any chronic illness, a medical alert bracelet is strongly encouraged.

TABLE 10–11. MEDICATIONS USED IN CHRONIC ADDISON'S DISEASE

Medication	Dosage	Precautions
Cortef (Hydrocortisone)	30 mg in divided doses (20 mg in morning, 10 mg in evening), is recommended; ideal dose should be adjusted for each patient	Fluid and electrolyte disturbances; hyperglycemia; infections; peptic ulcers; osteoporosis; behavioral disturbances Acute adrenal insufficiency with rapid withdrawal
Florinef acetate (Fludrocortisone acetate)	0.1 mg/d in combination with hydrocortisone Some patients may require 0.1 mg/wk to 0.2 mg/d, depending on disease severity and response to treatment	Same as above

■ CUSHING'S SYNDROME

General Characteristics

The word *syndrome* is often used when describing a disorder involving many different presentations. Cushing's syndrome involves adrenal hypersecretion. Refer to Figure 10–1 to review the location of the pituitary and adrenal glands.

The diagnosis of Cushing's syndrome can easily be made once the signs and symptoms have been recognized. The difficulty is in determining whether there is a pituitary or non-pituitary cause. Most patients with Cushing's *disease* present with an excess of adrenocorticotropic hormone (ACTH) and cortisol, which are regulated by the pituitary gland.[19] Others have adrenal disease or an ectopic (nonpituitary) ACTH-secreting neoplasm.[19] Still others may have exogenous Cushing's syndrome resulting from the use of steroid preparations such as dexamethasone.

Approximately 85% of patients with Cushing's disease have a pituitary tumor, of which most are microadenomas.[20] Unilateral adrenocortical neoplasms are found in the majority of patients with adrenal Cushing's syndrome. Ectopic ACTH production can be a result of a nonadrenal tumor, most of which are small-cell carcinomas of the lung. These lead to excess ACTH and cortisol production.[20] Ectopic corticotropin-releasing factor (CRF) is also a cause of Cushing's syndrome. CRF is a hypophysiotropic hormone that stimulates secretion of ACTH from the pituitary gland.[20]

Signs, Symptoms, and Diagnosis

Patients with Cushing's syndrome can present with a number of physical findings (Table 10–12), including a round plethoric face, truncal weight gain, and obesity. Obesity occurs mainly as a result of an increase in caloric intake, a metabolic tendency to spare fat, and a decrease in total lean body mass.[20] Men can experience impotence and women osteoporosis and abnormal menses. Clinical depression and occasionally psychotropic symptoms can occur. Occasionally hypertension is also exhibited. Most patients with ectopic ACTH production do not present with typical features of Cushing's syndrome.

Diagnosis can be achieved from testing the urine and serum ACTH levels and by CT. The 24-hour urine free cortisol test is done most frequently. An overnight dexamethasone suppression test is not performed routinely. Patients with adrenal

TABLE 10–12. CLINICAL FEATURES OF CUSHING'S SYNDROME
Centripetal obesity
Weakness or proximal myopathy
Hypertension
Easy bruising
Acne
Hirsutism
Skin hyperpigmentation
Osteoporosis
Psychologic changes
Oligo- or amenorrhea
Impotence
Pathologic fractures

From May et al.[20]

disease usually have very low ACTH.[19] Patients with pituitary Cushing's disease have ACTH levels that can be normal or markedly increased.[19] CT imaging helps to confirm and localize any potential tumors. False positive blood tests can occur as a result of obesity, alcohol abuse, depression, and the use of phenytoin and phenobarbital. One must also remember that cortisol and ACTH are stress hormones, and patients with acute illness may demonstrate increased levels and appear chemically to be exhibiting Cushing's syndrome but do not in fact have the condition.

Management

Surgical therapy is effective for most patients with pituitary Cushing's disease and for those with a single adrenal adenoma.[19] The prognosis for adrenal cancers is not good because of the difficulty involved with resection of these tumors. The initial cure rate for pituitary disease can be as high as 70%.[19] With proper treatment, a patient can show marked improvement in a few months. Left untreated, mortality and morbidity increase.

After selective resection of a pituitary adenoma, normal corticotropins are suppressed and require 6 to 36 months to recover normal function.[20] Hydrocortisone replacement therapy is necessary in the interim. Infections occur much more frequently because of the impairment of the immune system. This is due to increased cortisol secretion.

Life-style Changes

As previously discussed, men can experience impotence and transient infertility. Women can experience menstrual irregularities and hirsutism. This can play a major role for a couple who are trying to conceive. Female hirsutism can in itself cause many problems with self-image and -confidence. The most important information to relay is that there is treatment available and the majority will respond in a few months. There is no immediate way to resolve the obesity that may have taken months or years to develop; however, once treatment is initiated, the weight gain should begin to resolve. The clinician can educate the patient in regard to dietary considerations, even though this will probably be a lengthy process.

References

1. Karam JH. Diabetes mellitus and hypoglycemia. In: Tierney LM, McPhee SJ, Papadakis MA, eds. *Current Medical Diagnosis and Treatment.* Norwalk, Conn: Appleton & Lange; 1994:977.

2. Funnell MM, Merritt JH. The challenges of diabetes and older adults. *Nurs Clin North Am.* 1993;28:45–47, 57.

3. Kilo C, Williamson JR, Richmond D. Diabetes: the facts that let you regain control of your life. New York, NY: Wiley, 1987:20.

4. Wake MM. *Diseases. Endocrine Disorders.* Springhouse, Pa: Intermed Communications Inc; 1983:849–851. Nurses Reference Library.

5. Haas LB. Chronic complications of diabetes mellitus. *Nurs Clin North Am.* 1993;28:72–77.

6. Rae JL, Rankin SH. Revisiting nurse knowledge about diabetes: an update and implications for practice. *Diabetes Educator.* 1993;19:497–498.

7. Feingold KR, Gavin LA. The thyroid. In: Andreoli TE, Carpenter CCJ, Plum F, Smith LH. eds. *Cecil's Essentials of Medicine.* Philadelphia, PA: WB Saunders Co; 1986:450–460.

8. Orgiazzi JJ, Mornex R. Hyperthyroidism. In: Greer MA, ed. *The Thyroid Gland.* New York, NY: Raven Press; 1990:405–407.

9. Fitzgerald PA. Endocrine disorders. In: Tierney LM, McPhee SJ, Papadakis MA, eds. *Current Medical Diagnosis and Treatment.* Norwalk, Conn: Appleton & Lange; 1994:924–938.

10. Schimke RN. Hyperthyroidism. *Postgrad Med.* 1992;91:229–236.

11. Stocklist JR. Thyroid disease. *Med J Aust.* 1993;158:770–773.

12. Martinez M, Derkson D, Kapsner P. Making sense of hypothyroidism. *Postgrad Med.* 1993;93:134–145.

13. Laurberg P. Hypothyroidism. In: Greer, MA, ed. *The Thyroid Gland*, ed.. New York NY: Raven Press; 1990:498–500.

14. May ME, Vaughan ED, Carey RM. Adrenocortical insufficiency. In: *Adrenal Disorders.* Vaughan ED, Carey RM, eds. New York, NY: Thieme Medical Publishers Inc; 1989:171–191.

15. Howle S. I feel tired doctor. *Aust Fam Physician.* 1993;22:977–979.

16. Sheeler LR. Cushing's syndrome: easy to see, tricky to diagnose. *Cleve Clin J Med.* 1993;60:102–104.

17. May ME, Vaughan ED, Carey RM. Cushing's syndrome. In: *Adrenal Disorders.* Vaughan ED, Carey RM, eds. New York, NY: Thieme Medical Publishers Inc; 1989:147–171.

11

GASTROINTESTINAL DISORDERS

David P. Paar

■ HEPATITIS

General Characteristics

Hepatitis is an inflammatory condition of the liver (Fig. 11–1) that can be caused by viruses, drugs, and toxins. In addition, chronic autoimmune hepatitis is a disease of young and menopausal women with an etiology that is poorly understood. Viral hepatitis usually runs an acute, self-limited course; however, chronic hepatitis may occur following infection with hepatitis B virus (HBV) and hepatitis C virus (HCV).

There are five hepatitis viruses: hepatitis A virus (HAV), HBV, HCV, hepatitis delta virus (HDV), and hepatitis E virus (HEV). Hepatitis A, B, and C occur commonly in the United States.

HDV is an unusual virus because it requires the presence of HBV to reproduce and cause disease; it never occurs without coinfection with HBV. In the United States, HDV is uncommon but does occur in people who have multiple parenteral exposures, such as injecting drug users, hemophiliacs, and others who have received numerous blood transfusions.

HEV is also infrequently encountered in the United States. In developing countries, HEV is responsible for large epidemics of viral hepatitis in adults. Pregnant women who contract HEV have a high mortality rate. Table 11–1 gives the mode of transmission, incubation period, and mortality rate for each of the five hepatitis viruses.

Many drugs can cause hepatitis. Some of the more common ones include halothane, methyldopa, phenytoin, isoniazid, and acetaminophen when taken in large doses . The wild mushroom *Amanita phalloides* contains a potent toxin that produces severe hepatitis. Ethanol is another toxin that can cause acute and chronic hepatitis.

Signs, Symptoms, and Diagnosis

Acute viral hepatitis can be divided into incubation period, preicteric phase, icteric phase, and convalescence. Drug- and toxin-induced hepatitides do not have an incubation period, since these are not infectious diseases; otherwise, these resemble acute or chronic viral hepatitides.

Toward the end of the incubation period (Table 11–1) of acute viral hepatitis, the hepatic aminotransferases, aspartate aminotransferase (AST) and alanine aminotransferase (ALT), begin to rise. These peak at 100 times normal or higher in the early icteric phase and then return to normal in the convalescent phase. The preicteric phase is characterized by the onset of symptoms that include malaise, anorexia, nausea, right upper quadrant pain, and fever. These symptoms usually abate during the icteric phase, although malaise may persist well into the convalescent phase.

The onset of jaundice marks the beginning of the icteric phase. Bilirubin is excreted in the urine; therefore, many jaundiced patients pass dark-colored urine. Some patients with jaundice will complain of pruritus. Jaundice is not apparent until the serum bilirubin rises to 2.5 mg/dL; the serum bilirubin seldom rises above 20 times normal. Jaundice occurs in less than half the cases of acute viral hepatitis. In fact, most cases of acute viral hepatitis are asymptomatic or so mildly symptomatic that the patient passes off the illness as a cold or the flu.

Physical examination may show jaundice, mild hepatic enlargement with percussion tenderness, and small vascular spiders. Up to 1% of patients may develop fulminant hepatitis and hepatic failure. When this occurs, hepatic encephalopathy

115

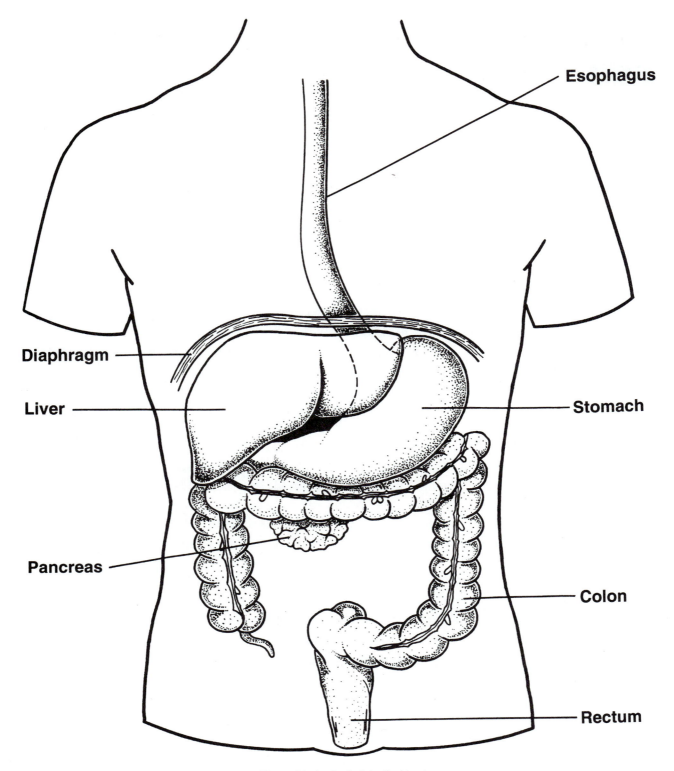

Figure 11–1. Gastrointestinal tract

TABLE 11–1. MODE OF TRANSMISSION, INCUBATION PERIOD, AND MORTALITY OF ACUTE VIRAL HEPATITIS

Virus	Mode of Transmission	Incubation Days	Mortality %
HAV	Fecal or oral; contaminated shellfish	20–37	0.0–0.2
HBV	Percutaneous; sexual	60–110	0.3–1.5
HCV	Percutaneous; sexual	35–70	? same as HBV
HDV	Percutaneous	? same as HBV	up to 20
HEV	Fecal or oral	10–56	1–2; up to 15 in pregnancy

ensues. Asterixis, seen in the flapping of the dorsiflexed hand, is the characteristic finding of hepatic encephalopathy. Fetor hepaticus is a peculiar, sweet smell of the breath that occurs with hepatic failure.

The convalescent phase is variable and is occasionally characterized by relapse of symptoms or jaundice. In general, malaise is the last symptom to abate during the convalescent phase. Table 11–2 shows the serologic tests that are used to distinguish between the different types of acute viral hepatitis.

The hallmark of recovery from acute HBV infection is clearance of hepatitis B surface antigen (HBsAg) from the serum, which coincides with development of antibody to HBsAg, anti-HBs (HBsAb). Patients with chronic HBV infection fail to develop HbsAb and therefore fail to clear HBsAg. By definition, chronic HBV infection occurs when HBsAg persists for longer than 6 months after acute HBV infection. Chronic hepatitis occurs 5% to 10% of the time following acute HBV infection and perhaps as frequently as 50% of the time following acute HCV infection. Chronic hepatitis is categorized as chronic persistent hepatitis (CPH) and chronic active hepatitis (CAH). Idiopathic autoimmune hepatitis is similarly classified. Liver biopsy is necessary to definitively diagnose CPH or CAH as well as to assess the degree of hepatic inflammation.

On liver biopsy, CPH is characterized by an inflammatory cell infiltrate that is limited to the portal triads; there is no hepatic parenchymal inflammation or cell death. CAH, on the other hand, is characterized by extension of the inflammatory cell infiltrate from the portal triad into the hepatic parenchyma. This may result in varying degrees of hepatocyte death. Bridging necrosis is the term used to describe the condition when the inflammation and hepatocyte death stretches from one portal triad to another.

Cirrhosis is the result of necrotic hepatocytes being replaced with fibrous connective tissue or scar. Fortunately the liver is able to regenerate when hepatocyte necrosis occurs. When inflammation and necrosis are severe, regenerating nodules occur in an irregular array, surrounded by areas of inflammation and cirrhosis. If inflammation and necrosis persist, the liver eventually loses the capacity to regenerate, and hepatic failure and ultimately death ensue. This occurs in approximately 12.5% of the cases of chronic HBV infection and perhaps 50% of the cases of chronic HCV infection.

Chronic hepatitis may be completely asymptomatic or may be characterized by asymptomatic periods alternating with periods of symptoms. Symptoms coincide with exacerbations of hepatic inflammation and include fatigue, fever, right

TABLE 11–2. SEROLOGIC TESTS USED TO DIAGNOSE VIRAL HEPATITIS

Virus	Test/Comment
HAV	anti-HAV IgM indicates acute HAV infection anti-HAV IgG indicates past HAV infection
HBV	HBcAb IgM ± HBsAg indicates acute infection HBsAb denotes past, resolved infection Persistence of HBsAg (>6 mo) indicates chronic HBV infection
HCV	Anti-HCV develops during convalescence; may indicate past, resolved infection or chronic infection When transaminases remain persistently elevated, chronic infection is likely
HDV	Anti-HDV indicates past or chronic infection
HEV	Anti-HEV indicates past infection

HBcAb, hepatitis B core antibody; HBsAg, hepatitis B surface antigen; IgG, immunoglobulin G; IgM, immunoglobulin M.

TABLE 11–3. INTERFERON DOSAGES FOR HEPATITIS B AND C

Medication	Dosage	Side Effects
Intron-A (interferon alfa-2b)	Adults: Hepatitis B: 5 million IU daily or 10 million IU 3 times weekly IM or SC for 16 weeks. Hepatitis C: 3 million IU IM or SC 3 times weekly for 24 wks. Children: under 18 yrs, not recommended.	Flu-like symptoms, liver disorders, fatigue, malaise, arthralgia, hematologic or visual disorders, uterine bleeding, CNS effects, syncope, GI upset, tinnitus, alopecia, sweating, rash, erythema, pruritus, local effects.

SC, subcutaneously.

upper quadrant pain, and sometimes jaundice. Elevations in hepatic transaminases up to 20 times normal and in serum bilirubin up to 5 times normal may occur during periods of disease activity. Chronic HBV infection is a major risk factor for the development of hepatocellular carcinoma. This usually occurs 10 to 20 years after acute infection with HBV. It is less clear whether HCV predisposes to hepatocellular carcinoma.

Patients with chronic hepatitis develop vascular spiders and palmar erythema. When cirrhosis is severe, proteins responsible for clotting and for maintaining serum oncotic pressure cannot be adequately synthesized. Ecchymoses, peripheral edema, and ascites are the result. Resistance to blood flow through the cirrhotic liver results in elevated portal venous pressures and splenomegaly. Dilated varices develop where portal and systemic blood flow join; these are located in the distal esophagus (bleeding esophageal varices), around the umbilicus (the so-called caput medusa), and in the anus (hemorrhoids). The enlarged spleen sequesters platelets, leading to petechiae and bleeding tendencies.

Management

The management of acute viral hepatitis is supportive. Bed rest at home is recommended during the period of acute symptoms. Antiemetics and intravenous fluids are administered as needed. In cases of fulminant hepatitis, support with intravenous fluids, electrolyte replacement, and blood products is mandatory. Hepatic encephalopathy is treated with a low-protein diet and either oral lactulose or neomycin to induce diarrhea and cleansing of the bowel. Sedatives should be avoided. Liver transplantation is an option for fulminant hepatic necrosis.

Chronic HBV and HCV can be treated with interferon-alpha. (Table 11–3) This results in a cure in about 35% to 40%

of the cases of chronic HBV infection; significantly fewer people with HCV are cured, but there is improvement in the disease for varying periods of time during and following interferon therapy. For HBV infection, interferon-alpha 5 million units subcutaneously per day for 4 months is recommended. The recommended dosage of interferon for chronic HCV infection is 3 million units subcutaneously three times per week for 6 months.

For prevention of hepatitis B, there are two different vaccines currently licensed for use in the United States. The recommended series of three intramuscular doses of vaccine induces protective immunity in greater than 90% of healthy adults. The Centers for Disease Control Immunization Practices Advisory Committee recommends vaccination of selected high-risk groups, including persons with occupational risk (health-care workers), clients and staff of institutions for the developmentally disabled, hemodialysis patients, recipients of certain blood products, household contacts and sex partners of HBV carriers, adoptees from countries where HBV infection is endemic, international travelers, injecting drug users, sexually active men and women, and inmates of long-term correctional facilities.

Life-style Changes

HAV often occurs in epidemics when water becomes contaminated with sewage. Outbreaks can be traced to eating uncooked shellfish, particularly oysters from contaminated waters. During reported outbreaks, people should heed advice not to eat raw shellfish or other contaminated foodstuffs from the area where the outbreak is occurring.

HBV and, to a lesser extent, HCV are sexually transmitted diseases. Safe-sex practices, including use of condoms and not sharing body fluids, may reduce the risk of infection.

■ PANCREATITIS

General Characteristics

The pancreas (Fig. 11–1) has both exocrine and endocrine functions. The exocrine function is to secrete into the intestine fluid that contains enzymes that aid in the digestion of fats, carbohydrates, and proteins. The endocrine function of the pancreas is to secrete insulin and glucagon, which are of primary importance in glucose metabolism.

Pancreatitis is an inflammatory condition of the pancreas that may be an acute or chronic process. Recovery from acute pancreatitis is often complete, with restoration of normal pancreatic function. However, chronic pancreatitis can lead to permanent pancreatic dysfunction, which results in malabsorption of foodstuffs. Table 11–4 lists the most common causes of pancreatitis.

Signs, Symptoms, and Diagnosis

Abdominal pain that radiates to the back is the most common symptom of acute pancreatitis. Nausea and vomiting also occur. On physical examination, hypoactive bowel sounds and abdominal tenderness are usually present. Patients may be febrile, tachycardic, and hypotensive. Uncommon signs of severe pancreatitis include a bluish discoloration around the umbilicus (Cullen's sign) and a blue to brown discoloration of the flanks (Turner's sign); these result from intra-abdominal hemorrhage that may complicate acute pancreatitis. The diagnosis of acute pancreatitis is usually confirmed by elevated amylase or lipase levels.

Chronic pancreatitis may present as either repeated relapses of acute pancreatitis, in which case each discrete episode is similar to acute pancreatitis, or as chronic damage, which is characterized by persistent pain or malabsorption. Diarrhea, flatus, abdominal discomfort, and weight loss are associated with malabsorption. Physical examination is frequently unremarkable and amylase and lipase levels are usually normal in those who suffer from chronic pancreatitis.

When the classic triad of pancreatic calcification (seen on abdominal radiograph or ultrasound), fatty stools, and diabetes mellitus are present, the diagnosis of chronic pancreatitis is obvious; however, this triad occurs in only one third of patients. A low serum level of trypsinogen (one of the measurable pancreatic enzymes) can establish the diagnosis. Other tests that either directly or indirectly stimulate the exocrine function of the pancreas include secretin or secretin-cholecystokinin stimulation, Lundh test meal, urinary N-benzoyl-L-tyrosyl-*p*-aminobenzoic acid test, and the pancreolauryl test. For a description of these, a standard internal medicine or gastroenterology textbook should be consulted.

Management

"Putting the pancreas to rest" is the aim of medical management of acute pancreatitis. This is accomplished by not feeding the patient. Intravenous fluids are necessary to maintain hydration and electrolyte balance. Analgesia is necessary for patient comfort. Nasogastric suction and antibiotics do not appear to add benefit in the management of acute, uncomplicated pancreatitis. Acute pancreatitis usually resolves within 1 week. When pain and elevation of amylase and lipase persist beyond this time period, complications should be sought. The complications of acute pancreatitis are listed in Table 11–5.

When chronic pancreatitis is associated with malabsorption and pain, supplementation with commercially available oral preparations of digestive enzymes will often correct the problem. Treatment with non-narcotic or narcotic analgesics may be necessary. Unfortunately, narcotic addiction is a common problem in patients with chronic pancreatitis. When pain is severe, evaluation with endoscopic retrograde cholangiopancreatography (ERCP) may reveal a surgically correctable lesion such as a stricture or obstruction of the pancreatic ducts.

TABLE 11–4. COMMON CAUSES OF ACUTE AND CHRONIC PANCREATITIS

Miscellaneous	Drugs
Gallstones	Alcohol
Abdominal surgery	Azathioprine
Abdominal trauma	Thiazide diuretics
Hypertriglyceridemia	Furosemide
Renal failure	Oral contraceptives
Heredity	Tetracyclines
Penetrating peptic ulcer	Pentamidine
Cystic fibrosis	Dideoxyinosine (ddI)

TABLE 11–5. INTRA-ABDOMINAL COMPLICATIONS OF ACUTE PANCREATITIS

Complication	Definition	Comment
Pseudocyst	Large collection of fluid contiguous with pancreas	Can be seen with abdominal CT scan or ultrasound Frequently necessary to perform a percutaneous aspiration to rule out active infection
Phlegmon	Inflammatory mass; not usually infectious	Can be seen with abdominal CT scan or ultrasound
Abscess	Usually arises from a preexisting pseudocyst or phlegmon	Can be demonstrated by abdominal CT or ultrasound Antibiotics and either percutaneous or surgical drainage are indicated

When chronic pancreatitis results in diabetes mellitus, hyperglycemia occurs, but the other complications of diabetes mellitus such as diabetic ketoacidosis, hyperosmolar coma, retinopathy, nephropathy, and neuropathy are rare. Elevated serum glucose can be controlled as outlined in Chapter 10.

Life-style Changes

Patients should avoid the precipitating causes of acute, recurrent pancreatitis such as alcohol or drugs. For those with chronic pancreatitis, alcohol and fatty meals should be avoided, since these commonly exacerbate the pain and malabsorption that occur.

■ IRRITABLE BOWEL SYNDROME

General Characteristics

Irritable Bowel Syndrome (IBS) is characterized by cramping abdominal pain and alternating constipation and diarrhea. IBS affects all age groups but is most common in young women. In many patients with IBS, subtle abnormalities in colonic motility have been detected; therefore, the disease should not automatically be attributed to an underlying anxiety disorder or depression.

Signs, Symptoms, and Diagnosis

The symptoms of IBS are intermittent and variable. They may be precipitated by a fatty meal or emotional stress. Crampy abdominal pain with either constipation or frequent, low-volume stools are seen. Many patients complain of mucus mixed with their stool. Nausea and vomiting are occasionally seen. Examination is usually remarkable for varying degrees of abdominal tenderness.

The differential diagnosis of IBS includes carcinoma of the colon, diverticulitis, lactose intolerance, and inflammatory bowel disease. If symptoms persist, a gastrointestinal (GI) work-up must be done to exclude these possibilities. This usually consists of an upper GI series with small bowel follow-through (SBFT) or upper endoscopy along with a barium enema or colonoscopy. The terminal ileum must be visualized to rule out inflammatory bowel disease.

Management

Reassurance and alteration of diet are the mainstays of therapy. Reducing fat in the diet and increasing dietary fiber are often helpful. Anticholinergic medications, such as dicyclomine hydrochloride (Bentyl), which reduce gut motility, may be used if dietary changes do not alleviate the problems (Table 11–6).

Life-style Changes

Reducing fat intake and increasing fiber intake may lead to improvement in symptoms. Emotional stress that precipitates symptoms should be avoided if at all possible.

TABLE 11–6. IRRITABLE BOWEL SYNDROME MEDICATIONS

Medication	Dosage	Precautions
Bentyl (Dicyclomine hydrochloride)	Adult: 20 mg qid to start, followed by 40 mg qid if tolerated and necessary Children: < 6 mo not recommended	Drowsiness; blurred vision; fever; heat stroke; incomplete intestinal obstruction
Donnatal (Phenobarbital, hyoscyamine sulfate, atropine sulfate, and scopolamine hydrobromide)	Adult: 1–2 tid or qid Child: varies with weight	Drowsiness; blurred vision; fever; heat stroke; incomplete intestinal obstruction; delayed gastric emptying; drug dependence; withdrawal symptoms
Levsinex Timecaps (Hyoscyamine sulfate)	Adult: 375–750 µg q 12 h to start, followed if necessary by 375 µg q 8 h up to 1500 µg/24 h Children (2–12 y): 375 µg q 12 h, up to 750 µg/24 h	Fever and heat stroke; drowsiness; blurred vision; incomplete intestinal obstruction
Librax (Chlordiazepoxide hydrochloride and clidinium bromide)	Adult: 1–2 caps tid or qid, before meals and at bedtime Children: not recommended	Drowsiness; confusion; drug dependence; withdrawal symptoms

■ DIVERTICULOSIS

General Characteristics

A diverticulum is a mucosal pouch that extends through a weak spot in the colon wall (Fig. 11–1) into the abdominal cavity. Diverticulosis refers to the existence of one diverticulum, or more. Diverticula occur most frequently in the left colon, perhaps because intraluminal pressure is greatest in this location; however, righted-sided diverticula also occur. Diverticula develop as part of the aging process. Eating a refined, low-fiber diet, and IBS are both associated with diverticular disease.

Diverticulitis describes the condition in which a diverticulum becomes infected as a result of obstruction from inspissated stool. This may progress to rupture, with resulting abscess formation or peritonitis.

Signs, Symptoms, and Diagnosis

Diverticulosis is usually asymptomatic, but it can result in chronic, recurrent abdominal pain and, rarely, gross rectal bleeding (hematochezia). Abdominal tenderness may be present, but there is no rebound tenderness, and temperature will be normal. Stool heme testing may show positive results. Diagnosis can be established with a barium enema or computed tomography (CT) scan of the abdomen.

Increased abdominal pain, diarrhea, and fever are associated with diverticulitis. Rectal bleeding is distinctly unusual. On examination there is localized tenderness, usually in the left lower quadrant, with rebound and frequently a palpable inflammatory mass. Rupture of the infected diverticulum can lead to more dramatic signs. CT scan of the abdomen or lower endoscopy are used to make the diagnosis of diverticulitis. Barium enema should be avoided, as this may predispose to colonic rupture.

Management

An increase in dietary fiber may reduce the symptoms associated with diverticulosis. If gastrointestinal bleeding occurs, hospitalization for monitoring and supportive care may be necessary. The bleeding usually halts spontaneously. In rare cases, surgical intervention is necessary to stop the bleeding.

Diverticulitis must be treated with antibiotics and some form of bowel rest. If the patient is not too ill, clear liquids and standard doses of oral amoxicillin or a first-generation cephalosporin can be administered on an outpatient basis. More severely ill patients should be hospitalized for complete bowel rest with nasogastric suctioning and intravenous antibiotics that should target gram-negative organisms and anaerobes. Regimens that include cefoxitin or cefotetan plus an aminoglycoside are usually employed. If the condition continues to progress despite medical therapy, surgical intervention may be necessary. An alternative to surgical therapy is percutaneous drainage of an abscess with CT or ultrasonic guidance.

Life-style Changes

Changing from a low-fiber to a high-fiber diet may be beneficial. One should also avoid eating foods which contain small seeds (eg, tomatoes, strawberries, popcorn, nuts, and other foods that break into small undigestible particles). These food products are likely to block off a diverticulum opening and cause diverticulitis.

PEPTIC ULCER DISEASE

General Characteristics

Peptic ulcer disease may involve the esophagus, stomach, and duodenum (Fig. 11–1). Regardless of the location, there is mucosal injury that leads to formation of an ulcer. Severe ulceration can lead to GI bleeding and perforation of the involved viscus.

Strictly speaking, peptic ulcer disease (PUD) refers to ulcers that are caused by the overproduction of gastric acid. However, evidence indicates that the etiology of ulcers is multifactorial, with gastric acid overproduction, infection of the mucosa with a bacterium called *Helicobacter pylori*, and certain drugs such as aspirin, nonsteroidal anti-inflammatory drugs (NSAIDs), or alcohol all contributing. Smoking tobacco contributes to or delays healing of PUD. Emotional stress may provoke PUD in some patients.

Signs, Symptoms, and Diagnosis

The characteristic pain of PUD is constant, mild to moderate, and aching or burning in nature. It occurs in the midepigastrium and is relieved with eating or antacids. It occurs at night or several hours after ingesting a meal. Nausea and vomiting are not prominent features. When an ulcer hemorrhages, hematemesis or melena occur.

On physical examination, abdominal tenderness may be present. The stool tests heme-positive if gastrointestinal bleeding is present. When bleeding is significant, pallor and hypotension are present.

The diagnosis can be established by upper GI series or upper endoscopy.

Management

Antacids, which neutralize stomach acids, and H_2 blockers, which prevent the secretion of gastric acid, promote healing of

TABLE 11–7. CURRENTLY AVAILABLE H_2 ANTAGONISTS

Drug	Dose
Tagamet (Cimetidine)	400 mg PO bid
Zantac (Ranitidine)	150 mg PO bid or 300 mg PO at bedtime
Pepcid (Famotidine)	20 mg bid PO or 40 mg PO at bedtime
Axid (Nizatidine)	150 mg PO bid or 300 mg PO at bedtime

Note: There is no intravenous form of nizatidine available, but the others may be given intravenously when necessary. PO, by mouth.

PUD. Although antacids are cheap and effective, they must be given seven times per day (1 and 3 hours after eating and at bedtime) to achieve maximal benefit. Some antacids contain a large amount of sodium, which may be undesirable in patients with concomitant congestive heart failure, renal failure, or hepatic insufficiency.

Drugs that inhibit gastric acid secretion by blocking histamine type 2 receptors (H_2 blockers) (Table 11–7) are commonly used to treat PUD. Other pharmacologic therapies such as sucralfate, omeprazole, and antibiotics (Table 11–8) are also employed.

If gastrointestinal hemorrhage occurs, hospitalization for monitoring, hydration, and transfusion of blood and blood products may be necessary. In this case, the H_2 blockers or omeprazole may be administered intravenously. Therapeutic endoscopy or surgery may be necessary to control massive GI hemorrhage.

Life-style Changes

Behavioral changes can significantly impact the rate of healing and recurrence of PUD. Smoking cessation, abstinence from alcohol, and avoiding aspirin or NSAIDs are all beneficial.

TABLE 11–8. THERAPIES OTHER THAN H_2 BLOCKERS FOR PEPTIC ULCER DISEASE

Therapy	Comment
Carafate (Sucralfate) 1 g PO qid	Promotes healing by binding to mucosal erosions
Amoxicillin 250–500 mg PO tid plus metronidazole 250 mg PO bid plus bismuth subsalicylate (Pepto-Bismol) tablets 2 PO qid	Eradication of *Helicobacter pylori* with this regimen prevents recurrent PUD; unclear if bismuth subsalicylate is a necessary component
Prilosec (Omeprazole) 20–40 mg PO bid	Acid pump inhibitor; short term treatment
Prevacid (lansoprazole) 15 mg PO qid	Acid pump inhibitor; short term treatment

PO, by mouth.

■ HIATAL HERNIA

General Characteristics

The esophagus passes through an anatomic defect, or hiatus, in the muscular diaphragm as it joins the stomach (Fig. 11–1). Hiatal hernia (HH) describes the condition in which the hiatus is enlarged, allowing a portion of the stomach to pass upward into the thoracic cavity. If the stomach is able to slide back and forth between the thoracic and the abdominal cavities, a sliding hiatal hernia is present. It is though that most cases of HH are asymptomatic. Peptic esophagitis, which is caused by gastric acid refluxing through an incompetent lower esophageal sphincter (reflux esophagitis), may accompany hiatal hernia and lead to symptoms.

Signs, Symptoms, and Diagnosis

Patients with peptic, or reflux, esophagitis complain of symptoms similar to PUD or heartburn. A bitter taste in the back of the throat or mouth (water brash) also occurs. The heartburn is frequently worse following meals or in the supine position, since these conditions promote esophageal reflux. Examination may be unremarkable or abdominal tenderness may be present.

The diagnosis may be apparent from the history when postprandial and supine symptoms occur. Upper GI series or upper endoscopy can confirm the diagnosis.

Management

When HH is associated with symptoms of reflux esophagitis, therapy is indicated. The same agents that are used to treat PUD are used to treat reflux esophagitis. In addition, avoidance of agents that relax the lower esophageal sphincter (Table 11–9) should be avoided. Drugs that promote gastroin-

TABLE 11–9. AGENTS THAT RELAX THE LOWER ESOPHAGEAL SPHINCTER

Fatty foods
Alcohol
Chocolate
Cigarettes

testinal peristalsis (prokinetic agents) and clearing of acid from the esophagus (Table 11–10) can be used alone or in combination with other medications.

When nighttime symptoms are prominent because of assuming the supine position, evening fasting and elevating the head of the bed with 15-cm blocks may provide additional benefit. If symptoms are severe and medical therapy fails, surgical intervention aimed at constructing a functional lower esophageal sphincter may provide benefit.

Life-style Changes

Avoiding agents that cause relaxation of the lower esophageal sphincter (Table 11–9), elevating the head of the bed on 15-cm blocks, and nighttime fasting can alleviate esophageal reflux. Weight loss may also help by decreasing the pressure that is exerted on the stomach by an obese abdomen.

TABLE 11–10. PROKINETIC DRUGS

Drug	Dose
Reglan (metoclopramide)	10–15 mg 30 min before eating and bedtime
Propulsid (cisapride)	10–20 mg PO qid

PO, by mouth.

12

Renal Disorders

Janice G. Curry
Jeffrey W. East
Joey D. Hobbs

■ RENAL CALCULI

General Characteristics

Renal calculi, or kidney stones, are generally caused by excessive urinary secretion of compounds of limited solubility. In 90% of cases, there is no identifiable cause of stones forming.[1,2] There are, however, some predisposing factors: alterations in urine pH, chronic urinary tract infections, structural abnormalities of the kidneys, chronic disease states, and dietary factors.[1,2]

The occurrence of renal calculi has a relationship to geographic location and industrialization, with a higher incidence of stones in industrialized countries.[3] Urolithiasis in the United States and other technologically developed countries most commonly occurs in the upper urinary tract, whereas bladder stones are more common in less developed countries (Fig. 12–1). There is also a higher incidence of stone formation in the southeastern United States.[4] Men are more likely to suffer from stone formation than women, with a higher incidence in the third through fifth decades of life.

Kidney stones are generally classified by the type of crystals that form the stone. There are four main types of crystals that accumulate to form stones: calcium, struvite, urate, and cystine. Calcium and cystine stones are primarily caused by overexcretion of calcium, uric acid, oxalate, or cystine. Uric acid stones are primarily caused by an abnormally low urine pH but can also be caused by overexcretion of uric acid. Struvite stones are produced only by bacteria such as *Proteus* species or, less often, *Pseudomonas, Klebsiella*, or enterobacteria that possess the enzyme urease and are therefore the result of urinary tract infection (Table 12–1).[4]

Signs, Symptoms, and Diagnosis

The clinical history may help in determining the cause of stone formation. Important areas in the history are outlined in Table 12–2.[5] Certain occupations, such as those involving manual labor in hot environments, may cause large fluid loss from perspiration or respiration, which may cause the urine to concentrate.[4] Also, easy access to fluids and bathroom facilities may not be possible in some occupations. Dietary factors such as an excessive intake of dietary protein, calcium, or foods high in oxalate may encourage stone formation. Some medications such as calcium channel blockers, theophylline, and excessive vitamin and mineral supplements may also predispose one to stone formation. As long as stones remain attached to the renal papillae, where they usually form, there may be no symptoms except hematuria. When they become free to move in the urinary stream, stones can produce pain from acute obstruction of the renal collecting system anywhere from the ureteropelvic junction to the ureterovesical junction. The pain is caused by increasing pressure and consequent dilation of the kidney and urinary collecting system. This pain is known as renal colic. It begins suddenly, increases in intensity, and remains constant. Nausea and vomiting may be present and are generally attributed to the pain of renal colic. Flank pain on the side of the affected kidney is also common. In addition, there may be dysuria, urgency, and frequency.

Frequently, stones are asymptomatic and are discovered on routine x-ray for another condition. Except for uric acid stones, renal stones are radiopaque. Generally calcium stones present as small, densely radiopaque objects; cystine stones are

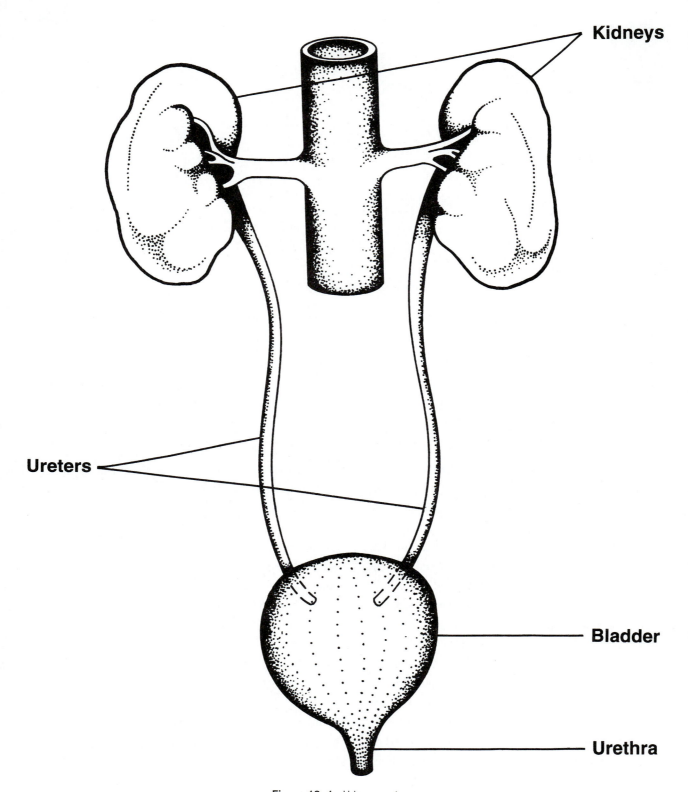

Figure 12–1. Urinary system

TABLE 12–1. PREVALENCE AND FREQUENCY OF RENAL CALCULI

Type of Stone	Approximate Frequency (%)	Sex Ratio Men:Women
Calcium	74	3:1
Struvite	15	1:5
Uric acid	7	variable
Cystine	3	1:1

From Gillenwater et al.[4]

TABLE 12–2. HISTORICAL ASPECTS THAT AID IN DIAGNOSIS OF RENAL CALCULI

Sex
Family history
Geographic residence
Occupation
Fluid intake
Diet
Medications
Previous stone passage
Interventional procedures
Previous stone formation
Urinary tract infections
Chronic medical conditions

slightly less radiopaque and have soft edges; struvite stones often form branching "staghorn" calculi.[5]

The laboratory evaluation may reveal hematuria, bacturia, hypercalcemia, and possibly crystalluria. A compete metabolic work-up should be done for patients with recurrent stone formation.

Management

Asymptomatic stones may pass from the body without notice. Others may be painful but will still pass on their own. It is not uncommon for a procedure called lithotripsy to be used to break up the stone through the use of high-frequency sound waves. The broken stone can then be passed through the ureters with little discomfort. On rare occasions the stone has to be surgically removed. A complete analysis of the stone should be done if at all possible. Once the stone has been analyzed, correcting the underlying metabolic disorder is the primary management goal.[6] This may be accomplished by dietary modifications, medications, or a combination of both. Adequate hydration is not only a treatment concern but is also a mainstay for prevention of further stone formation.

Life-style Changes

Depending on what type of stone is identified, there may be dietary limitations or modifications. For example, if a calcium stone is found, dietary calcium should be limited, which can be accomplished by eliminating dairy products and excessive protein from the diet. Oxalate-rich foods may also need to be limited. Foods high in oxalate are tea; coffee; colas; most green, leafy vegetables excluding lettuce; and berries.[5] If struvite stones are diagnosed, it may be necessary to keep the patient on an antibiotic regimen for the prevention of urinary tract infections. Regardless of the type of stone, it is imperative that the patient be educated on the need for increased fluid intake to keep the urine as dilute as possible.

■ ACUTE GLOMERULONEPHRITIS

General Characteristics

The kidney's major function is classically described as "filtering" because of its ability to eliminate wastes and toxins through the production of urine. The glomerulus is a specialized part of the kidney cell, or nephron, that is responsible for forming filtrate and maintaining a proper fluid balance. Acute glomerulonephritis is the inflammation of the glomerular system secondary to an immune response. Although the etiology and classification of acute glomerulonephritis is lengthy and variable, most of these diseases have an immunologic origin and a similar clinical picture (Table 12–3). Poststreptoccal glomerulonephritis (PSGN) is the most common type and is the focus of this segment. Acute glomerulonephritis usually develops 6 to 20 days after a group A beta-hemolytic streptococcal infection of the oropharynx or skin (eg, impetigo), at a rate of less than 5% and 25% to 50% respectively. This disease is more common in children ages 2 to 12 years old but may occur in older children and adults. PSGN can occur sporadically or in epidemic form, depending on the strain of the bacteria. The rates of males and females with PSGN is related to the type of infection, season, and the patient's geographic location.[7]

Signs, Symptoms, and Diagnosis

The clinical presentation of poststreptococcal glomerulonephritis varies from subclinical symptoms to acute renal failure. The majority of patients present with an abrupt onset of hematuria (typically described as dark- or "smoky"-colored urine), edema (especially facial), and increased blood pressure. Patients may complain of generalized malaise, gastrointestinal symptoms, decreased urine output, flank discomfort, weight gain, and occasionally headache, seizure, and a low-grade fever. It is important on the physical examination for clinicians to note any skin lesions and evidence of fluid overload (eg, dyspnea, periorbital and peripheral edema, tachycardia, and tachypnea). The diagnosis of PSGN is made by identifying the typical clinical characteristics as well as the signs of recent streptoccal infection. Usually a renal biopsy is not necessary to make the diagnosis. A urine analysis will likely have white blood cells (WBCs), red blood cells (RBCs), casts, and possibly a positive culture for streptococcus. The streptozyme

TABLE 12–3. EXAMPLES OF CONDITIONS ASSOCIATED WITH GLOMERULONEPHRITIS

Diseases Involving Immune Complexes
  A. Postinfection
       Poststreptococcal
       Visceral abscess
  B. Collagen vascular disease
       Lupus nephritis
       Henoch-Schönlein purpura
  C. Primary renal disease
       I_GA nephropathy
       Membranoproliferative glomerulonephritis
  D. Other
       Goodpasture's syndrome
Diseases Without Immune Complexes
     Polyarteritis
     Wegener's granulomatosis
     Idiopathic glomerulonephritis

From Schrier.[6]

test and antistreptolysin O (ASO) titer are useful serologic markers for confirming a recent streptococcal infection.

The clinical features of PSGN occur secondary to inflammatory response at the level of the glomeruli. In response to bacterial infection, circulating antibodies react with the glomeruli, eventually causing damage to the glomerular membranes. This causes the glomeruli to be less selectively permeable, meaning that the glomeruli lose their ability to control what substances are filtered. As a result of changing osmotic forces, blood and protein are lost in urine as fluid enters tissue spaces, resulting in edema and hematuria.[7] Except for the immunopathologic aspect, the pathophysiology in PSGN and that in the other types of glomerulonephritis are essentially the same.

Management

The majority of patients with poststreptococcal glomerulonephritis completely recover within 1 to 3 weeks without specific therapy. The acute phase of the disease typically lasts 4 to 10 days. Ninety-five percent of children will spontaneously recover, including those requiring a brief dialysis during the acute illness.[7] Adults, especially the elderly, are at higher risk for developing complications such as chronic renal failure.

Since this disease is considered to be self-limiting, only supportive therapy is warranted. However, some patients may require salt restriction, antihypertensive medication, diuresis, or temporary dialysis. Appropriate antibiotic therapy should be used when bacterial cultures are positive. Steroids have not been shown to be effective in PSGN but are used in some glomerular disorders.

Life-style Changes

Patients may be concerned about continuing problems with urination after experiencing oliguria during the acute illness. The majority of patients with PSGN recover full function (ie, normal urine stream) within weeks and do not experience further problems. However, some patients develop intermittent proteinuria and visible hematuria, which may persist for months. Unless these patients continue to have evidence of worsening renal function (increased serum blood urea nitrogen [BUN] and creatinine), they are not likely to develop chronic renal failure. They should be reassured that most patients recover without significant treatment measures and that continuing dialysis is rarely indicated.

■ PYELONEPHRITIS

General Characteristics

Acute pyelonephritis is a serious, potentially life-threatening urinary tract infection involving kidney tissue. When evaluating a patient complaining of urinary tract infection symptoms, it is critical for a clinician to distinguish a bladder infection (cystitis) from pyelonephritis.

The most common cause of pyelonephritis is the bacterium *Escherichia coli,* occurring in approximately 90% of all cases.[8] Bacterial colonization of the urethra extends further up the urinary tract by retrograde migration, eventually causing inflammation of renal tissue (Fig. 12–1). Other causative organisms are listed in Table 12–4.

Urinary tract infections occur more commonly in young women and the elderly. Other predisposing factors for pyelonephritis include pregnancy, diabetes, neurologic disorders (eg, neurogenic bladder), and a history of kidney stones and recurrent cystitis. Patients with Foley catheters, abnormal urinary tracts, or who are hospitalized are at a higher risk for infection as well.[9]

Signs, Symptoms, and Diagnosis

Because they present similarly clinically, it is often difficult to differentiate pyelonephritis from cystitis. Patients with pyelonephritis usually appear ill, presenting with an acute onset of fever, chills, flank pain, malaise, and myalgias. Other possible symptoms include dysuria, urinary frequency, nausea, vomiting, and signs of dehydration. Patients with cystitis or subclinical pyelonephritis typically complain only of dysuria, frequency, urgency, and suprapubic discomfort (Table 12–5).[9]

A definitive diagnosis can be made with a urine analysis. Both upper and lower urinary tract infections cause pyuria and bacteriuria; however, WBC casts are seen only in pyelonephritis. A positive urine culture and Grams' stain, as well as leukocytosis seen on a complete blood count (CBC) support the diagnosis. Additional studies that may be useful are intravenous pyelography (IVP), a plain abdominal radiologic film, ultrasonography, computed tomography (CT), and radionuclide scintigraphy.[8]

The differential diagnoses include pelvic inflammatory disease, cystitis, renal calculi, as well as the other causes of an acute abdomen.

Management

Patients with acute pyelonephritis can be treated in the hospital or as outpatients, depending on the severity of the illness. Toxic and dehydrated patients, or those at high risk for complications (eg, young children, the elderly, pregnant women, diabetics, men, and immunocompromised hosts), should be admitted for fluid replacement and intravenous antibiotics.[7]

Outpatients should receive 2 weeks of a single oral antibiotic that is adjusted according to urine culture and sensitivities. Table 12–6 lists the oral agents recommended for outpatient treatment. Initial intravenous antibiotic coverage in inpatients depends on the urine Gram's stain and the patient's clinical history. Combination therapy with intravenous antibiotics should be considered for immunocompromised patients and those with nosocomial infections.[8] After identifying an organism and its sensitivities, a 10- to 14-day course of an oral

TABLE 12–4. CAUSES OF ACUTE PYELONEPHRITIS

Type of Organism	Cases [%]
Escherichia coli	85–90
Proteus mirabilis	2–5
Klebsiella	2–5
Staphylococcus saprophyticus	2–5
Mycoplasma hominis	1
Ureaplasma urealyticum	1
Pseudomonas species	1
Staphylococcus aureus	less than 1
Candida albicans	less than 1
Mycobacterium tuberculosis	less than 1

From Guibert et al.[8]

TABLE 12–5. COMPARISON OF SIGNS AND SYMPTOMS OF PYELONEPHRITIS AND CYSTITIS

Pyelonephritis	Cystitis
Fever	Frequency
Flank pain	Dysuria
CVA tenderness	Urgency
Nausea, vomiting	Suprapubic pain
Leukocytosis	
WBC casts	

CVA, costal vertebral angle; WBC, white blood cell.

TABLE 12–6. ORAL ANTIBIOTICS FOR TREATMENT OF PYELONEPHRITIS

Trimethoprim and sulfamethoxazole (Bactrim)
Ampicillin (Omnipen)
Cephalexin (Keflex)
Amoxicillin and clavulanate potassium (Augmentin)
Ciprofloxacin hydrochloride (Cipro)
Olfloxacin (Floxin)

From Tenner et al.[9]

antibiotic can be started in patients who respond to parenteral therapy. Aminoglycosides, third-generation cephalosporins, or a sulfonamide are the drugs of choice, such as ceftriaxone (Rocephin), ceftazidime (Fortaz), trimethoprim and sulfamethoxazole (Bactrim), gentamicin (Garamycin), and tobramycin (Nebcin). Ampicillin is also used, especially if an *Enterococcus* infection is suspected.

Despite appropriate management, severe complication can occur in patients with pyelonephritis such as sepsis, persistent fever, renal abscess, hydronephrosis, renal papillary necrosis, acute renal failure, hypertension, and renal scarring.

In general, after 3 to 5 days of therapy, a patient should improve clinically. Repeat urine cultures are needed 2 to 4 weeks after completion of therapy. Any signs of relapse should be investigated further to determine drug adherence and tolerance and culture sensitivities.[3]

Life-style Changes

Most patients with pyelonephritis respond well to routine therapy and do not suffer significant life-style changes. However, some patients may develop recurrent infections and will require prophylaxis with an antibiotic. Patients who suffer serious complications such as a renal abscess will require extensive follow-up care. Female patients should be educated about the proper methods used to decrease the risk for urinary tract infections as described in the cystitis life-style changes section.

■ CYSTITIS

General Characteristics

Cystitis is a urinary tract infection (UTI) localized at the bladder (Fig. 12–1). It is usually due to bacterial infection but may be the result of viral or fungal infections, toxic chemicals, drugs, or radiation.[10] In most cases, cystitis is caused by organisms reaching the urinary tract by the ascending route. Anatomic and mechanical factors can contribute to the development of UTIs by promoting urinary stasis, retention, and bacterial colonization. Most UTIs are caused by bacteria, with the most common being *Escherichia coli* (Table 12–7).[6] Cystitis is more common in women than men. There is also an age-related prevalence associated with cystitis (Table 12–8).[11]

There are other high-risk groups and risk factors for cystitis including sexually active young women, especially when pregnant, men with prostatic obstruction, diabetics, persons with catheters, using barrier contraceptives such as diaphragms, and engaging in sexual intercourse.

Signs, Symptoms, and Diagnosis

The main symptoms of cystitis are fever, frequency, dysuria, urgency, hematuria, and suprapubic tenderness.[4] Not all of these symptoms are consistently present, and once again age may be an important factor in determining which symptoms are present. For example, in children there may be significant fever, whereas in the elderly population, fever is quite often absent. Children who cry on micturition, complain of vague abdominal pains, or have foul-smelling urine should be suspected of having cystitis. In the elderly population, any acute onset of mental status change should alert the clinician to possible cystitis. Flank

TABLE 12–7. MICROBIAL PATHOGENS OF CYSTITIS

Microorganism	Percentage of Urine Cultures
Escherichia coli	50–90
Klebsiella or *Enterobacter*	10–40
Proteus, Morganella, Providencia	5–10
Pseudomonas aeruginosa	2–10
Staphylococcus epidermidis	2–10
Enterococci	2–10
Candida albicans	1–2
Staphylococcus aureus	1–2

From Schrier[6]

TABLE 12–8. INCIDENCE AND PREVALENCE OF CYSTITIS

Group	Prevalence (%)	Sex Ratio Male: Female
Neonatal	1	1.5:1.0
Preschool	2–3	1:10
School age	1–2	1:30
Reproductive age	2.5	1:50
Elderly living at home	20	1:10
Over 80 living at home	30	1:2
Elderly in hospitals or chronic care facilities	30	1:1

From Tanagho et al.[11]

pain is relatively uncommon in cystitis and suggests either renal calculi or pyelonephritis.[12] Cystitis may also be asymptomatic.

Other than clinical findings, the most useful and cost-effective means of diagnosing cystitis is urinalysis. Microscopic examination of the urine may reveal pyuria and frequently the causative agent. Protein and glucose may be present; however, other conditions (eg, diabetes mellitus and nephritis) may also be responsible for these results. Pyuria in the absence of bacteria should always suggest tuberculosis until proven otherwise.[10] Cultures are generally not indicated in uncomplicated cystitis; however, they should be obtained for all the following patients: adult men, women over 50 years, children, immunosuppressed patients, patients with indwelling catheters, elderly, patients with recurrent infections, and those with underlying medical disorders.[7] It is also important to note that good patient instruction is vital for the collection of an uncontaminated urine specimen.

Management

Antibiotics are the mainstay of therapy for cystitis (Table 12–9). Significant dehydration may also occur, especially in children and the elderly, and may require intravenous fluid supplementation. Selection of appropriate antimicrobials has become difficult with the increasing number of available agents. Choice of antibiotic should be based on a knowledge of the prevailing sensitivity pattern of the common urinary tract pathogens and the conditions under which the infection was acquired.[7] Fortunately, in most cases there are several satisfactory agents, in which case the most economical choice is best. The length of therapy varies, depending on the severity and length of the in-

TABLE 12–9. SELECTED ANTIBIOTICS FOR CYSTITIS

Medication	Dosage	Precautions
Floxin (Ofloxacin)	200 mg q 12 h; continue therapy for 3 d for cystitis caused by *Escherichia coli* or *Klebsiella pneumoniae*, 7 d for cystitis caused by other organisms	Hypersensitivity; pseudomembranous colitis; neurologic effects; blood glucose disturbances; phototoxicity; arthropathy
Maxaquin (Lomefloxacin hydrochloride)	400 mg q 24 h for 10 d	Hypersensitivity; pseudomembranous colitis; neurologic effects; phototoxicity; arthropathy
Noroxin (Norfloxacin)	400 mg q 12 h for 3 d (uncomplicated infections caused by *E. coli, K. pneumoniae,* or *Proteus mirabilis*); 7–10 d (uncomplicated infections caused by other organisms); 10–21 d (complicated infections)	Crystalluria; dizziness; light-headedness; CNS effects; hypersensitivity; CNS stimulation; pseudomembranous colitis; phototoxicity
Bactrim (Trimethoprim and sulfamethoxazole)	2 tabs or 1 DS tab q 12 h for 10–14 d	Hypersensitivity; bone marrow suppression; crystalluria; urolithiasis

CNS, central nervous system.

fection as well as the condition of the patient (eg, is the patient pregnant, elderly, immunosuppressed, or is this a recurrent infection?). A single-dose regimen has been proven successful in nonpregnant women who are at low risk. The 3-day antibiotic regimen is more widely accepted by patients and clinicians and is indicated for symptoms that have not been present for over 3 days. A 7-day regimen is indicated if symptoms have been present for over 3 days, during pregnancy, if an underlying medical condition exists, if there is an underlying urologic abnormality, or if there is a history of recurrent cystitis or renal calculi.

Life-style Changes

There are several things that can be done to help prevent cystitis. Drinking plenty of fluids—at least eight 8-ounce glasses of fluid daily. Women should make sure they wipe themselves from the front to the back to avoid contamination of the urethral entrance with bacteria from the bowel. Vaginal deodorants, bubble baths, and other irritating substances should be avoided. If a woman uses a diaphragm, she should consider using a smaller size or switching to an alternative means of birth control. Women who have frequent cystitis should drink a glass of water prior to intercourse and urinate immediately after intercourse. This helps flush out any bacteria that may have been accidentally pushed into the vagina. Drinking cranberry juice has been recommended in conjunction with antibiotic use. It is thought to be beneficial because of the increased acid content, which makes it difficult for bacteria to adhere to the bladder mucosa.

■ URINARY INCONTINENCE

General Characteristics

It is estimated some 8 to 12 million Americans may suffer from urinary incontinence. Approximately 40% of females aged 45 to 64 suffer from incontinence to some degree. Until recently, women have been reluctant to seek medical help for their affliction, largely because of the widely held misconception that the condition was merely a part of aging and that little treatment existed. In the United States alone, some $10 billion dollars per year is reportedly spent on products to help patients cope with incontinence.[13]

Urinary incontinence is, by definition, involuntary loss of urine, but the amount of urine loss and precipitating factors vary greatly. Although incontinence can occur at any time in a woman's life, women in postmenopausal years are more susceptible, secondary to declining estrogen levels and subsequent thinning of urinary tract tissues. Incontinence produces an array of psychologic and social stigmas. Social withdrawal, low self-esteem, and depression are common among sufferers.

Signs, Symptoms, and Diagnosis

The mechanics of voluntary urination need to be understood in order to comprehend the pathology of involuntary loss. The bladder wall consists of the detrusor muscle, a smooth muscle responsive to parasympathetic stimulation, which permits bladder contraction (Figs. 12–2, 12–3A). Beta-adrenergic stimulation, in conjunction with inhibitory sympathetic activity, causes bladder relaxation. Brain-stem signals initiate bladder contraction. Bladder continence is maintained via alpha-adrenergic stimulation to cause smooth muscle tone and contraction of the urethra (Fig. 12–3B). Voluntary urination is accomplished when detrusor contraction, urethral relaxation, and contraction of pelvic floor muscles via the pudendal nerve are performed in concert.

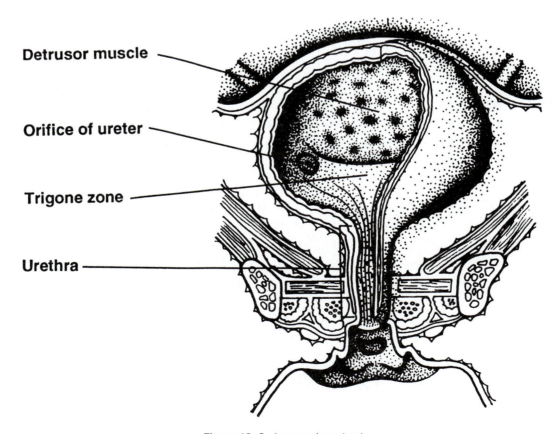

Detrusor muscle

Orifice of ureter

Trigone zone

Urethra

Figure 12–2. Lower urinary tract

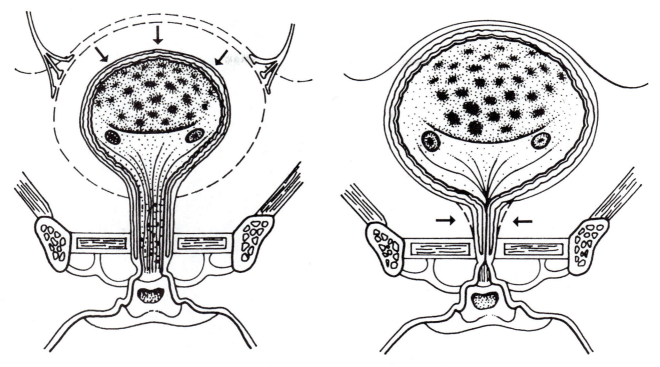

Figure 12–3. A. Parasympathetic stimulation causes detrusor contraction. B. Alpha-adrenergic stimulation causes bladder neck contraction.

Incontinence can be acute or chronic in nature. Acute or transient forms may be caused by drug side effects, infection, delirium, anxiety, depression, atrophy, or restricted mobility. Once recognized, this condition is usually easily reversible. Chronic incontinence consists of four types: stress, urge, overflow, and functional. A mixture of these types may be present.

Stress incontinence is the most common type and occurs with increased intra-abdominal pressure from coughing, sneezing, laughing, or bending. The loss of urine is variable, but it is important to note that the urine loss ceases after the stimulating event ceases. "Intrinsic sphincter deficiency" is the prime cause of this condition. Sphincter deficiency occurs with hypermobility of the bladder neck, or the neck drops out of normal position, is weakened, and becomes scarred open. Stress incontinence may also be caused by decreased estrogen levels during menopause or with bladder prolapse resulting from weakened ligaments and muscles. Physical examination may reveal a protrusion (cystocele) of the anterior vaginal wall, urethra, or bladder (Fig. 12–4). Cystoceles have three grades (Fig. 12–5), and grades 1 and 2 are nonspecific and may or may not be associated with incontinence. A Valsalva's maneuver in standing or supine position with a full bladder may demonstrate stress incontinence. A postvoid residual urine volume measurement will always yield less than 100 mL.

Urge incontinence is the inability to withhold urine flow long enough to reach the bathroom. The amount of urine is variable. Common causes include hormonal deficiency, UTI, bladder inflammation, spinal nerve root pathology, or spinal cord injury. Constipation or fecal impaction may also be the cause.

Overflow incontinence is the accidental loss of urine secondary to a chronically full bladder. The urge to void is usually absent; this is common in women with a cystocele. Bladder outlet obstruction and neuropathy secondary to diabetes is also a common cause of overflow incontinence. Urine loss is associated with exertion, standing, or bending. Postvoid residual urine volume is usually greater than 100 mL.

Functional incontinence is usually associated with restricted mobility. Other causes include UTI, delirium, atrophic vaginitis, and medicine side effects. When the mobility restriction is corrected, the incontinence can be resolved.

Diagnosis depends on a detailed history including urologic, medical, gynecologic, and neurologic information. Current medications and previous surgical procedures are important to note. A urinary voiding diary is very important to help classify the type of incontinence. This should include time and

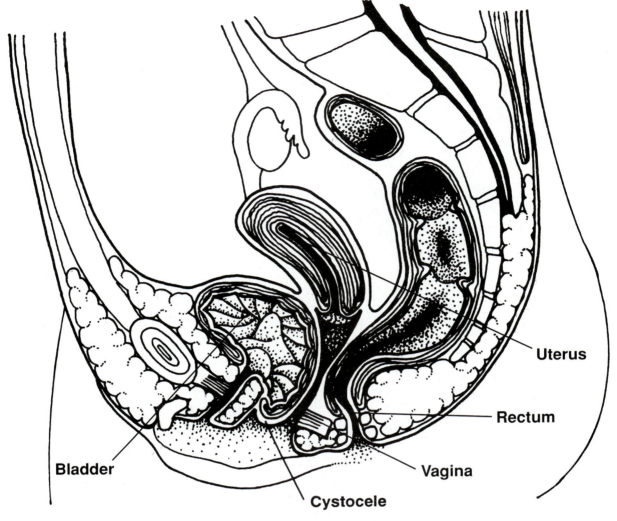

Figure 12–4. Cystocele

amount of fluid intake and urine loss, if urge was present, and any activity engaged in during the incontinent event. Physical data should be obtained from a complete gynecologic, rectal, pelvic, and abdominal examination. Mental status should also be assessed. Urinalysis, postvoid residual urine volume, and serum levels of BUN and creatinine should be obtained. Ultrasound of the kidneys may be needed to rule out renal blockage. Urodynamic studies are useful to evaluate bladder function. If a cystocele is present, referral to a urologist for a cystourethrogram may be necessary.

Management

Stress incontinence is initially treated nonpharmacologically with pelvic floor exercises and biofeedback. Drug therapy (Table 12–10) may be used in conjunction with these mea-

sures and usually includes an alpha agonist, which increases smooth muscle tone. Phenylpropanolamine is the usual drug of choice. Pseudoephedrine and ephedrine have also been employed. Imipramine, a tricyclic antidepressant, is used for its anticholinergic action, but care must be exercised to monitor side effects such as postural hypotension, sedation, and constipation. Topical estrogen may be mildly helpful. Finally, surgery may be considered for resistant cases.

Urge incontinence is also treated with nonpharmacologic methods. Drugs that have been used to treat this condition include propantheline and imipramine. These drugs work via anticholinergic activity. Bladder relaxants, which inhibit bladder spasm, include oxybutynin, flavoxate, and dicyclomine. Estrogen replacement therapy has proven moderately helpful in urge incontinence.

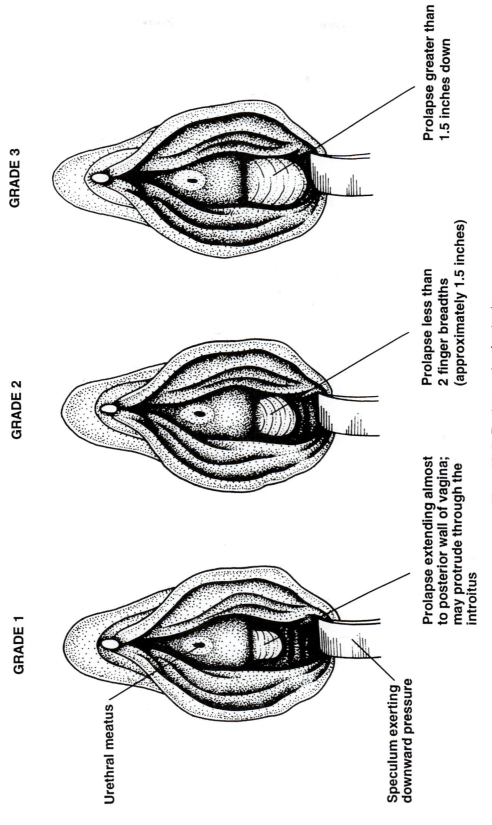

GRADE 1

GRADE 2

GRADE 3

Urethral meatus

Speculum exerting downward pressure

Prolapse extending almost to posterior wall of vagina; may protrude through the introitus

Prolapse less than 2 finger breadths (approximately 1.5 inches)

Prolapse greater than 1.5 inches down

Figure 12–5. The three grades of cystocele

TABLE 12–10. MEDICATIONS FOR THE TREATMENT OF URINARY INCONTINENCE

Drug	Dosage
Stress Incontinence	
Phenylpropanolamine	25–50 mg q 6–8 h
Pseudoephedrine	60 mg q 6–8 h
Imipramine	25–100 mg at bedtime
Estrogen intravaginal cream	2 g 2 times/wk
Urge Incontinence	
Oxybutynin	2.5–5.0 mg q 8 h
Flavoxate	100–200 mg q 6–8 h
Imipramine	25–100 mg at bedtime
Estrogen intravaginal cream	2 g 2 times/wk
Overflow Incontinence	
Bethanechol	20–100 mg q 6 h
Terazosin	1–10 mg/d
Prazosin	3–12 mg in divided doses, q 8–12 h

Overflow incontinence treatment with medication is considered only after correction of outflow obstruction. Self-catheterization and double voiding are helpful. When medications are used, a cholinergic agent is employed, such as bethanechol. Bethanechol is contraindicated in patients with hyperthyroidism, peptic ulcer disease, or asthma. Alpha-adrenergic agents such as prazosin and terazosin have some use in pharmacologic therapy.[14]

Life-style Changes

Patients should maintain an adequate fluid intake of six to eight glasses of water per day to prevent excessive urine concentration, which may cause bladder irritation. No fluid intake several hours before bedtime is important. Avoiding spicy foods such as citrus fruits, caffeine, alcohol, chocolate, and aspartame (NutraSweet) may prove helpful. Frequent urination is also important.

Two organizations exist for patients to help them cope with this condition:

Help for Incontinent People (HIP)
PO Box 544
Union, S.C. 29379
1-800-579-7900

The Simon Foundation
PO Box 835
Wilmette, IL 60091
1-800-237-4666

References

1. Resnick MI, Caldamore AA, Spirnak JP. *Decision Making in Urology*, 2nd ed. Hamilton, Ont: BC Decker Inc; 1991: 52–55.
2. Resnick MI, Pak CYC, eds. *Urolithiasis: A Medical and Surgical Reference*. Philadelphia, Pa: WB Saunders Co; 1990: 155–171.
3. Abuelo JG, ed. *Renal Pathophysiology—The Essentials*. Baltimore, Md: Williams & Wilkins; 1989:190–198.
4. Gillenwater JY, Grayhack JT, Howard SS, et al. *Adult and Pediatric Urology*. Vol 1. St. Louis, Mo: Mosby Yearbook Inc; 1991:275–324, 403–434.
5. Davidson AJ, Hartman DS, eds. *Radiology of the Kidney and Urinary Tract*. Philadelphia, Pa: WB Saunders Co; 1994: 435–452, 607–648.
6. Schrier RW, ed. *Manual of Nephrology*. 3rd ed. Boston, Mass: Little Brown & Co Inc; 1990:89–118.
7. *Cystitis Pyelonephritis, Nephrolithiasis*. Denver, Colo: Microdmedics Inc; 1975–1994, 85. Emergindex Clinical Review.
8. Guibert J, Meyrier A. Diagnosis and drug treatment of acute pyelonephritis. *Drugs*. 1992;44:356–357.
9. Tenner SM, Yadven MW, Kimmel PL. Acute pyelonephritis. *Postgrad Med*. 1992;91:261–268.
10. Asscher AW, Moffat DB, eds. *Nephro-Urology*. Chicago, Ill: Year Book Medical Publishers Inc; 1984:69–82, 99–106.
11. Tanagho EA, McAninch JW. *Smith's General Urology*. Norwalk, Conn: Appleton & Lange; 1992:195–307.
12. Cameron S. *Kidney Disease: the Facts*. 2nd ed. New York, NY: Oxford University Press; 1986:27–47, 68–83.
13. Pegg JF. Urologic incontinence in the elderly: pharmacologic therapies. *Am Fam Physician*. 1992;45:1763–1769.
14. Whitmore KE, Burgio KL. Urinary incontinence: practical management strategies. *Menopause Manage*. 1994 (May/June):14–20.

Neurologic Disorders

Angela Wegmann

■ SEIZURE DISORDERS

General Characteristics

Epilepsy is a condition characterized by recurrent seizures that result from pathologic, hypersynchronous discharges of cerebral neurons. Epilepsy can be either a primary disorder of unknown cause or a symptom of an underlying pathologic condition. Conditions that may cause a seizure disorder include head trauma, birth defects, central nervous system infections, tumors, and vascular disease. Despite a thorough work-up, no treatable source for seizures is found in 26% to 47% of patients.[1] This is known as primary epilepsy and is thought to be caused by genetic predisposition.

Seizures may be classified into three types: partial, generalized, and unclassified. Partial seizures are characterized by localized symptoms originating from a focal lesion of the brain. Generalized seizures consist of bilateral bodily involvement or have no focus. Unclassified seizures do not fit into the other categories and usually do not involve loss of consciousness.

Signs, Symptoms, and Diagnosis

Most seizures consist of three phases: the aura, ictus (the seizure itself), and the postictal state (Table 13–1). The aura can present as unusual tastes or smells, a sense of déjà vu, dizziness, headache, or aphasia. The ictal phase varies in duration and type of activity, depending on the type of seizure. The postictal phase usually consists of amnesia of the event, confusion, and somnolence. Diagnosis includes determining seizure type and etiology. Because the attack is rarely witnessed by the patient's health care provider, evidence of type of seizure activity comes from patient and observer history. A physical and neurologic examination helps to identify any evidence of un-derlying disease. Laboratory studies such as hematologic and immunologic studies, blood chemistries, and cerebrospinal fluid analysis should be performed. The electroencephalogram is one of the most helpful diagnostic tests and will reveal either focal or symmetrical disturbances. Studies such as computed tomographic (CT) scan or magnetic resonance imaging (MRI) with contrast enhancement should also be included, especially for patients in whom seizures started after childhood or whose examination suggests a focal abnormality.

Management

Once a reversible cause has been ruled out, the treatment consists of pharmacologic management of seizure activity (Table 13–2). Accurate diagnosis of seizure type is essential because certain medications may ameliorate some types of seizures but not others. Valproic acid and phenobarbital may be used for most seizure types. Other commonly used medications are phenytoin, carbamazepine, clonazepam, and primidone. Most patients will need to remain on medication for life. Some experts advocate a trial off medication if a patient has had full suppression of seizures for about 2 to 5 years.[2]

Frustration and depression are frequently experienced by seizure patients and should be treated with counseling, support groups, and medication if necessary. Patients considering having children should be counseled that the risk of their child having one or more seizures in their lifetime is 4% to 10%.[2]

Life-style Changes

Life-style changes for the seizure patient are numerous and revolve around safety. The goal of these changes is to maintain

TABLE 13–1. CHARACTERISTICS OF COMMON SEIZURE TYPES

Type	Aura	Duration	Loss of Consciousness	Ictus
Simple partial	No	30 s–several minutes	Not usually	Ranges from twitching to jerking or paresthesias of one limb or psychic sensations such as déjà vu
Complex partial	Yes	15 s–8 min	Usually just blunting	Automatisms such as lip smacking or aimless walking
Tonic-clonic (grand mal)	Usually	1–2 min	Yes	Body rigidity followed by jerking of head and limbs, incontinence, and stertorous breathing
Absence (petit mal)	No	2–15 s	No	Blank stare or fluttering of eyelids

s, second.

the highest level of functioning while minimizing potential for injury. In general, activities should be planned ahead of time in order to consider potential safety hazards.

- Activities like swimming or cooking while alone should be avoided.
- A shower or bath seat with safety straps should be used to avoid falls into water.
- Seat belts should always be used when traveling.
- A medical alert bracelet should be worn at all times.

- Patient should avoid driving unless approved by a health care provider.
- Counter and furniture edges should be padded.
- Storage items should be placed at accessible heights to avoid climbing.
- Ironing should be avoided whenever possible.
- Throw rugs should be removed.
- Family members and friends need to be taught to recognize seizure activity and to move nearby hazardous objects when it occurs. They should also be taught to assist if choking occurs.

TABLE 13–2. COMMON ANTICONVULSANTS

Generic Name	Trade Name	Seizure Type	Common Side Effects
Carbamazepine	Tegretol	Tonic-clonic Complex partial Simple partial	Lethargy, dizziness, ataxia, diplopia
Phenytoin	Dilantin	Tonic-clonic Complex partial Simple partial	Blurred vision, gingival hyperplasia, ataxia, rash
Phenobarbital		Tonic-clonic Partial	Drowsiness, irritability, excitability, cognitive impairment
Valproic acid	Depakene	Absence Tonic-clonic	Hair loss, tremor, nausea or vomiting, increased appetite

■ STROKE

General Characteristics

Stroke, or cerebrovascular accident (CVA), is the third leading cause of death in the United States as well as a frequent cause of physical and mental disability. Strokes are caused by either hemorrhagic or ischemic changes in the brain that lead to infarction. The resulting neurologic impairment can last days, weeks, or permanently; the specific deficits vary depending on the size and location of affected cerebrum. While several factors (Table 13–3) are associated with higher risk for stroke, hypertension appears to be the predominant risk factor. Although the overall mortality rate is significant at 36%, it has in recent years declined.[1] This is thought to be due in part to the improving treatment of hypertension.

Ischemic stroke appears to be far more common than hemorrhagic. Nearly 80% of all strokes are due to ischemia from either a thrombus or an embolus.[3] The single most common cause of stroke is thrombus formation secondary to atherosclerosis (Fig. 13–1). The peak incidence occurs between ages 60 to 80.[1] Only about 20% of strokes are caused by hemorrhage.[3] The peak age range is 50 to 80 years and is usually associated with hypertension and rupture of microaneurysms.[1]

Nearly 25% of acute stroke patients die during hospitalization. Among the survivors, approximately 40% make considerable neurologic recovery. Patients who suffer from hemorrhagic stroke seem to have a better chance of functional recovery. Indicators of poor prognosis are advanced age, coma, extensive brain-stem damage, and severe heart disease.[4]

Signs, Symptoms, and Diagnosis

Specific symptoms of stroke are determined by the site and size of the infarction. The classic presentation is contralateral

TABLE 13–3. RISK FACTORS FOR STROKE

Advanced age
Hypertension
Diabetes
Prior history of stroke or transient ischemic attack (TIA)
Obesity
Heart disease
Cigarette smoking (controversial)
Cocaine use

hemiparesis and hemianesthesia (Table 13–4). Variations of aphasia, apraxia, and visual defects are also common.

Thrombotic strokes typically are preceded by one or more transient ischemic attacks (TIAs). Neurologic signs often occur suddenly and maximize within a few minutes. Embolic strokes occur most often in patients with a previous history of heart disease, especially chronic atrial fibrillation. Onset is frequently at night or during routine activity. These also evolve quickly, with the neurologic deficit being maximal at onset. In contrast, an altered mental status that progresses over several hours and is preceded by severe headache and vomiting usually indicates hemorrhagic stroke.

Diagnosis requires a careful history and physical examination. A detailed neurologic examination may help to localize the lesion, but cerebral imaging by CT scan or MRI is the best method to visualize cerebral contents. Numerous laboratory tests may be helpful to determine the etiology and risk factors for stroke. An electrocardiogram (ECG) and echocardiogram should be performed if underlying heart disease is suspected. Cerebrospinal fluid examination is done only when it is necessary to rule out infection, subarachnoid hemorrhage, or vasculitis. Cerebral angiogram remains the "gold standard" in patients with cerebrovascular symptoms; however, it carries significant risk.

Management

Management in the acute phase and over the long term is determined by the etiology and clinical severity of the stroke. No currently available therapy will reverse neurologic damage that has occurred; therefore, initial management is directed at maintaining vital functions and preventing worsening of the deficit. Appropriate treatment of risk factors with antihypertensives and antiarrhythmics should be started early and continued chronically. Aspirin and anticoagulation with heparin should be initiated immediately in patients with ischemic infarction. Intra-arterial injection of thrombolytic agents such as streptokinase and urokinase has shown encouraging results but is still being studied. Surgical intervention may be considered for some patients, depending on the location, size, and etiology of their lesion as well as their overall clinical status.

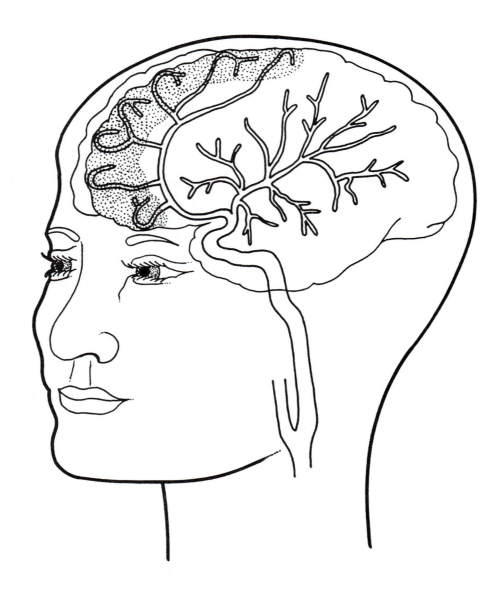

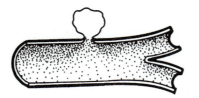

**Stroke from
hemorrhage**

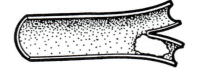

**Stroke from
blood clot
(thrombus)**

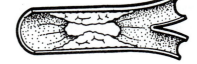

**Stroke from
clogged artery
and clot**

Figure 13–1. Different types of stroke

TABLE 13–4. COMMON SIGNS OF STROKE

Right Hemisphere	Left Hemisphere
Left hemiparesis	Right hemiparesis
Spatial-perceptual deficits	Aphasia
Dysarthria	Dysphagia
Dysphagia	Right-side neglect
Left-side neglect	Apraxia
Apraxia	Right visual field deficit
Left visual field deficit	
May deny or underestimate deficits	

Long-term management takes a multidisciplinary approach. Elimination or reduction of risk factors is essential. Occupational therapy helps patients relearn activities of daily living and become as autonomous as possible. Physical therapy and passive range-of-motion (ROM) exercises help prevent spasticity of paralyzed limbs, while active ROM exercises strengthen unaffected extremities. Assistive devices for ambulation such as canes, walkers, or short leg braces may be useful. Splinting of affected limbs intermittently during the day and continuously at night helps to prevent debilitating contractures. Speech therapy can improve communication and comprehension in patients with speech and language impairments. If necessary, arrangements should be made for home nursing visits or meal deliveries. Other patients who cannot be cared for at home should be considered for nursing home placement. Family members and caregivers should be reminded that too much assistance can cause a patient to become dependent and lose any skills gained from therapy.

Life-style Changes
Certain life-style changes will be necessary to reduce or eliminate risk factors and to prevent another stroke. These include:

- Smoking cessation
- Treatment of hypertension
- Weight loss for obese patients
- Some form of routine exercise
- Daily anti-platelet aggregation therapy
- Rehabilitation with occupational, physical, and speech therapies

■ HEADACHES

General Characteristics

Chronic or recurring headache is among the most common complaints encountered in clinical practice. Approximately 60% of men and 75% of women will experience at least one significant headache per month.[5] While most headaches occur independent of any underlying disorder, headache can also be a symptom of serious disease. Tumors, abscesses, hematomas, and meningitis will cause pain by distension or inflammation of pain-sensitive tissues in the cranium. These are infrequent causes of headache and are differentiated by daily, worsening pain and neurologic signs.

The most common type of headache is the tension-type headache and it accounts for approximately 90% of all headaches.[6] The etiology is poorly understood; however, many experts believe that tension headaches are caused by sustained muscle contraction of pericranial muscles. These headaches are often exacerbated by stress and can be accompanied by analgesic overuse, chronic depression, or anxiety.

Migraines are the second most common type and account for approximately 6% of all headaches.[6] The etiology of migraines is also a source of controversy, but the most widely accepted model is that pain is caused by a cycle of vasospasm and vasodilation of cranial blood vessels. The disorder is generally considered hereditary and affects women 3:1 over males as a result of the aggravating influences of estrogen. The onset of migraines is usually within the first three decades of life.

Cluster headaches, another type of vascular headache, are characterized by clustering bouts of severe and debilitating pain alternating with periods of quiescence. Although the attacks are relatively brief, they may cause fear, panic, or agitation in many sufferers. Cluster headaches affect approximately 1% of the general population, predominantly men.[7] The exact mechanism of these headaches is unknown but appears to be multifactorial.

Signs, Symptoms, and Diagnosis

The major distinguishing features between four common types of headaches can be seen in Table 13–5. The diagnosis of each of the common headaches is relatively straightforward. Tension-type headaches can be diagnosed on the basis of detailed history and physical examination. With a classic history and normal physical examination, laboratory and radiographic studies are generally unnecessary.

The diagnosis of vascular headaches (migraine and cluster) can also be based predominately on history and physical examination. A patient who gives a typical history for migraine, has a normal neurological examination, and experienced the onset of headaches before age 40 does not require adjunctive tests. If the clinical presentation is atypical or onset is after age 40, other causes should be ruled out by obtaining a CT scan or an MRI.

Cluster headaches, like migraines and tension-type ones, can be presumptively diagnosed by their distinct history. Physical examination is normal except during the headache, when changes such as ptosis, miosis, and lacrimation may be seen.

Sinus headache can be diagnosed by a consistent history and sinus tenderness on examination. The diagnosis may be confirmed by CT scan or sinus x-rays.

Management

Treatment of tension-type headaches usually involves a combination of modalities. The principal conservative treatment is to reduce stress and muscle contractions by hot or cold packs, respite from stressors, regular exercise, or relaxation therapy. Pharmacologic therapy depends on whether the headaches are episodic or chronic. Analgesic treatment should be initiated with the least addictive and least potent medication and then adjusted accordingly. Muscle relaxants can be added for synergistic effect. Narcotics in general should be avoided. Chronic tension-type headaches are more difficult to manage than episodic headaches and may require the addition of an antidepressant agent or even psychotherapy.

Pharmacologic treatment of migraine is either prophylactic or abortive. Prophylactic therapy is used to minimize the frequency of attacks in patients who suffer from two or more headaches per week. Abortive therapy is used to either reverse or control the headache once the attack has begun and is appropriate for those who suffer from fewer than two attacks per week. The addition of metoclopramide for abortive treatment can improve absorption of oral analgesics and suppress gastrointestinal symptoms.

TABLE 13–5. COMMON HEADACHES

Type	Presentation	Occurrence	Treatment
Tension	No prodrome Bilateral, bandlike Variable intensity Gradual onset Dull, aching, nonthrobbing	Intermittent or daily May last several hours to several days	Topical hot or cold packs Relaxation therapy NSAIDs Muscle relaxants Antidepressants
Migraine	Prodrome or aura Unilateral or bilateral Moderate to severe intensity Throbbing Often associated with nausea and vomiting	One to 10 attacks/mo May last 4–24 h	Abortive: Ergotamines Sumatriptan Narcotics NSAIDs Prophylactic: TCAs Propranolol Lithium carbonate
Cluster	Explosive onset, frequently from sleep Unilateral, periorbital Severe intensity Associated with lacrimation, and nasal congestion on the affected side	One to 6 attacks/d Clusters last 3–16 wk Usually occur at same time each day	Symptomatic: Oxygen Ergotamines Sumatriptan Intranasal lidocaine Prophylactic: Verapamil Steroids Lithium carbonate Valproic acid
Sinus	Unilateral or bilateral Usually superficial to affected sinus Mild to moderate intensity Dull, pressurelike Often associated with nasal congestion and purulent drainage		Antibiotics NSAIDs Decongestants Nasal steroids

NSAIDs, nonsteroidal anti-inflammatory drugs; TCAs, tricyclic antidepressants.

Treatment of cluster headaches is complicated by the brevity and incapacitating effect of the attacks. Symptomatic treatment is generally not effective because the attack is over before most oral medications begin to work. The basic treatment strategy is prophylaxis, with symptomatic treatment secondary.

Sinus headache caused by acute or chronic sinusitis is treated with antibiotics, nasal steroids, and decongestants.

Life-style Changes

Life-style changes for chronic sufferers of tension-type headaches include: respite from stressors, regular physical activity, and relaxation techniques such as biofeedback.

Life-style changes for migraine sufferers are basic strategies to reduce the frequency of attacks and include:

- Special diets that eliminate tyramine-rich food such as aged cheese and chocolate

- Regular meals, three times a day
- Avoiding alcohol, caffeine, and monosodium glutamate (MSG)
- Discontinuation of smoking
- Regulated daily routines
- Regular exercise
- Stress reduction with relaxation training
- Women should discontinue exogenous estrogen, including birth control pills if possible

Life-style changes for cluster headaches include:

- Avoiding alcohol, especially during clustering
- Discontinuation of smoking
- Carrying extra "insurance" treatment (steroids) while traveling or away from medical care
- Avoiding nitrates in food or medications

There are no significant life-style changes for sinus headaches.

■ ALZHEIMER'S DISEASE

General Characteristics

Alzheimer's disease is the most common cause of dementia in the elderly. It is estimated that the disease affects 2 million Americans and results in 100,000 deaths annually. The prevalence approximates 6% in persons age 60, 10% in persons ages 75 to 85, and 20% in those older than 85.[8] Men and women are equally affected.

Alzheimer's disease is described as a chronic and progressive dementia associated with neuronal degeneration, amyloid plaques, and decreased neurotransmitter production. The cause is unknown but several factors have been implicated, including viruses, environmental toxins, and genetic predisposition. Family history is a major factor; however, risk varies greatly. The disease appears to be inherited in an autosomal dominant pattern in about 15% to 20% of families.[9]

Signs, Symptoms, and Diagnosis

Clinical presentation of Alzheimer's can vary considerably. The earliest sign is forgetfulness, especially of recent events. Inability to remember names and misplacing objects are common. The patient may compensate by avoiding tasks that reveal his or her impairments.

With time, the patient has increasing difficulty with tasks that require planning and judgment. Inability to concentrate and cope with multiple stimuli causes frustration. Social withdrawal and depression are common. Alterations in mood, personality, and behavior can be manifested by aggression, pacing, or repeated questioning.

Gradually the patient loses his or her ability to perform activities of daily living without supervision. Comprehension of written and spoken language declines. Communication becomes difficult. Agitation, anxiety, and nighttime awakening may be seen. He or she may mistake his mirror image for a real person.

In the latter stages the patient no longer recognizes family members, his body parts, or himself. Verbal communication stops and patients become bedridden and incontinent. Activity consists of small purposeless movements. Death occurs on the average 6 to 10 years after the onset of disease, usually from superimposed infection.[8]

Definitive diagnosis of Alzheimer's can only be made by brain biopsy. Clinical diagnosis is made by a lengthy series of examinations and tests to rule out other causes of dementia. A history, physical examination, and neuropsychologic interview should be performed. Diagnostic tests including chest x-ray, electroencephalogram, CT or MRI (Figures 13–2 and 13–3) of the head, serologic tests for syphilis, thyroid, hepatic and renal functions, and cerebrospinal fluid analysis are necessary to exclude other conditions. Figure 13–3 demonstrates cerebral atrophy on an MRI, a common manifestation.

Management

Since no cure is currently available, management is directed at improving quality of life, minimizing cognitive and physical disability, and supporting caregivers. A newly approved drug called tacrine hydrochloride (Cognex) (Table 13–6) has been shown to improve cognition and slow the rate of decline in some patients.[10] The drug should be started in the early stages of disease, and patients must be closely monitored for signs of hepatotoxicity. Symptomatic relief with anxiolytics or antidepressants is recommended for patients who experience anxiety, agitation, or depression. Treatment with anxiolytics should be limited to short-term use. Care should be taken with prescribing benzodiazepines and tricyclic antidepressants, as drug effects can be amplified in these patients, causing increased confusion. Patients who develop seizures in late stages are treated with anticonvulsant drugs such as carbamazepine (Tegretol). Insomnia should be managed with nonpharmacologic approaches such as avoiding stimulants or naps during the day. If these methods are unsuccessful, short-term use of benzodiazepines at bedtime is appropriate. Supervised, regular physical activity is recommended. Support groups and even referral to professional counseling if needed is recommended for family members and caregivers. Caregivers must be reminded that the disease will cause progressive changes in intellect, personality, and motor function.

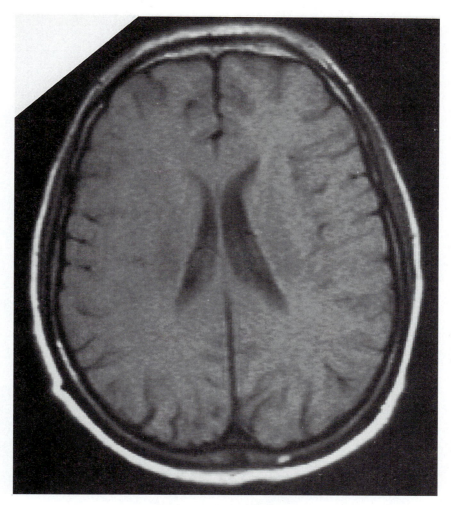

Figure 13–2. Normal MRI of brain

Life-style Changes

Numerous life-style changes will be necessary to provide a safe environment and improve quality of life. Distractions should be kept at a minimum. Caregivers should remove mirrors, photos, radios, and televisions from the individual's room. Limiting the numbers of different food items at mealtime will also help. To promote orientation, calendars and clocks should be placed in all rooms and the day and the activity about to be performed by the patient be announced. (Example: Today is Monday and we are going to have lunch now.) Repetitive tasks such as folding clothes or weeding should be assigned to eliminate anxiety about decision making. The caregiver should avoid assigning more than one task at a time. (Example: Brush your hair and get dressed). The patient should avoid fatigue by taking frequent rests throughout the day. A schedule should be made and followed with as little deviation as possible. It is best to do the same activities at the same time each day. Avoiding changes in schedule, environment, or caregiver will prevent anxiety. Medications should be stored out of reach. For safety, stairways should be barricaded and rails should be mounted on tubs and near toilets. The patient should wear an identification bracelet at all times. Adult day care should be considered for eligible patients to provide activity and socialization. Occasional respite for caregivers is essential.

More information can be obtained from:

Alzheimer's Association
70 E Lake Street, Suite 600
Dept N 92
Chicago, IL, 60601
1-800-621-0379

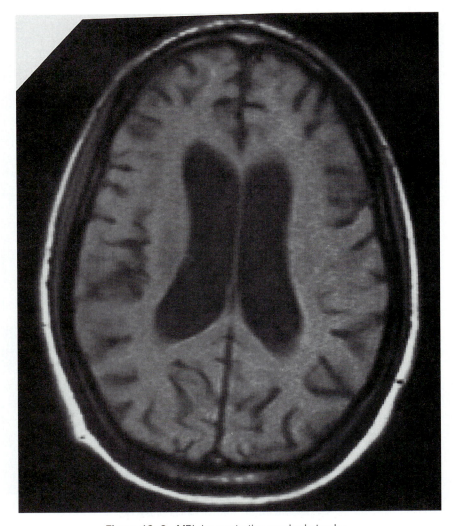

Figure 13–3. MRI demonstrating cerebral atrophy

TABLE 13–6. ALZHEIMER'S THERAPY

Medication	Dosage	Precautions
Cognex (Tacrine hydrochloride)	10 mg qid for at least 6 wk to start, then increase to 20 mg qid, providing there are no elevations in liver transaminases; titrate to 30 and 40 mg qid at 6 wk intervals on basis of tolerance	Transaminase elevations; neutropenia; seizure activity; bladder outflow obstruction

References

1. Stajich JM. Common neurologic disorders. *Physician Assist* 1990;14(suppl):53–58.
2. Andreoli TE, Carpenter CC, Plum F. Epilepsy. *Cecil Essentials of Medicine*. Philadelphia, Pa: WB Saunders Co; 1986: 760–770.
3. Claroni JB. Rehabilitating the stroke patient. *J Am Acad Physician Assist* 1993;6:179–194.
4. Andreoli TE, Carpenter CC, Plum F et al. Cerebrovascular disease. *Cecil Essentials of Medicine*. Philadelphia, Pa: WB Saunders Co; 1986:739–750.
5. Saper JR, Silberstein S, Gordon CD. *Handbook of Headache Management*. Baltimore, Md: Williams & Wilkins; 1993: 93–121.
6. Hendler N, Kozikowski JG, Schlesinger R. Diagnosis and treatment of muscle tension headaches. *Physician Assist*. 1991; 15(12):72–83.

7. Mastrangelo R. Chronic headache. *Advance.* 1993(October):11–12.

8. Chui HC. Clinical update on Alzheimer's disease. *J Am Acad Physician Assist.* 1990;3:231–239.

9. Szwabo P, Tideeiksaar R. Alzheimer's disease and senile dementia. *Physician Assist.* 1991;15(9):19–29.

10. Segal-Gidan FI, Chui HC. Alzheimer's disease and related dementias. *Clinician Rev.* 1994;4(1):65–88.

Neoplastic Disorders

Marvis J. Lary
Debra D. Davis
Richard D. Muma

■ LUNG CANCER

General Characteristics

Lung cancer is a disease of relatively modern times. Although the prevalence has increased over the last six decades, it was not until the 1950s that epidemiologic studies convincingly linked smoking—especially cigarette smoking—to the rising death rate attributed to lung cancer. The American Cancer Society projects that close to 200,000 new cases of lung cancer will be diagnosed this year, accounting for 18% of new cancers in men and 12% in women. Most patients present between the ages of 50 and 70. Fewer than 5% of lung cancer patients are under 40 years of age.[1,2]

Cigarette smoking is the most important cause of lung cancer in both men and women in the United States. Ionizing radiation, asbestos, heavy metals, and industrial carcinogens are established but less potent pulmonary carcinogens. Lung scars, air pollution, and genetics are also implicated, but the data supporting these associations are not conclusive. Primary lung cancer in nonsmokers is uncommon.

Squamous cell carcinoma and adenocarcinoma are the most common types of bronchogenic carcinoma and account for about 30% to 35% of primary tumors each. Small-cell carcinoma and large-cell carcinoma account for about 20% to 25% and 15% respectively (Table 14–1).

Signs, Symptoms, and Diagnosis

The clinical features of lung cancer depend on the primary cancer itself, its metastases, systemic effects of the cancer, and other coexisting medical problems. Only 10% to 25% of pa-

tients are symptomatic at the time of diagnosis of lung cancer. Symptomatic lung cancer is generally advanced and often not resectable. Initial symptoms include nonspecific complaints such as cough, weight loss, dyspnea, chest pain, and hemoptysis, which are associated with other disorders.

All patients with suspected lung cancer should receive a complete blood count (CBC), liver function tests, and measurement of serum electrolytes and calcium in addition to a chest radiograph. Chest radiography demonstrates abnormal findings in nearly all patients with lung cancer. Computed tomography (CT), magnetic resonance imaging (MRI), and ultrasound may also be used diagnostically. Definitive diagnosis requires cytologic or histologic evidence of cancer. Sputum cytologic examination may prevent the need for a bronchoscopy or other invasive procedure. Tissue for histologic confirmation of lung cancer may be obtained by various techniques, including bronchoscopy, percutaneous needle aspiration, or lymph node biopsy. Thoracotomy is occasionally necessary to diagnose lung cancer when simpler cytologic and histologic evaluations are negative.

Management

The main treatment options in lung cancer include surgery, chemotherapy, and radiation therapy. Laser photoresection is sometimes performed on obstructing central tumors to relieve dyspnea and control hemoptysis. Surgery remains the treatment of choice for patients with non–small-cell carcinoma. Unfortunately, only about 25% of patients with lung cancer are

TABLE 14–1. BROAD CLASSIFICATIONS FOR LUNG CANCER

Type of Cancer	Characteristics
Small-cell carcinomas (15%–25%)	Rapid growth and early metastases; thus lower cure rate
Non–small-cell carcinomas (75%–85%)	Varying growth rates and metastatic tendencies; include adenocarcinoma, squamous cell carcinoma, large-cell carcinoma
Miscellaneous tumors (2%–3%)	Carcinoid tumors, adenoid cystic carcinoma, mucoepidermoid carcinoma; varying growth rates and metastatic tendencies

appropriate candidates for surgery. Contraindications to surgery include extrathoracic metastases; tumor involving the trachea, carina, or proximal main-stem bronchi; tumor involving the esophagus or pericardium; poor general health; and extensive involvement of the chest wall. Elderly patients with severe chronic obstructive pulmonary disease (COPD) are especially likely to be functionally inoperable.

The type and location of lung cancer determines whether patients receive adjuvant therapy (chemotherapy, radiation therapy, or both) during the postoperative period. Combination chemotherapy is the treatment of choice for small-cell carcinoma, and radiation therapy is often used to palliate symptoms such as cough, hemoptysis, pain from bone metastases, and dyspnea from bronchial or tracheal obstruction.

Lung cancer patients must be followed closely with complete history, physical examination, chest radiographs, CBC, and blood chemistries every 2 to 3 months during the first 2 years and every 4 to 6 months subsequently. The overall 5-year survival rate for lung cancer is 10% to 15%. Determinants of survival include the stage of disease at the time of presentation, the patient's general health, age, histologic type of tumor, tumor growth rate, and type of therapy.

Life-style Changes

Lung cancer can be very disabling, depending on the stage of the disease, the patient's general health and age, and the type of therapy used. Activity level and quality of life depend on how compromised the respiratory system is from surgery or chronic disease.

Patients need attentive care from their health care provider and family. Community support services, such as the American Cancer Society, can help patients identify needed resources such as medical supplies, transportation for health care, and if needed, hospice services.

■ BREAST CANCER

General Characteristics

Each year about 180,000 women develop breast cancer, resulting in about 46,000 deaths. It is startling to realize that one in nine women will develop breast cancer in their lifetime. There are many risk factors involved in the development of breast cancer; however, it is important to realize that in the majority of women who develop it, age is the only risk factor. The incidence of breast cancer clearly increases with age, and screening programs have demonstrated clear benefit for screening women over 50 years of age (Table 14–2).[3]

Identification of very-high-risk women is important and may lead to more aggressive screening programs earlier in life. Although women who have a first-degree relative with breast cancer represent only 5% of all those who develop breast cancer, they are clearly at high risk. A personal history of breast cancer also increases a woman's risk for future breast cancer.

Signs, Symptoms, and Diagnosis

Health care practitioners should instruct their patients on the proper technique for breast-self examinations (BSE) and encourage them to perform BSE monthly. Populations who do perform BSE have been noted to detect breast cancer at an earlier stage and have a decreased mortality of approximately 10% to 20% over women who do not perform BSE. Health care practitioners are encouraged to perform thorough breast ex-

aminations of their patients annually at the time of physical examination and health screening (Table 14–3). This is a good opportunity to question patients about their compliance with BSE and to reevaluate their technique.

Mammography is the only method available to consistently detect breast cancer before it is clinically apparent. Although mammography is a fairly sensitive means of detection, it does carry a 10% to 20% false negative rate. Mammography can detect cancers as small as 0.2 cm in diameter, usually 3 to 5 years before they are palpable. Because breast cancers detected by mammography are at an earlier stage, they have a higher overall cure rate than those detected by examination only. Detection of breast cancer at an earlier stage leads to approximately 30% reduction in cancer mortality at 10 years.

Clinical symptoms of breast cancer detected by patients may include discharge from the nipple, or a palpable mass (usually painless), or an area of increased "thickening" (Figure 14–1). In addition, patients may notice a dimpling or "orange peel" appearance of their breast. Any such signs should be brought to the attention of a practitioner so that further diagnostic procedures can be initiated.

The diagnosis of breast cancer may be suggested by the presence of a hard, irregular dominant mass or by suspect mammographic findings; however, confirmation of the diagnosis depends on histologic examination of tissue obtained by needle aspiration, needle biopsy, or incisional or excisional biopsy.[4,5]

Management

Once the diagnosis of breast cancer has been established, the stage of the disease must be determined before treatment can be undertaken. In a patient with clinical stage I disease without symptoms of metastasis, chest x-ray, mammography, CBC, and blood chemistry (SMA-12) are sufficient. In patients with

TABLE 14–2. RISK FACTORS ASSOCIATED WITH BREAST CANCER

Degree of Risk	Factor
High risk	1st degree relative (mother, sister, daughter) with breast cancer Personal history of breast cancer or biopsy-proven atypical hyperplasia Age (most breast cancer occurs after age 40; increasing incidence with age)
Moderate risk	Menarche before age 12 Menopause after age 50 Nulliparity Over age 30 at first full-term pregnancy Previous history of endometrial, ovarian, or colon cancer
Other risk factors	Diet high in animal fats Obesity (greater than 20% over ideal weight) Alcohol consumption

TABLE 14–3. AMERICAN CANCER SOCIETY BREAST CANCER SCREENING GUIDELINES

Age 40	BSE, annual breast examination, screening mammography every 1–2 yr
Age 50	BSE, annual breast examination, screening mammography every yr

BSE, breast self-examination.

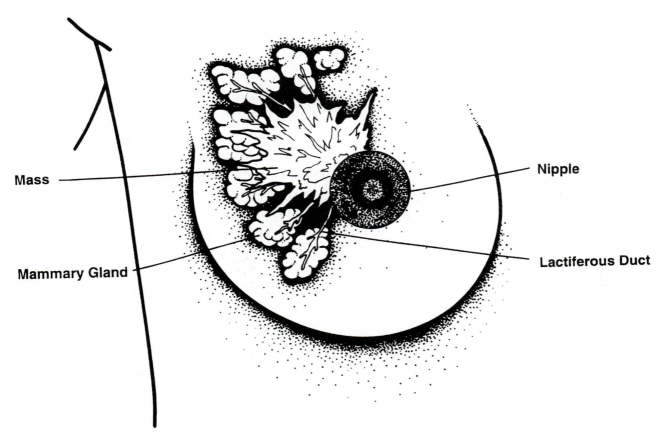

Mass

Mammary Gland

Nipple

Lactiferous Duct

Figure 14–1. Cancer of the breast

stage II disease, a bone scan is sometimes recommended, and for patients with stage III or IV disease, bone scans are recommended as well as other tests required to assess symptoms or abnormal laboratory values.

Treatment for breast cancer has changed dramatically over the past 20 years. It is now known that for stage I and II, more conservative surgical treatment is just as effective as the once employed radical mastectomy. Depending on the stage of the disease, treatment ranges from a simple lumpectomy to a modified radical mastectomy with adjuvant chemotherapy or radiation therapy.

For metastatic breast cancer, the two major kinds of systemic therapy are endocrine manipulation and cytotoxic chemotherapy. The hormone receptor status of the patient's tumor is of paramount importance in choosing the treatment. Only about 30% of all breast cancers are hormone-dependent and respond to endocrine therapy. Bilateral oophorectomy or the antiestrogen tamoxifen may be indicated for premenopausal women.

Life-style Changes

There are no changes in the activity level for women with a history of breast cancer. However, women who have undergone a mastectomy may need help adjusting to an altered body image. For some women, breast reconstruction may be appropriate to augment psychologic adaptation; for others, special garments and prostheses are available. Local support groups are helpful for mastectomy patients and their families, particularly in the first few weeks and months following surgery. Whatever approach is taken for rehabilitation, it is essential to employ a sensible and attentive manner in dealing with a patient's emotional concerns.

■ COLORECTAL CANCER

General Characteristics

In the United States, colorectal cancer is the second most common cause of cancer mortality after lung cancer. Fortunately, in recent years, both incidence and mortality rates have begun to decline. This decline in incidence may, in part, reflect improved public and professional health awareness and improved primary prevention, including better nutrition and, possibly, removal of colorectal tumors. In addition, as more patients with invasive colorectal cancer are being cured, their quality of life is also improving, thanks to improved surgical technique and more effective rehabilitation.[3,6]

In the United States, an individual has about a 1 in 20 lifetime risk of developing colorectal cancer, but the risk increases with age. The incidence rate for those under 65 years of age is 19 per 100,000, but among those over 65 years of age, it is 337 per 100,000. Only about 3% of colorectal cancers occur in persons under age 40, although initiating and promoting events may be occurring at this time.

Adenocarcinoma is the most common cancer of the colon and rectum. Lymphoma, carcinoid, melanoma, fibrosarcoma, and other types of cancer occur rarely. The treatment of all is essentially the same.

Although variations in incidence can be correlated with migration patterns, economic development, family size, and other environmental and social conditions, the most salient risk factor for colorectal cancer is diet. Dietary fat, particularly animal fat, is associated with high risk, and dietary fiber, particularly insoluble or grain fiber, is associated with low risk.

Signs, Symptoms, and Diagnosis

Symptoms vary, depending on the location of the cancerous lesion in the colon (Fig. 14–2); however, a persistent change in the customary bowel habits should alert the practitioner to investigate the colon. Bright-red rectal bleeding is a cardinal diagnostic point. Hemoccult-positive stool is a more subtle and frequent presentation. Patients may have early vague abdominal discomfort, which may progress to cramplike pain. Some patients experience increasing constipation with short bouts of diarrhea. Occasionally, the first sign is acute colonic obstruction. A small amount of bright-red blood with bowel movements is common, and anemia is found in about 20% of cases.

At times a mass is palpable and about half of patients give a history of weight loss.

A peroxidase test (Hemoccult) is the most widely used screening test for fecal occult blood. Although simple, convenient, and inexpensive, the test has a false-positive rate of 2% to 3%, a false-negative rate 20% to 31%, and predictive values for adenomas and cancer 22% to 58%. Digital examination of the rectum detects only those tumors within reach of the examining finger, perhaps 10% to 15% of all colorectal cancers. Digital rectal examination also is useful for examination of the cul-de-sac in women and of the prostate in men. Endoscopy and radiography remain the ultimate diagnostic procedures for identifying cancer of the colon (Table 14–4).

Management

Approximately 85% of patients diagnosed with colorectal cancer can have an operation intended for cure. Even patients deemed to have incurable cancer often have palliative resection to abort anemia, prevent obstruction, and reduce the risk of invasion of adjacent organs such as the bladder. A preoperative carcinoembryonic antigen level (CEA) is obtained for baseline data and used to follow up the patient's progress after surgery. The best indicator of prognosis after surgery is the depth of invasion of the primary tumor.

Colorectal cancer is responsive to radiation therapy; however, because the colon is adjacent to the radiosensitive small intestine and kidneys, adjuvant radiation therapy has proven most applicable to rectal cancer.

After surgery for colon cancer, chemotherapy with fluorouracil (5-FU) and levamisole for one year has reduced recurrence rates by 39%, cancer related deaths by 32%, and overall death rates by 31%.

Five-year, disease-free survival rates for colorectal cancer are generally equivalent to cure rates and depend on the stage of the disease. About 85% of all recurrences are evident within 3 years after the primary surgery. Patients are normally seen at 3-month intervals for 3 years, and annually thereafter. If they had an elevated CEA level before surgery, they should have the CEA level checked at each visit. After a curative operation, an elevated preoperative CEA level usually reverts to normal within 6 weeks. Periodic endoscopy should be per-

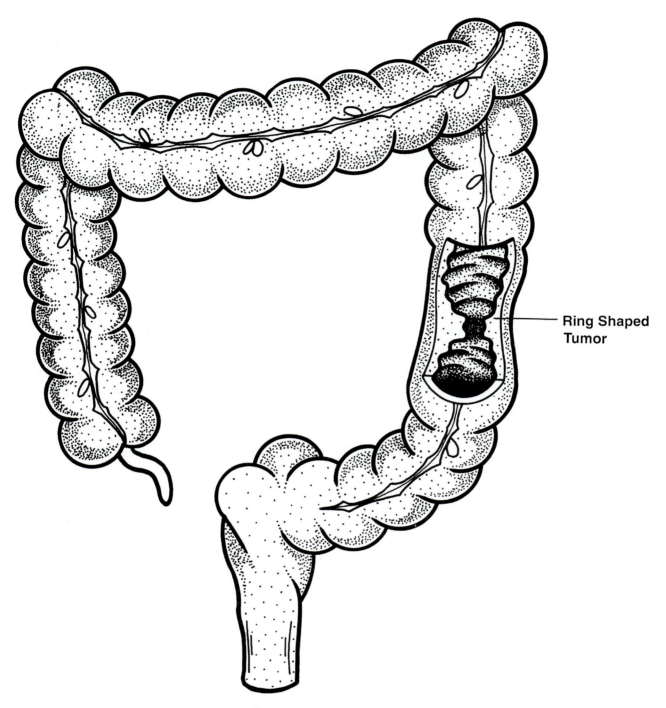

— Ring Shaped
Tumor

Figure 14–2. Cancer of the colon

TABLE 14–4. AMERICAN CANCER SOCIETY RECOMMENDATIONS FOR COLORECTAL CANCER SCREENING

Population	Starting Age	Procedure	Frequency
Asymptomatic, no risk factors	40	Digital rectal exam	Annually
	50	Fecal occult blood	Annually
	50	Sigmoidoscopy, preferably flexible	q 3–5 yr
First-degree family members of patient with colorectal cancer diagnosed under age 55	35–40	Colonoscopy or double-contrast barium enema X-ray	q 5 yr

formed, with the frequency depending on the type and stage of the lesion. Annual chest x-rays should be obtained for all patients.

Life-style Changes

The aim of curative treatment is to restore the patient to normal social, physical, and sexual function, while preserving life expectancy. Enterostomal therapists and the use of new devices help patients with a colostomy to achieve independence and comfort. Instruction in colostomy management should begin as soon as possible after surgery, while the patient is still hospitalized. Access to psychosocial services, such as local support groups for colostomy patients, is helpful to the patient and his or her family.

Patients require consultation with a nutritionist, since significant dietary changes are usually necessary after colon surgery. The patient's ongoing nutritional state plays a significant role in the recovery and lifelong health of the patient.

■ TESTICULAR CANCER

General Characteristics

Testicular cancer is uncommon in relation to other cancers such as those of the breast and lung. Approximately 5000 cases occur annually in the United States. Although uncommon, testicular cancer is the most common solid tumor in males aged 15 to 35, most occurring in Caucasian individuals. Early detection by monthly testicular self-exams can decrease the morbidity and mortality associated with the disease[7].

The etiology is unclear; however, several factors have been noted in relation to the disease. For example, undescended testes that are not corrected in early childhood have been related to an increased incidence in the development of the tumor. Previous trauma to the testes is also a frequent association. In addition, a higher incidence has been reported in twins, suggesting the presence of genetic factors.

There are several types of testicular tumors. Lymphomas are the most common primary testicular neoplasm in men over the age of 55 and germ-cell tumors (seminoma, teratoma, embryonal carcinoma, or yolk sac tumor) are seen in young men.

Signs, Symptoms, and Diagnosis

The most common presenting sign of a testicular tumor is a painless and firm testicular mass (Fig. 14–3). Although painful masses have been reported, this finding should prompt one to investigate the presence of other conditions, such as epididymitis or testicular torsion. Some patients have no mass and present with metastatic disease (eg, retroperitoneal lymph node, lung, and brain involvement); hence, their symptoms may be back pain, shortness of breath, and seizures. If a tumor is suspected and other causes have been ruled out, immediate surgical exploration consisting of a high inguinal orchiectomy (removal of testicle) should be initiated, and subsequent biopsy of the mass performed. It is not recommended to do a biopsy of the mass before removal because testicular cancers proliferate rapidly and if there are treatment delays, the risk of spreading to other organs is increased.

Management

Management depends on the stage of the tumor and whether the tumor has spread to other organ systems; therefore, staging

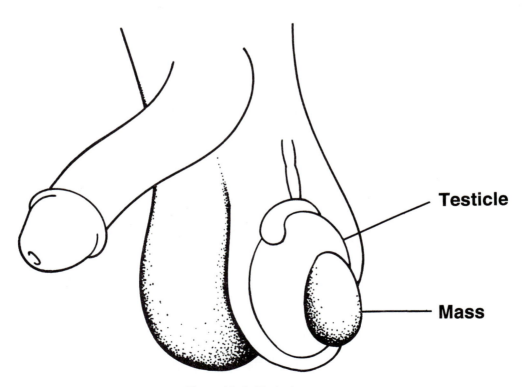

Figure 14–3. Testicular cancer

should be done soon after diagnosis (Tables 14–5 and 14–6). Staging first consists of determination of tumor markers, alpha-fetoprotein (APP) and human chorionic gonadotropin (hCG), as both are generally elevated in advanced disease. They are also useful in determining whether the tumor has recurred after treatment. Chest radiograph and CT of the chest, abdomen, and pelvis as well as bipedal lymphangiography are all routine and used to rule out metastatic disease. Some experts use lymphangiography when a retroperitoneal lymph node dissection is not done. Others believe that a lymph node dissection has both diagnostic and therapeutic value and should be done, especially in patients diagnosed with non-seminomatous tumors.

Seminomas are usually limited to the testes and retroperitoneal lymph nodes and are very responsive to radiation therapy. Therefore, radiation therapy is administered, after surgery, to the involved and adjacent areas. Those with stage A and B disease achieve a 90% cure rate. Those with stage C disease require additional treatment similar to those with nonseminomatous lesions, and their cure rate is slightly lower. Nonseminomatous germ-cell tumors are very proliferative and carry a poorer prognosis; thus, extensive chemotherapy is required. For those with metastatic lesions, after surgery,

TABLE 14–5. STAGING SYSTEM FOR TESTICULAR CANCER

Stage	Involvement	Recurrence Rate (%)
A (I)	Confined to the testis	10
B (II)	Retroperitoneal nodes	50
C (III)	Supradiaphragmatic or visceral	80

TABLE 14–6. STEPWISE MANAGEMENT OF TESTICULAR CANCER AFTER SURGERY

Step	Procedure	Order
1	Determine tumor markers	Alpha-fetoprotein (AFP) and human chorionic gonadotropin (hCG)
2	Determine stage of tumor	Chest x-ray; computed tomography of chest, abdomen, and pelvis, bipedal lymphangiography
3	Determine appropriate therapy	Radiation and/or chemotherapy

chemotherapy (eg, *cis*-platinum, vinblastine, actinomycin D, bleomycin, and cyclophosphamide) is usually required once a month for 3 to 4 months. Most of these cases achieve at least a 50% cure rate. For those with local disease, surgery is recommended with a retroperitoneal lymph node dissection, and in some cases adjuvant chemotherapy, leading to a cure rate of approximately 90%.

Life-style Changes

Concerns may be expressed about the possibility of posttreatment life-style changes including impotence, decreased or absent ejaculation, and sterility. Since surgery usually involves the removal of one testicle, potency, ejaculation, and fertility will be maintained. However, in rare cases, a radical lymph node dissection is required, which may lead to a "dry" ejaculation and subsequent sterility. Another concern may be the appearance of the scrotum after surgery. In most cases, a testicular prosthesis that looks anatomically correct is put in place.

■ PROSTATE CANCER

General Characteristics

The number of prostate cancer cases reported has increased markedly in recent years. Prostate cancer is the most common cancer in men in the United States other than skin cancer. Autopsy studies have shown that as many as 70% of men in their 80s have evidence of prostatic cancer. Nonetheless, only 6% to 8% of men have clinically detectable prostatic cancers in their lifetime.[3]

Black patients are more likely than white patients to be diagnosed with metastatic prostate cancer. Four factors have been cited as possible etiologic factors in prostate cancer. These include genetic predisposition, hormonal influences, dietary and environmental factors, and infectious agents. While genetic and environmental influences play a role in etiology of prostate cancer, male hormones play an essential role as a tumor promoter. The majority of prostatic cancers are adenocarcinomas that arise from prostatic acinar cells, are hormonally sensitive, and grow rapidly in the presence of male hormones.[8]

Signs, Symptoms, and Diagnosis

Many patients with prostatic cancer are asymptomatic; others have symptoms that cannot be distinguished from those of benign prostatic hypertrophy (BPH), ie, frequency, dribbling, nocturia. An occasional patient presents with bone pain resulting from metastases or with evidence of uremia as a result of urethral or bilateral ureteral obstruction. Some patients with prostate cancer present with an incidentally discovered nodule found on rectal examination performed as part of a routine physical examination (Fig. 14–4).

The most widely used tumor marker for prostatic cancer is the prostate-specific antigen (PSA). The upper limit of normal for PSA is 4 ng/mL. Levels above 10 ng/mL are almost always due to prostate cancer. Transrectal ultrasound is useful in evaluating prostatic cancer; however, 20% of prostatic tumors will be missed by ultrasound even though they are palpable on rectal examination. The fine-needle aspiration technique is widely used for prostate biopsy to confirm the diagnosis of prostate cancer.

Grading (Gleason system) of prostatic tumors ranges from grade I (well-differentiated) to grade V (undifferentiated). The Gleason grading system correlates well with tumor size, likelihood of metastases to pelvic lymph nodes, and PSA levels. Staging of the tumor is also critical (Table 14–7).

Patients with low-stage disease have a long-term survival rate of 80% to 90%. For patients with metastatic disease, the 5-year survival rate ranges from 40% to 50%.

Management

In stages A and B of prostate cancer, it is generally agreed that comparable results are achieved with surgical resection and radiation therapy. Newer surgical procedures that are "nerve sparing" are much less likely to cause impotence. The incidence of incontinence following radical prostatectomy varies from 0.5% to 11%.

Several options are available for the management of metastatic cancer of the prostate: bilateral orchiectomy has demonstrated effectiveness, testosterone levels can be decreased by estrogen administration, or a transurethral resection (TUR) may be done to prevent urinary obstruction and combined with hormonal therapy. Chemotherapy for metastatic prostate cancer has proven to be relatively ineffective; however, there are some newer drugs that are still in the experimental stages.

Patients with prostate cancer require continued medical attention with regular PSA, chest x-ray, bone scans, and other studies depending on the stage and grade of the cancer.

TABLE 14–7. STAGING SYSTEM FOR PROSTATIC CANCER

Stage	Tumor
A	Tumor is microscopic and not palpable upon rectal examination
B	Tumor is palpable on rectal examination
C	There is extracapsular extension of the tumor
D	Represents metastatic disease and may be further categorized depending on whether it is confined to the pelvis

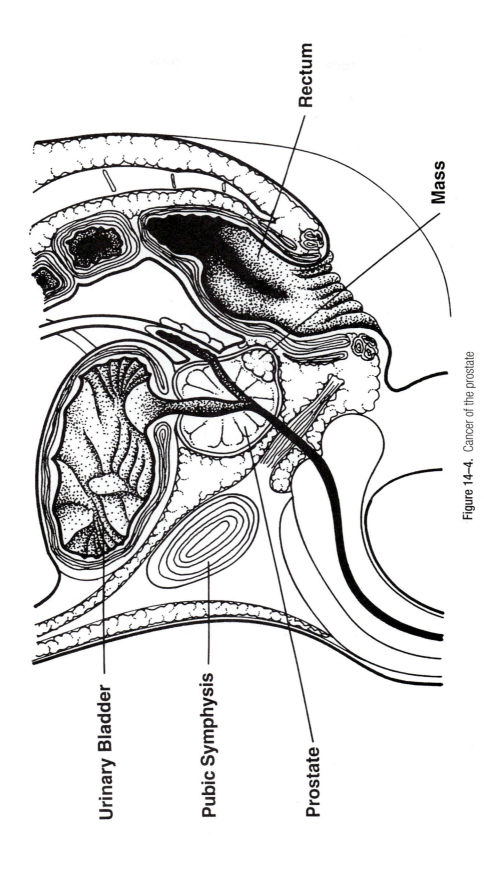

Rectum

Mass

Urinary Bladder

Pubic Symphysis

Prostate

Figure 14–4. Cancer of the prostate

Life-style Changes

For patients with low-stage prostate cancer, there may be no life-style changes. Patients with metastatic disease may experience some degree of incontinence or impotence as a result of more aggressive treatment. The incidence of these complications has been reduced dramatically in recent years as a result of improved surgical techniques. Counseling may be needed for patients and their mates if sexual dysfunction is present.

The majority of patients with prostate cancer are asymptomatic and have no life-style change.

■ SKIN CANCER

General Characteristics

Skin cancer is the most common type of cancer in the United States. Over half a million cases are newly diagnosed each year. Of those cases, approximately 9100 result in death. Skin cancer is a preventable disease. With the appropriate education and screening, a significant impact can be made to reduce morbidity and mortality.

Exposure to ultraviolet radiation is by far the greatest risk factor. This occurs either through sun exposure or through tanning devices. The body's primary defense to UV radiation is melanin. Melanin, produced by melanocytes in the epidermal layer of the skin, gives the skin its pigment (Fig 14–5). Tanning occurs when the melanocytes are stimulated through direct response to UV radiation exposure to produce pigment,

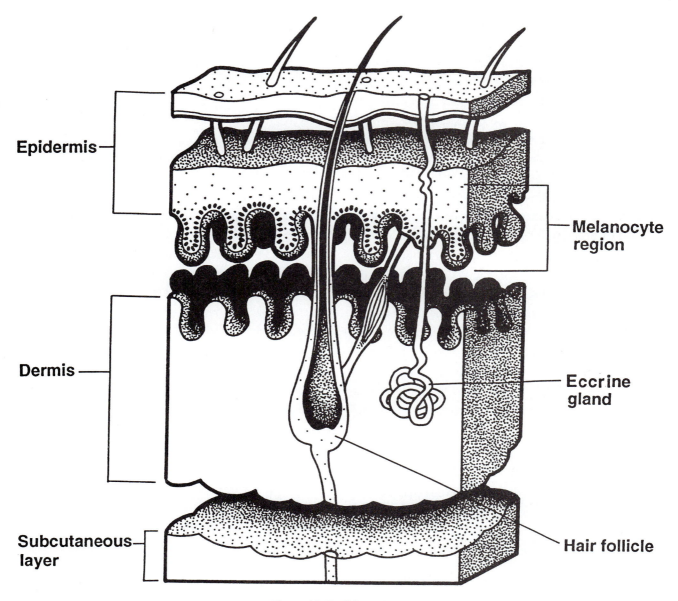

Epidermis

Melanocyte region

Dermis

Eccrine gland

Subcutaneous layer

Hair follicle

Figure 14–5. Skin anatomy

thereby providing protection for the skin. The ability to produce melanin varies among individuals. Fair-skinned individuals are not able to produce melanin to the same degree as darker-skinned individuals and thus do not have the protection from UV radiation injury that darker-skinned individuals have. Erythema of the skin, in response to sun exposure (sunburn), is the earliest sign of UV radiation damage to the skin and is inversely proportional to the amount of melanin present in the skin. It is this type of damage that predisposes people to skin cancer.

Individual skin types are classified on the basis of their tendency to burn or tan with sun exposure (Table 14–8). Those with skin type I have a higher risk for developing skin cancer. Individuals with skin type VI are at lower risk. Other risk factors for the development of skin cancer include chemical exposure to petroleum products such as tar and mineral spirits, trauma to the skin such as a burn, skin ulcers, and a family history of skin cancer. The presence of certain types of precancerous skin lesions is also a risk factor (Table 14–9).

Most skin cancers fall into two categories: melanoma and nonmelanoma. Melanoma has gained the most attention and produces the greatest fear among people; however, nonmelanoma types of skin cancer, which include basal cell carcinoma (BCC) and squamous cell carcinoma (SCC), are much more common. The vast majority of nonmelanoma-type cancers are BCCs.[9–11]

Signs, Symptoms, and Diagnosis

Nonmelanoma skin cancers occur in chronically sun-exposed areas such as the face, neck, and hands. Melanoma, on the other hand, is associated with intense, intermittent sun exposure. Severe blistering sunburns that occur in childhood are believed to predispose individuals to melanoma later in life. Melanoma most commonly occurs on the trunk and extremities.

TABLE 14–8. CLASSIFICATION OF SKIN TYPES

Skin Type	Reaction to Sun Exposure
I	Always burns, never tans
II	Usually burns, tans with difficulty
III	Sometimes burns, usually tans
IV	Rarely burns, tans easily
V	Never burns, olive base to skin
VI	Never burns, black skin

TABLE 14–9. RISK FACTORS IN THE DEVELOPMENT OF SKIN CANCER

Age (>age 40 for BCC and SCC, >age 15 for melanoma)
Tendency to burn easily (skin types I, II)
Chronic sun exposure
History of severe, blistering sunburns
Geographic location (near the equator or high altitudes)
Family history of skin cancer
Chemical exposure to arsenic, petroleum products
Sites of chronic infection
Trauma (such as thermal or radiation burns)
Immunosuppression
Premalignant skin lesions
   Actinic keratosis
   Bowen's disease
   Congenital nevi (large nevi >1 cm that have been present since 1st yr of life, or giant bathing trunk nevus
   Dysplastic nevus syndrome
   Leukoplakia
   Lichen sclerosis et atrophicus

BCC, basal cell carcinoma; SCC, Squamous cell carcinoma.

BCC, sometimes known as a rodent ulcer, is characterized by a pearly-white papule with telangiectatic vessels. As the lesion progresses, it becomes larger and more nodular. It is frequently accompanied by ulceration and bleeding in the center. Sites of predilection include the face, ears, neck, or bald scalp (Fig. 14–6). Because it rarely metastasizes, BCC has also been referred to in the past as a nonmalignant form of skin cancer; however, BCC can cause significant morbidity and even death by direct invasion of underlying tissues such as bone and brain.

SCC varies in its appearance. It can present as a papule, nodule, or plaque. The lesion is usually reddish in color or whitish on an erythematous base. It is usually indurated. It is often accompanied by ulceration, erosion, or crusting. Common sites of predilection for SCC are the border of the lower lip (Fig. 14–7) and the back of the hands, which are rather uncommon sites for BCC. SCC can also be found on the mucous membranes and the anogenital region. Lesions in this region as well as on the lower lip tend to be more aggressive and metastasize more frequently. Because of the propensity to metastasize, regional lymph nodes should be palpated as part of the evaluation for SCC.

Melanoma usually presents as a mole that has undergone recent change or is irregular in shape, color, or size (Fig.

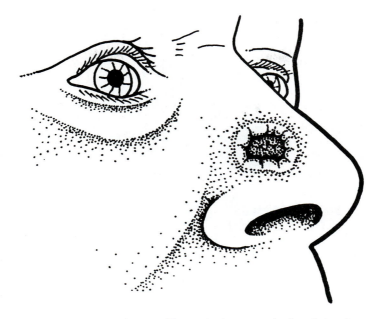

Figure 14–6. Basal cell carcinoma on the nose: The center is commonly ulcerated and covered with a crust.

14–8). Melanoma can also arise in the absence of a previous lesion or from a large congenital nevus or dysplastic nevus. The mnemonic using letters A, B, C, and D is frequently used in the evaluation of suspected lesions (Table 14–10). Other signs suggesting malignancy in a nevus include itching, ulceration, bleeding, and tenderness. Melanoma commonly occurs on the back in both males and females, and on the legs in females. The growth of melanoma occurs in two stages. Radial or horizontal growth occurs early on, with vertical growth in the later stages. Generally, the more vertical growth that has occurred, the worse the prognosis (Fig. 14–9).[12–13]

Diagnosis and Management

The decision as to which type of biopsy is indicated for a specific skin lesion is determined by the size, location, and cell type of that lesion.

In general, biopsies are either incisional or excisional. An incisional biopsy is one in which a portion of the lesion is

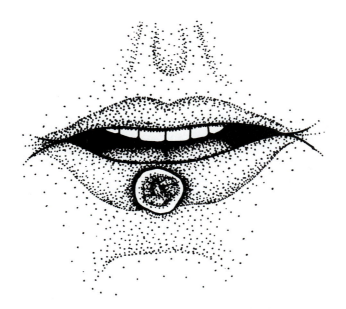

Figure 14–7. Squamous cell carcinoma: The sun-exposed lip is a common site.

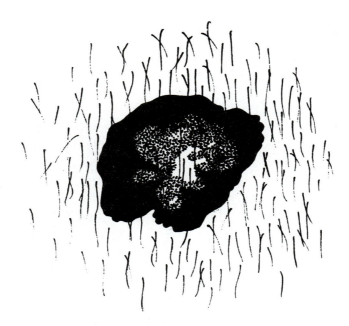

Figure 14–8. Superficial spreading melanoma: the color variation and scalloped and notched outline should alert the examiner to the possibility of malignancy.

removed and sent for pathologic examination. Based on the histologic examination, further treatment can then be decided. An excisional biopsy involves removing the entire lesion and is usually curative as well. Most procedures are of the excisional type.

The punch biopsy is an example of an incisional biopsy (Fig. 14–10). This procedure is used in surgically sensitive areas or with very large lesions. It provides a cylindrical tissue sample that is 3 to 4 mm in depth. The advantages are that it requires only a small amount of local anesthesia and usually requires no suture closure. The disadvantage is that it may not provide an accurate estimate of a lesion's depth when the depth varies within a lesion. If possible, the biopsy should be taken from the deepest part of the lesion.

A shave biopsy is a method for removing lesions and obtaining tissue for pathologic study. After infiltration of the surrounding area with a small amount of lidocaine, the lesion is shaved from the skin, with the scalpel held parallel to the skin.

TABLE 14–10. THE ABCD OF MALIGNANT MELANOMA

A—Asymmetry (rather than round or oval)
B—Border irregularity
C—Color variation (change in color or different colors within the lesion)
D—Diameter (large nevus, greater than 1 cm in diameter)

Shave biopsies are useful in the management of superficial, elevated lesions.

Electrodessication and curettage are useful for small tumors (2 cm or less in size). This procedure involves anesthetizing the area locally prior to beginning the procedure and using a curette to scoop out the lesion. An electrode is then used in contact with the skin to create tissue charring and control hemostasis.

Mohs' microscopic surgery is another technique used for certain types of skin tumors. Tumors that are poorly differentiated or with poorly demarcated borders, tumors that are of long duration, or tumors situated where it is important to preserve as much healthy tissue as possible are good candidates for Mohs' surgery. The procedure involves removing tissue in horizontal layers. The procedure is repeated until a tumor-free plane is reached.

Surgical excision involves removing the entire lesion with at least a 1/2- to 1-cm elliptical margin around the lesion. Complete surgical excision is the only recommended means of management for melanoma. The pathologist reports the depth of the lesion by both the Breslow and the Clark methods. The Breslow method is based on the millimeter depth of the lesion, whereas the Clark method is based on the depth of the lesion with respect to which layer of the skin or subcutaneous tissue is involved. The melanoma is then staged, based on whether the

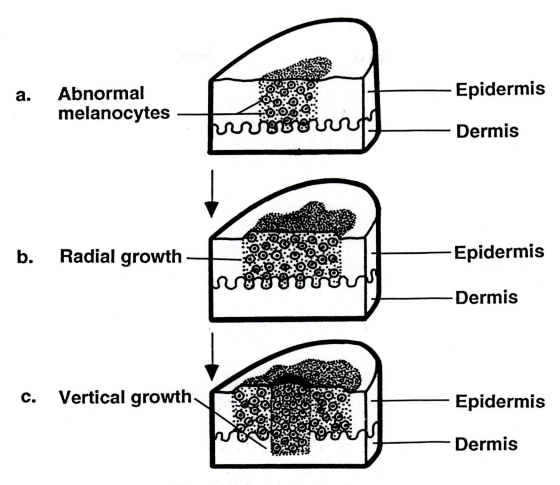

a. **Abnormal melanocytes** — Epidermis — Dermis

b. **Radial growth** — Epidermis — Dermis

c. **Vertical growth** — Epidermis — Dermis

Figure 14–9. Growth phase of a melanoma

lesion is localized, whether there is regional lymph node involvement, or whether evidence of distant metastasis is present.

Radiation therapy is also sometimes used in the treatment of BCC and SCC if the patient is a poor surgical candidate or when preservation of surrounding tissue is of vital importance.[14]

Life-style Changes

Prevention of skin cancer can be accomplished through regular screening and, most importantly, through avoidance of UV radiation exposure. Patients should be taught how to recognize potentially cancerous lesions and to do self-examination on a regular basis. Primary care providers should make a complete skin examination part of routine well care check-ups.

Patients with skin types I through IV should be encouraged to regularly use preventive measures that minimize UV radiation exposure such as sunscreens and protective clothing.

Many brands of sunscreens are now available. Patients should be told to use a sunscreen that provides both UVA and UVB radiation protection. Ideally, it should be applied 30 minutes prior to sun exposure and reapplied frequently when sweating or swimming. Waterproof sunscreens are also now available and do not need to be reapplied as often. A sunscreen with a minimum sun protective factor (SPF) of 15 should be used. Some dermatologists recommend using a sunscreen with an SPF of 25 to 30 on the face. Parents of young children should be taught to apply sunscreen whenever sun exposure will occur. Direct sun exposure between the hours of 10:00 AM and 2:00 PM should be avoided as much as possible.

Patients should be cautioned regarding the use of the popular tanning beds. Today's tanning beds are designed to provide UVA exposure rather than UVB. The belief was previously held that UVB radiation was carcinogenic and UVA was not. It is now thought that UVA penetrates more deeply and po-

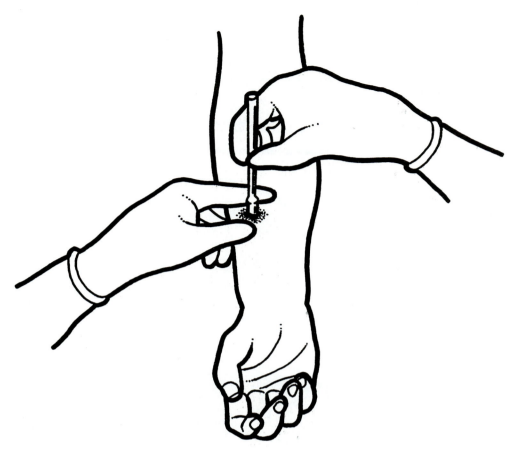

Figure 14–10. A. Punch Biopsy. Punch is placed perpendicular to the skin and advanced with moderate pressure while rotating it back and forth between thumb and forefinger.

tentiates the effects of UVB radiation. The effects of the two are cumulative.

If a tan is necessary, bronzing gels are available that provide the appearance of a tan. The effect is both safe and immediate. Through adequate screening, early recognition, and education regarding prevention, the incidence and the morbidity and mortality resulting from skin cancer can be decreased.[15–17]

References

1. Harvey JC, Beattie EJ. Clinical symposia. *Lung Cancer*. 1993; 45(3):2–32.
2. Stauffer, JL. Pulmonary diseases. *Current Medical Diagnosis & Treatment*. Tierney LM, McPhee SJ, Papadakis MA (eds). Norwalk, Conn: Appleton & Lange; 1994;241–250.
3. Cancer statistics 1994. *CA: Cancer J Clin*. 1994;44(1):7–60.
4. Women's health issues and the Physician Assistant; cancer detection and treatment. Presented at the Third Annual National Satellite Videoconference for Veterans Administration and Dept. of Defense Physician Assistants; April 27, 1994; Dept. of Veterans Affairs, Durham Regional Medical Education Center, Durham, NC
5. Stereotactic breast biopsy. *CA: Cancer J Clin*. 1994;44(3):172–189.
6. *Healthy People 2000: National Health Promotion and Disease Prevention Objectives*. Washington, DC: US Government Printing Office; 1990. US Dept of Health and Human Services publication PHS 91-50212.
7. Tanagho EA, McAninch JW. *General Urology*. Englewood Cliffs, NJ: Prentice-Hall Inc; 1992.
8. Prostate cancer. *CA Cancer J Clin*. 1994;45(3):134–176.
9. Browder JF. Photoaging: cosmetic effects of sun damage. *Postgrad Med*. 1993;93(8):75–92.
10. Habif TP. Nevi and malignant melanoma. In: *Clinical Dermatology: A Color Guide to Diagnosis and Therapy*. 2nd ed. St Louis, Mo: CV Mosby Co; 1990;551–580.
11. Hunter JA, Savin JA, Dahl MV. Skin tumours. In: *Clinical Dermatology*. Oxford, England: Blackwell Scientific Publications; 1989;180–211.
12. Habif TP. Premalignant and malignant skin tumors. In: *Clinical Dermatology: A Color Guide to Diagnosis and*

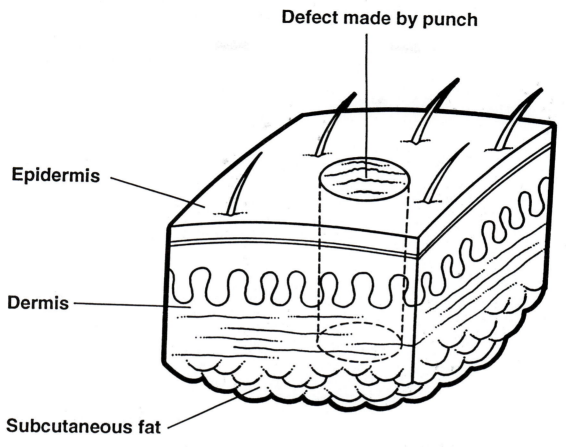

Defect made by punch

Epidermis

Dermis

Subcutaneous fat

Figure 14–10. B. Cross sectional view of punch biopsy site.

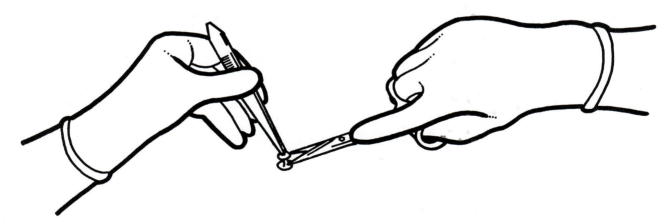

Figure 14–10. C. Specimen is lifted with tissue forceps and pedicle clipped with iris scissors to free.

Therapy. 2nd ed. St. Louis, Mo: CV Mosby Co; 1990:519–549

13. Hacker SM, Flowers FP. Squamous cell carcinoma of the skin: will heightened awareness of risk factors slow its increase? *Postgrad Med*. 1993;93(8):115–126.

14. Hacker SM, Browder JF, Ramos-Caro FA. Basal cell carcinoma: choosing the best method of treatment for a particular lesion. *Postgrad Med*. 1993;93(8):108–111.

15. McGrann J. (1994). Saving their skins: diagnosis, management and preventing skin cancer. *Advance, PA*. 1992;2(5):10–12.

16. Muglia JJ, McDonald CJ. Skin cancer screening: the PA's role in early diagnosis. *Physician Assist*. 1994;18(1):21–32.

17. Shenefelt PD. Cancer epidemiology, prevention and screening. In: Herold AH, ed. *Primary Care*. Philadelphia, Pa: WB Saunders Co; 1992;19:557–573.

15

Obstetrics and Gynecology

Teresa A. Newman
Marvis J. Lary

■ PREGNANCY

General Characteristics

Pregnancy is the most common cause of amenorrhea in women of childbearing age. Ideally, all women should have preconception care before pregnancy, although this usually does not happen. All women should be encouraged to obtain prenatal care soon after pregnancy is documented.

Sign, Symptoms, and Diagnosis

Fatigue is the universal symptom of pregnancy.[1] Women may also complain of nausea, vomiting, breast tenderness and engorgement, or urinary frequency without dysuria.

There are presumptive, probable, and possible signs of pregnancy (Table 15–1).[1] Some of these signs may also be seen in conditions other than pregnancy. While a pregnancy test is used to diagnose pregnancy, a positive test does not mean there is a viable pregnancy. Pregnancy tests can be positive with a molar pregnancy (hydatidiform mole), missed abortions, and tumors.

Management

A thorough history and physical should be performed on the first prenatal visit with particular attention to previous pregnancies, family history, and any complaints with the current pregnancy. If the patient has any risk factors (eg, 35 years and older or 16 years and younger), closer follow-up is necessary.

Prenatal laboratory specimens (Table 15–2) should be drawn on the first visit as well as a Pap smear and gonorrhea

TABLE 15–1. SIGNS OF PREGNANCY

Presumptive Signs of Pregnancy
- Bluish discoloration of the vulva, vagina, and cervix (Chadwick's sign)
- Dark line down the midline of the lower abdomen (linea nigra)
- Dark pigmentation under the eyes and over the nose (chloasma)

Probable Signs of Pregnancy
- Uterine enlargement
- The palpable connection between the cervix and the fundus as the uterus begins to soften (Hegar's sign)
- Ballottement of the fetus
- Palpable uterine contractions
- Positive pregnancy test

Positive Signs of Pregnancy
- Fetal heart tones, which may be heard with Doppler as early as 10 wk
- Palpable fetal movement

TABLE 15–2. PRENATAL LABORATORY TESTS PERFORMED ON FIRST VISIT

Complete blood count
Rh factor, blood type, and antibody screen
Rubella titer
Serologic test for syphilis
Complete urinalysis
Hepatitis B surface antigen
Pap smear
Gonorrhea culture of the cervix
Chlamydia culture of the cervix
Sickle cell screen (if indicated)
Urine drug screen (if indicated and with consent)
HIV testing (if indicated and with consent)
Diabetes screening before 24 wk if patient has risk factors

and chlamydia cultures taken of the cervix.[1] At approximately 16 weeks, an alpha-fetoprotein (AFP) blood test should be offered to evaluate for spinal deformities such as spina bifida. Diabetes screening should be performed on every pregnant woman between 24 and 28 weeks. If the patient has any risk factors for diabetes, screening should be done on the first visit.[1]

The patient should be instructed to take prenatal vitamins daily. Danger signals (Table 15–3) should be reviewed with the patient. She should be instructed to notify the clinician if she develops any of these complaints.

Return appointments should occur once a month until the patient is at 28 weeks, then every 2 weeks until she is at 36 weeks, and every week thereafter. If birth is past due, further assessment of the fetus is necessary. A nonstress test and ultrasound should be ordered if the birth is past due. Return appointments usually include an assessment of blood pressure, weight, urine evaluation for protein and glucose, fundal height, and fetal heart tones. The patient should be asked if there are any discomforts or concerns. Specific attention should be paid to danger signals (Table 15–3).

TABLE 15–3. PREGNANCY DANGER SIGNALS

Vaginal bleeding
Vaginal leaking of fluid
Severe abdominal pain
Edema of the face and hands or persistent edema of the feet and ankles
Severe headache not relieved with acetaminophen
Decreased fetal movement
Significant change in well-being

■ VAGINITIS

General Characteristics

Nearly every woman at some time in her life experiences a vaginal infection. During pregnancy and at midcycle there is an increase in vaginal secretions of cervical mucus, exudates from Bartholin's and Skene's glands, and transudates from the vaginal squamous epithelium and exfoliated squamous cells.[2] This normal vaginal discharge has no odor, but some women may mistake this for a vaginal infection.

Most vaginal infections are caused by bacteria (bacterial vaginosis, nonspecific vaginitis), fungi (candidiasis), and protozoa (*Trichomonas vaginalis*).[2,3] However, the clinician should always keep sexually transmitted diseases in the differential diagnosis when the chief complaint is vaginal discharge.

Signs, Symptoms, and Diagnosis

When taking a history, the clinician must remember to ask about hygiene and sexual practices along with the characteristics of the discharge (amount, color, odor, and character).[2,3] The patient may or may not be able to describe the characteristics, but she should be able to remember if she has changed soaps, detergents, fabric softeners, and perfumes that could be a secondary irritant when they come in contact with vaginal secretions. She may also complain of vaginal or vulvar itching and burning.

On physical examination of the vulva and vagina, the clinician should note any erythema, edema, or petechiae. The most important part of the examination for vaginal infections is the microscopic examination. A sample of the discharge should be taken from the vagina with a cotton-tipped applicator and suspended in 2 mL of normal saline.[2] A small amount of this solution should be placed on a glass slide, covered with a coverslip, and examined under the microscope. If fungi, such as *Candida*, are suspected, the clinician should place a small amount of 10% to 20% potassium hydroxide on a glass slide with the vaginal discharge and examine under the microscope looking for hyphae and spores.[2] Risk factors for developing candidiasis include pregnancy, oral contraceptive use, antibiotic use, and diabetes. Table 15–4 shows the differences among the three most common vaginal infections.

Management

The management of bacterial vaginosis is oral metronidazole 500 mg twice daily for 7 days (Table 15–5).[2,3] Clindamycin 300 mg twice daily for 7 days and tetracycline 500 mg four times daily for 7 days may also be used but not in pregnancy or for nursing mothers. Metronidazole is classified as a Pregnancy Category B drug in the 1995 *Physicians' Desk Reference* and should not be used in the first trimester and with caution in the second and third trimester. Nursing mothers should not use metronidazole unless they stop nursing during the treatment. During pregnancy, ampicillin 500 mg four times a day for 7 days may be used. Since bacterial vaginosis may be sexually transmitted, the patient's partner(s) should also be treated in the same manner.[2,3] When taking metronidazole, the patient should abstain from alcohol, since the drug acts like disulfiram.

TABLE 15–4. DIFFERENTIAL DIAGNOSIS OF VAGINITIS

Characteristic	Bacterial Vaginosis	Candidiasis	Trichomonas
Discharge			
Amount	moderate	variable	moderate
Color	gray-white	white	yellow-green
Odor	fishy	none	slight
Character	thin	thick, curdy	frothy
Symptoms			
Itching	none	moderate–severe	none–severe
Burning	none–slight	slight–severe	slight
Physical Exam			
Erythema	none	moderate–severe	slight–severe
Petechiae	none	none	on cervix
Microscopic	Clue cells	Hyphae with hydroxide potassium	*Trichomonas*

TABLE 15–5. SELECTED MEDICATIONS FOR VAGINITIS

Medication	Dosage	Side Effects
Flagyl (metronidazole)	*Bacterial vaginosis*, 500 mg bid for 7 days. *Trichomonas*, 2 grams orally one day therapy, or 250 mg tid for 7 days.	Seizures, peripheral neuropathy, leukopenia, nausea, vomiting with alcohol ingestion, headache, anorexia, diarrhea, cramps, constipation, metallic taste, rash, dysuria, dyspareunia, joint pain.
Sumycin (tetracycline)	500 mg qid for 7 days (bacterial vaginosis).	Nausea, dizziness, rash, blood dyscrasias, superinfection, pseudotumor cerebri, photosensitivity, increased BUN, hepatotoxicity.
Cleocin (clindamycin)	300 mg bid for seven days (bacterial vaginosis).	Pseudomembranous colitis, diarrhea, GI upset, rash, anaphylaxis, jaundice, renal dysfunction, blood dyscrasias, polyarthritis, superinfection.
Omnipen (ampicillin)	500 mg qid for seven days (bacterial vaginosis).	Superinfection, anaphylaxis, urticaria, GI upset, blood dyscrasias.
Gyne-Lotrimin (clotrimazole 1% cream)	1 insert vaginally at bedtime for 7 days (fungal vaginitis).	Vaginal itching, irritation, rash, abdominal cramps, bloating, urinary frequency, dyspareunia.
Diflucan (fluconazole)	150 mg orally once (fungal vaginitis).	GI upset, headache, dizziness; hepatotoxicity (rare).

Candidiasis, also known as monilia and yeast, may be managed with topical antifungal agents: miconazole, clotrimazole, butoconazole, or terconozole used vaginally for 3 to 14 days.[2,3] Patients who have frequent recurrences should be evaluated for diabetes and immunosuppression if they are not using oral contraceptives or antibiotics. Prophylactic treatment for candidiasis should be considered if an antibiotic is given to women susceptible to candidiasis.

Management of *Trichomonas* vaginitis consists of oral metronidazole, which may be given as a 1-day therapy in a 2 g dose or 1 g in the morning and 1 g at bedtime, or as 250 mg three times daily for 7 days.[2,3] All the same precautions should be used as for bacterial vaginosis when the patient is pregnant.

■ MENOPAUSE

General Characteristics

Menopause is the cessation of menses, or the last menstrual period in a woman's life. The transitional period between ovulatory cycles and the menopause, during which progressive loss of ovarian function occurs, is known as the climacteric, or perimenopausal period. The term *postmenopausal* or *menopausal* refers to the time after the menopause. During this time, a woman usually experiences various endocrine, somatic, and psychologic changes.

The median age at menopause is 50 to 51 years, and the average life expectancy of women in the United States at birth is 79 years; therefore, approximately one third of a woman's life is spent after menopause. The average age at menopause does not appear to be related to the age at menarche, social or economic conditions, race, parity, height, or weight. The age at menopause may be affected by smoking, however. Cigarette smokers experience earlier spontaneous menopause than do nonsmokers.[4,5]

Signs, Symptoms, and Diagnosis

Soon after an adolescent woman has her first menstrual cycle, regular, predictable menstrual cycles are established and continue until about 40 years of age. At around age 40, the number of ovarian follicles becomes substantially depleted and subtle changes occur in the frequency and length of menstrual cycles. The frequency of ovulation decreases gradually over a period of years prior to menopause. As the changes in the reproductive cycle take place, there are concomitant changes in the plasma concentration of follicle-stimulating hormone (FSH) and luteinizing hormone (LH). During the perimenopausal years, women begin to experience signs and symptoms of estrogen deficiency (Fig. 15–1).[4,5]

Although there is a wide variation of symptoms among women, the hot flash is usually the first physical manifestation of ovarian failure, occurring in over 95% of women during the perimenopausal and menopausal years. Hot flashes may be accompanied by diaphoresis, especially at night. Estrogen replacement will resolve hot flashes within 3 to 6 weeks or if left untreated, hot flashes will usually resolve spontaneously within 2 to 3 years. Other signs and symptoms of menopause include sleep disturbances, vaginal dryness and genital tract atrophy, and mood changes. Estrogen deficiency also causes thinning of the skin, hair shedding, and changes in nail texture. Coronary artery disease becomes a greater risk to women as estrogen levels decrease. Prior to menopause, women have significantly lower incidence of cardiovascular disease than do men; however, after menopause, women have the same risk factors as men unless they receive estrogen replacement.[4–6]

Osteoporosis is the most important health hazard associated with menopause. If left untreated, osteoporosis is one of the most devastating diseases of aged women. Estrogen deficiency is believed to be the major cause of bone loss in women. Bone loss after menopause appears to proceed at a rate of 1% to 2% per year.[4] Refer to Chapter 17 for further information on osteoporosis.

Management

Because the signs and symptoms of menopause result from declining estrogen production, estrogen replacement therapy obviates most of these changes. Before implementation of estrogen replacement, each woman must be evaluated, with careful consideration given to her age, health status, current symptoms, past medical and family history. Contraindications to estrogen replacement must be ruled out. They include undiagnosed vaginal bleeding, certain types of carcinoma of the breast, thromboembolic disease, and metastatic endometrial carcinoma.

There are a number of estrogen preparations available through various routes of administration, including oral, transdermal, transbuccal, transvaginal, and parenteral (Table 15–6). Although there are a number of regimens used for estrogen replacement, the two primary ones are unopposed estrogen and estrogen with cyclic progestin. Dosages of estrogen range from 0.3 mg to 2.5 mg daily and may be taken continuously or cyclically. The minimal dosage to maintain bone mass has been determined to be 0.625 mg daily. Progestin may be given only 10 days each month in doses of 5 to 10 mg or may be given in smaller doses of 2.5 mg every day. Health care providers must decide which treatment regimen and route of administration is most appropriate for each of their menopausal patients. It cannot be assumed that all women can be treated the same way.[4–7]

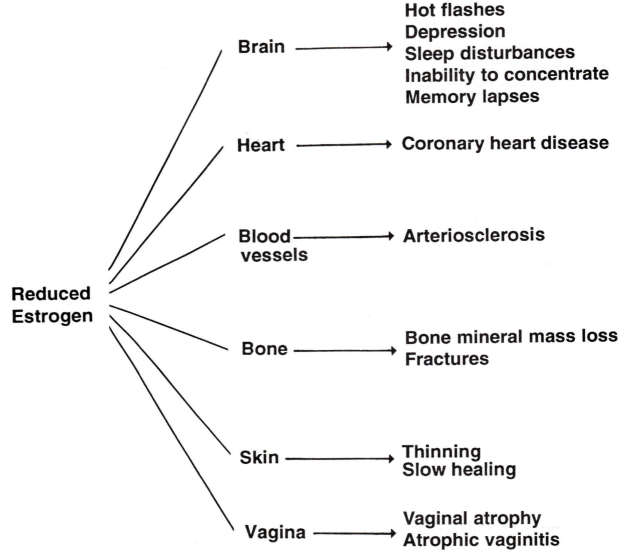

Figure 15–1. Effects of reduced estrogen levels on various target tissues and their clinical manifestations in the postmenopausal woman

Menopausal women must be encouraged to have regular Pap smears and mammograms and to practice a healthy life-style with attention given to diet (including calcium intake), exercise, and a positive outlook on life.

Life-style Changes
Menopause signals the presence of midlife. This in itself can cause some women to feel depressed or "old." Menopause occurs in a women's life when many women are experiencing a number of other significant changes, such as children leaving home or perhaps health problems for themselves or a mate. Life-style changes are not directly related to menopause as much as to other changes that take place for women in midlife.

The "ease" with which women pass through the perimenopausal period is reflective of the individual's general health and overall satisfaction with other components of life. Menopause should be thought of as a normal physiologic function in a woman's life cycle rather than a pathologic event to be dreaded.

TABLE 15–6. SELECTED MENOPAUSAL MEDICATIONS

Medication	Dosage	Side Effects
Estraderm (estrogen patch)	initially one 0.05 mg/day patch twice a week applied to trunk (avoid breasts and waistline). Maintenance: administer cyclically (3 wks on, 1 wk off).	Increased risk of endometrial cancer or hyperplasia, gallbladder disease, thromboembolic disorders, hepatic tumors. Irritation at application site, fluid retention, breakthrough bleeding, mastodynia, nausea, abdominal cramps, headache, migraine, dizziness, intolerance to contact lenses, increased size of uterine fibromyomata.
Ogen (estrogen vaginal cream)	0.625–5 mg daily, given cyclically (3 wks on, 1 wk off).	Nausea, vomiting, breakthrough bleeding, edema, weight changes, swollen and tender breasts, hypertension, mental depression, intolerance to contact lenses, hair loss or hirsuitism, changes in libido, increased size of uterine fibromyomata, chloasma. Increased risk of estrogen-dependent carcinoma, gallbladder disease, thromboembolic disorders, hepatic tumors.
Estratab (estrogen tablets)	Given cyclically (3 wks on, 1 wk off). Menopausal symptoms: 0.625–2.5 mg daily.	GI upset, dysmenorrhea, breakthrough bleeding, migraine, edema, swollen and tender breasts, mental depression, changes in libido and weight, hypertension.
Depo Estradiol	1 cc IM every 30 days	Dysmenorrhea, breakthrough bleeding, migraine, edema, swollen and tender breasts, mental depression, changes in libido and weight, hypertension.

Reference

1. Hacker NF, Moore JG, eds. *Essentials of Obstetrics and Gynecology*. 2nd ed. Philadelphia, Pa: WB Saunders Co; 1992: 12–87.

2. Gunning J. Vaginal and vulvar infections. In: Hacker NF and Moore JG, eds. *Essentials of Obstetrics and Gynecology*. 2nd ed. Philadelphia, Pa: WB Saunders Co; 1992:377–380.

3. Beckmann CRB, Ling FW, Barzansky BM, et al. *Obstetrics and Gynecology for Medical Students*. Baltimore, Md: Williams & Wilkins; 1992:263–267.

4. Beckmann CRB, Ling FW, Barzansky BM et al. Menopause. In: *Obstetrics and Gynecology for Medical Students*. Baltimore, Md: Williams & Wilkins; 1992;343–348.

5. Clarke-Pearson DL, Dawood MY. Menopause. In: *Green's Gynecology*. Boston, Mass: Little Brown & Co Inc; 1990:457–471.

6. Gant NF, Cunningham GF. Menopause. Estrogen replacement. In: *Basic Gynecology & Obstetrics*. Norwalk, Conn: Appleton & Lange; 1993:192–195.

7. Andreoli TE, Bennett JC, Carpenter CJ. Female endocrinology. In: *Cecil Essentials of Medicine*. Philadelphia, Pa: WB Saunders Co; 1993:493–501.

16

Infectious Diseases

Tammy Becker
Sandee Roquemore

■ SEXUALLY TRANSMITTED DISEASES

Sexually transmitted diseases (STDs) are diseases that are primarily transmitted through sexual contact. They can also be transmitted to the fetus during pregnancy or at delivery. The term *sexually transmitted disease* can be used to describe any of more than 20 different disease entities. Five of these, gonorrhea, chlamydia, syphilis, genital herpes, and condyloma, are discussed here (Table 16–1).

■ *Gonorrhea*

General Characteristics

Gonorrhea is a reportable sexually transmitted disease caused by *Neisseria gonorrhoeae*. Infection may occur at any mucosal site. The most prevalent sites of infection are the cervix in women, and the urethra in men. However, infection can also occur in the rectum, pharynx, or conjunctiva.

Signs, Symptoms, and Diagnosis

Signs and symptoms may differ in men and women. Men commonly present with urethritis, causing dysuria and purulent penile discharge. Symptoms generally appear 2 to 7 days after exposure. If symptoms are left untreated in men, epididymitis may develop, causing unilateral scrotal pain. Anorectal gonorrhea may present with rectal discharge, pain, or tenesmus (spasmodic contraction of the anal sphincter).[1] This is a common presentation in homosexual men.

The female patient may be totally asymptomatic. If symptoms are present, they may include vaginal discharge, genital itching, or dysuria. The major complication associated with untreated gonorrhea in women is pelvic inflammatory disease (PID), resulting from the ascent of *N. gonorrhoeae* to the upper genital tract. Signs and symptoms of PID may include fever, vaginal discharge, abdominal tenderness to palpation, and adnexal tenderness.[1]

Neonatal gonococcal ophthalmia may be present in infants born to infected mothers. Conjunctival infection may produce a purulent conjunctivitis, appearing 2 to 5 days after delivery. Ocular complications may spread locally or systemically.[2]

Diagnosis is made by a Gram's stain examination of the discharge. A gonococcal culture can be obtained from any mucosal site suspected to be involved. At the present time, serologic testing for gonorrhea cannot differentiate past from present infection. Every patient suspected of having gonorrhea should have serologic testing for syphilis and a culture obtained for chlamydia.

Management

The treatment of choice for uncomplicated gonorrhea is ceftriaxone plus doxycycline (Table 16–2). Doxycycline is used because coinfection with chlamydia is common. Neonatal gonococcal ophthalmia should be treated with intravenous aqueous crystalline penicillin G for 7 days.[3] The most common cause of treatment failure is repeated exposure by the asymptomatic partner; therefore partners should also be treated. Posttreatment cultures should be obtained to confirm treatment response.

TABLE 16–1. COMMON SEXUALLY TRANSMITTED DISEASES

Clinical Syndrome	Infectious Agent	Microscopic Examination	Incubation Period
Gonorrhea	*Neisseria gonorrhoeae*	gram (−) negative intracellular diplococcus	2–7 d
Syphilis	*Treponema pallidum*	spirochete	weeks to months
Herpes	Herpes simplex virus (HSV)	multinucleated giant cell	2–20 d
Chlamydia	*Chlamydia trachomatis*	obligate intracellular bacteria	1–3 wk
Condyloma	Human papilloma virus (HPV)	noncapsulated DNA viruses	months to years

TABLE 16–2. CDC RECOMMENDATIONS FOR THE TREATMENT OF SEXUALLY TRANSMITTED DISEASES

Clinical Syndrome	Recommended Therapy		Pregnancy
	Drug of Choice	*Other Choices*	
Gonorrhea	Ceftriaxone 125 mg IM plus doxy-cycline 100 mg PO bid × 7 d	Ciprofloxacin 500 mg PO single dose or spectinomycin 2.0 g IM or cefixime 400 mg PO single dose or ofloxacin 400 mg PO single dose. Doxycycline 100 mg PO bid × 7 d should be given in addition to the above.	Pregnant women should use ceftriaxone 125 mg IM plus ery-thromycin base 500 mg PO qid × 7 d
Chlamydia	Doxycycline 100 mg PO bid × 7 d or Azithromycin (Zithromax) 1.0 g PO single dose	Erythromycin base 500 mg PO qid × 7 d or erythromycin ethyl-succinate 800 mg qid × 7 d or ofloxacin 300 mg bid × 7 d or sulfisoxazole 500 mg qid × 10 d (inferior to other regimens)	Pregnant women should use ery-thromycin base 250 mg PO qid × 14 d or erythromycin ethyl-succinate 800 mg PO qid × 7 d or amoxicillin 500 mg tid × 7 d (if erythromycin ethylsucci-nate can't be tolerated)
Genital herpes (HSV)	Acylovir (Zovirax) 200 mg PO 5×/d × 7–10 d	Herpes resistant to acyclovir: fos-carnet 40 mg/kg IV (infuse over 2 hr) q 8 h × 21 d	Acyclovir has not been adequately tested in pregnant or lactating women
Condyloma acuminatum	Podophyllin in tincture of benzoin applied topically wkly × 4 wk	Interferon-alfa 2-b 1.0 million u into lesions 3 ×/wk × 3 wk or cryotherapy with liquid nitrogen or electrocautery or trichloro-acetic acid (TCA) or podofilox applied bid × 3 d	Cervical warts should not be treated until Pap smear results are available. Avoid therapy with podophyllin and podofilox during pregnancy.
Syphilis	Early primary, secondary, latent <1 yr: penicillin G benzathine 2.4 million u IM. >1 yr: penicillin G benzathine IM q wk × 3	Doxycycline 100 mg bid × 2 wk or tetracycline 500 mg qid × 2 wk	There is no alternative therapy to penicillin during pregnancy; if allergic, hospitalize for de-sensitization
Symptomatic neurosyphilis	Aqueous crystalline penicillin 2–4 million u IV q 4 h × 10–14 d	Penicillin G procaine 2.4 million u IM daily × 10–14 d plus probenecid 500 mg PO qid × 10–14 d	There is no alternative therapy to penicillin during pregnancy; if allergic, hospitalize for de-sensitization.

From MMWR.[5]

bid, twice a day; IM, intramuscularly; IV, intraveous; PO, by mouth; qid, four times a day; tid, three times a day.

■ *Chlamydia*

General Characteristics

Chlamydia is the most common sexually transmitted bacterial infection. It is caused by *Chlamydia trachomatis*, an intracellular bacterium. Incubation period is estimated at 1 to 3 weeks in men. Because women are often asymptomatic, the incubation period is difficult to assess.[1] Untreated chlamydial infections can persist for years.

Signs, Symptoms, and Diagnosis

Like gonorrhea, chlamydial infection is often asymptomatic. The man with chlamydia will usually present with urethritis; however, proctitis is also possible if the patient has participated in receptive anorectal intercourse. Chlamydia, or nongonococcal urethritis (NGU), is characterized by pyuria, mucopurulent penile discharge, dysuria, urinary frequency, and urethral pruritus. Ascending infections can occur if the condition is left untreated.[1]

The cervix is the most common site of infection in women. Approximately 70% of female patients are asymptomatic. Mucopurulent endocervical discharge, friability of the cervix (bleeding induced easily), and cervical edema may be present.[1] Because of its asymptomatic nature, chlamydia may be left untreated, which can lead to infertility resulting from tubal scarring.

Conjunctivitis and pneumonitis are the most common clinical manifestations in neonates infected with chlamydia. Purulent conjunctivitis presents 5 to 12 days after delivery. Pneumonitis may present with cough, congestion, tachypnea, and rales. The patient is usually afebrile.[2]

Culture is necessary to make the diagnosis of chlamydial infection. Tissue cultures are obtained from mucosal secretions, which are then inoculated on a special medium in the laboratory. Serologic testing is of little value at the present time.

Management

The most widely accepted treatment for chlamydia is doxycycline, with erythromycin being the drug of choice for allergic patients (Table 16–2). Sexual partners should also be treated. Oral erythromycin in four divided doses for 14 days is recommended in infants with chlamydial conjunctivitis or pneumonitis.[3] Posttreatment cultures should also be obtained to confirm treatment response.

■ *Syphilis*

General Characteristics

Syphilis is an STD caused by *Treponema pallidum*. It is capable of infecting virtually any organ system in the body. The infection enters through minor skin or mucosal lesions and becomes a systemic disease shortly after infection. Incubation period is approximately 10 to 90 days after exposure.[4] Syphilis is divided into four stages: primary, secondary, latent, and tertiary syphilis. It is during the latent stage that a patient will be seropositive but demonstrate no clinical manifestations.

Signs, Symptoms, and Diagnosis

Primary syphilis usually presents with a painless ulceration known as a chancre (Fig. 16–1). There is generally lymphadenopathy associated with the primary lesion. The chancre is most often located in the genital area but may also appear on the oropharynx, anorectal area, breast, or fingers. It appears as a superficial ulceration with indurated margins.[4] Healing will occur without therapy, and the disease therefore may go undetected.

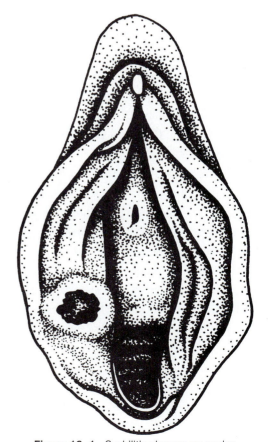

Figure 16–1. Syphilitic chancre on vagina

Secondary syphilis generally presents as a diffuse maculopapular rash with constitutional symptoms, weeks to months after the primary lesion has healed. Classic presentation involves the soles and palms. Lesions may also be present on mucosal membranes.

Latent syphilis may develop after resolution of the secondary lesions. In this stage there are no clinical signs or symptoms, and can go undetected for many years.

Tertiary syphilis can develop when latent syphilis is left untreated. Virtually any organ system may be involved. When the cardiovascular system becomes involved, the outcome can be fatal. Lesions may develop on the aorta resulting in aneurysm. If neurologic manifestations are present, neurosyphilis should be ruled out.

Syphilis during pregnancy most commonly results in spontaneous abortion. Successfully completed pregnancies are complicated by prematurity or intrauterine growth retardation (IUGR). Early congenital syphilis may present with rhinitis, pneumonia, or failure to thrive, usually beginning within the first 3 months. Nasal discharge becomes thick and even hemorrhagic. Like adult syphilis, congenital syphilis can affect multiple organ systems.[2]

Diagnosis of syphilis can be made through serologic testing. There are two major types of tests available. Direct methods include the fluorescent treponemal antibody absorption (FTA-ABS) and the microhemagglutination assay for antibodies to *T. pallidum* (MHA-TP). Indirect methods include the rapid plasma reagin (RPR) and the Venereal Disease Research Laboratory (VDRL).[5]

The RPR is the most widely used antibody test for initial screening. It is highly sensitive but has less specificity than the other tests. The FTA-ABS is used for confirmation of disease. Once a diagnosis of syphilis has been established and treatment undertaken, the RPR titer can be repeated to ascertain therapeutic response. If neurosyphilis is suspected, a lumbar puncture should be performed. Indirect testing of the cerebrospinal fluid (CSF) by VDRL is a highly specific means of diagnosing syphilis. The VDRL is the only standard test that can be used with CSF.[5]

Management

The management of syphilis clearly depends on staging. Primary, secondary, or early latent syphilis of less than 1 year's duration require a single intramuscular injection of penicillin G. If the duration of disease is greater than 1 year, three weekly injections of intramuscular penicillin G are required (Table 16–2). With tertiary syphilis, intravenous penicillin is required (Table 16–2). There is no satisfactory alternative therapy to penicillin for the treatment of syphilis in pregnancy. Desensitization is recommended in penicillan allergic pregnant women with syphilis. Penicillin is also used in neonates with syphilis. Serologic tests should be performed at months 3, 6, and 12 to measure response in adults as well as in neonates.[3]

■ Genital Herpes

General Characteristics

Genital herpes is the most common cause of genital ulceration. It is caused by herpes simplex virus (HSV), which can be further differentiated into HSV I and HSV II. Either of these may cause genital disease; however, HSV II is more often the causative agent. The incubation period ranges from 2 to 20 days after exposure.[4] Lesions may appear on the penis (Fig. 16–2), scrotum, anorectal area, labia, vagina, cervix, or oropharynx. The initial herpes infection is usually acquired during sexual contact.

Signs, Symptoms, and Diagnosis

Primary herpes lesions may be associated with fever, headache, malaise, myalgias, arthralgia, and inguinal lymphadenopathy, peaking 3 to 4 days after the onset of lesions. The lesions may appear as groups of vesicles on an erythematous base, which may evolve into pustules and eventually ulcerate.[4] The lesions tend to be painful, and often edema and erythema are present in the surrounding areas. Secondary infection can be a problem in the immunocompromised patient.

After the skin is inoculated with the herpes virus, it then spreads to the peripheral nerve endings and eventually makes its way to the dorsal root ganglia. A persistent but subclinical infection remains at this site. The virus can then reactivate to cause recurrent disease. Recurrent lesions tend to be less painful, with virtually no constitutional symptoms. A prodrome of burning, paresthesias, or itching may be present prior to eruption.[4]

Neonatal HSV is most often symptomatic and can be fatal. It may be localized to the skin, eyes, or mouth; disseminated, involving multiple organ systems; or it may present as encephalitis with or without localized infection. A vesicular

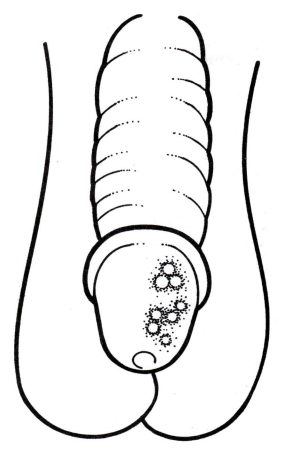

Figure 16–2. Genital herpes

rash is pathognomonic for HSV infection. With disseminated infection or encephalitis, symptoms may include irritability, seizures, poor feeding, respiratory distress, temperature instability, or shock.[2]

Definitive diagnosis can be made by a viral culture of the ulcerated area or from the fluid of a vesicle. The culture should then be transported immediately to the laboratory or stored at 4°C to preserve the virus.[6] Tzanck smear is useful but not as sensitive as culture for a definitive diagnosis. If herpes encephalitis is suspected, a lumbar puncture should be performed. Serologic and other viral cultures should be obtained to rule out other causes of infection.

Management

Herpes simplex is a chronic disease for which there is no cure available. Active lesions are treated with a 10-day course of acyclovir (Zovirax). Recurrent lesions are treated in the same manner. If a patient is prone to numerous recurrences,

maintenance therapy with acyclovir is recommended (Table 16–2).[3]

■ *Condyloma Acuminata*

General Characteristics

Condyloma, or genital warts, is caused by human papilloma virus, or HPV. There are at least 40 different types of HPV. Experts now believe that there are strong associations between the presence of HPV infection and neoplastic disorders. This has been studied for many years in association with cervical or vulvar cancers. Studies are now underway to determine if there is a possible link to carcinoma of the male genital tract and anus.[4]

Signs, Symptoms, and Diagnosis

Condyloma usually present with soft, fleshy growths that may coalesce into large masses (Fig. 16–3). These warty lesions are often characterized as cauliflower lesions because of their flowerlike appearance. The most common sites involved are the vulva, perirectal area, penis, vagina, cervix, urethra, or the oropharynx. These lesions may get so large that they interfere with sexual intercourse, urination, or defecation.

Diagnosis is most often made by physical examination since these lesions are so characteristic; however, occasionally a biopsy is performed to make a definitive diagnosis.

Management

Current treatments available for condyloma acuminatum include cryosurgery with liquid nitrogen, podophyllin applied topically, laser ablation, and interferon applied intralesionally. Although podophyllin continues to be the most popular treatment, lesions tend to recur. Intralesional interferon is undergoing extensive research as treatment for condyloma (Table 16–2).[3]

Life-style Changes for Sexually Transmitted Diseases

STDs can be prevented by modifying sexual behavior. Groups at highest risk for the development of STDs include sexually active adolescents, patients of low socioeconomic status, patients who have had a recent change in sexual partner, patients with multiple sexual partners, and patients who fail to use bar-

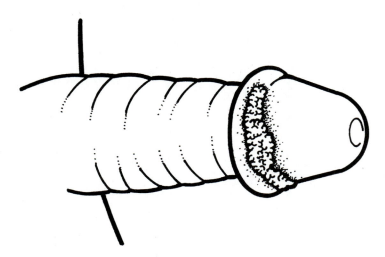

Figure 16–3. Venereal wart

rier methods of contraception (eg, condoms). The use of latex condoms should be encouraged; however, patients should be counseled that they are not 100% effective. Adding a spermaticide containing nonoxynol 9 is thought to render condoms more effective at preventing STDs as well as pregnancy. Abstinence continues to be the best way to prevent STDs.

■ HIV AND AIDS

General Characteristics

Acquired immunodeficiency syndrome (AIDS), was first recognized in 1981 when numbers of homosexual men were diagnosed with *Pneumocystis carinii* pneumonia (PCP). AIDS is the end of a spectrum of diseases caused by the human immunodeficiency virus (HIV). The virus was first isolated in 1985. HIV is a member of the retrovirus family, which means that it replicates in reverse fashion. The viruses in this family use an enzyme, reverse transcriptase, to change their genetic information from RNA to DNA.

HIV can be transmitted through contaminated blood products and clotting factor concentrates, through sexual contact, perinatally from an infected mother to infant, and by needle sharing through injection of intravenous drugs. HIV results in a systemic infection and can be found in a number of body fluids including blood, semen, bone marrow, lymph tissue, vaginal secretions, CSF, stool, tears, urine, sweat, and saliva. Although HIV has been isolated in these body fluids, there is no documentation of transmission of HIV through tears, saliva, or sweat. Once HIV has been transmitted to an individual, it infects helper T lymphocytes (CD4 cells or T4 cells). These cells are specifically in charge of orchestrating the individual's immune system. The immune system is responsible for protecting the body from certain opportunistic infections and neoplasms. Most patients live up to 10 years after initial infection before signs or symptoms of advanced disease are noted.

Signs, Symptoms, and Diagnosis

The symptoms associated with HIV or AIDS are truly dependent upon the stage of the disease. Upon initial exposure to the virus, seroconversion normally takes place within 6 to 12 weeks, although it can take months. Seroconversion is usually associated with a self-limited, mononucleosislike viral illness. Symptoms may include fever, malaise, headache, anorexia, nausea, and generalized lymphadenopathy. Signs associated with initial exposure may be hepatosplenomegaly or oral candidiasis. After the initial illness, most patients live for years without any signs or symptoms of infection. Although the patient may be clinically asymptomatic, the virus may be actively replicating and invading the immune system. During this asymptomatic period, the patient can infect others.

Lymphadenopathy associated with HIV infection may be noted by the patient or during routine physical examination. Persistent generalized lymphadenopathy (PGL) is defined as palpable lymph nodes 1 cm or larger, found in two or more extrainguinal sites, persisting for longer than 3 months. These enlarged nodes must not be attributable to any concurrent illness except HIV infection (Table 16–3).

As the HIV infection progresses, constitutional symptoms such as fever, weight loss, fatigue, diarrhea, night sweats, headaches, and lymphadenopathy may appear intermittently. These symptoms are referred to as AIDS-related complex (ARC). As the immune system becomes further compromised, other signs may appear. These include oral candidiasis, oral hairy leukoplakia, and varicella zoster virus (shingles). Nu-

TABLE 16–3. 1993 REVISED CLASSIFICATION SYSTEM FOR HIV INFECTION AND EXPANDED AIDS SURVEILLANCE DEFINITION FOR ADOLESCENTS AND ADULTS*

CD4 Levels	(A) Symptomatic, Acute (Primary) HIV or PGL†	(B) Symptomatic, Not (A) or (C) Conditions‡	(C) AIDS-Indicator Conditions§
(1) >500	A1	B1	C1*
(2) 200–499	A2	B2	C2*
(3) <200; AIDS indicator T-cell count	A3*	B3*	C3*

PGL, persistent generalized lymphadenopathy.
*C1-3, A3, and B3 illustrate the expanded AIDS surveillance case definition. Persons with AIDS-indicator conditions (categories C1–C3) as well as those with CD4 T-lymphocyte counts less than 200 cells/mm³ (categories A3 and B3) are now reportable as AIDS cases in the US and territories, effective January 1, 1993.
†Clinical category A includes acute (primary) HIV infection.
‡Examples include bacillary angiomatosis, oral candidiasis, vulvovaginal candidiasis, cervical dysplasia, cervical carcinoma in situ, constitutional symptoms or diarrhea lasting longer than 1 month, oral hairy leukoplakia, herpes zoster involving at least two distinct episodes or more than one dermatome, idiopathic thrombocytopenia, listeriosis, pelvic inflammatory disease, peripheral neuropathy.
§See Tables 16–4 and 16–5.
Adapted from the Centers for Disease Control and Prevention. 1993 revised classification system for HIV infection and expanded surveillance case definition for AIDS among adolescents and adults. Morb Mortal Wkly Rep. 1992;41(RR-17):1–19.

merous skin conditions that are associated with HIV infection may develop. These include seborrheic dermatitis, fungal rashes, and a nonspecific, generalized, pruritic, papular rash.

The development of an opportunistic infection is a poor prognostic sign. This signifies further deterioration of the immune system. Opportunistic infections are a selective group of disease processes that only invade when the immune system is no longer capable of protecting the body (Tables 16–4 and 16–5).

Diagnosis of HIV infection is usually made by the detection of antibody to HIV. The most common test used is the enzyme-linked immunosorbent assay (ELISA). If this test is repeatedly reactive, a confirmatory test is performed. The most widely used confirmatory test is the Western Blot. It also detects antibody to HIV. During the acute infection, or seroconversion, standard HIV tests are negative because the virus is present but antibodies have not developed. It may take up to 1 year before antibodies are present and can be detected. During the initial infection, p24 antigen (HIV antigen) may be present and could be used to suggest HIV infection.

The diagnosis of HIV-related illnesses can be facilitated if the clinician has a recent CD4 level. For example, patients with CD4 levels greater than 500 cells/mm^3 are not expected to have any AIDS-defining illnesses. They are, however, susceptible to diseases that any HIV-negative person could have. As the CD4 levels fall below 500 cells/mm^3, certain disease processes should be included in the differential (Tables 16–4 and 16–5). The patient should be evaluated for these disease processes at each clinic visit. Remember that normal and abnormal laboratory values may vary for each laboratory.

The CD4 levels are not only used to help the clinician evaluate for the development of opportunistic infections but also to classify patients into groups designated by the Centers for Disease Control (CDC) (Table 16–3).

Management

The management of a patient with HIV infection is dependent on the status of the patient's immune system. CD4 determinations are an important part of the decision-making process. On initial diagnosis of HIV infection, two CD4 determinations

TABLE 16–4. OPPORTUNISTIC INFECTIONS

Infection	Presenting Symptoms	Diagnosis
Pneumocystis carinii pneumonia (PCP)	fever, cough, shortness of breath (SOB)	chest x-ray demonstrating bilateral interstitial infiltrates; definitive diagnosis: fiberoptic bronchoscopy with bronchoalveolar lavage (BAL)
Histoplasmosis	fever, weight loss, malaise, anemia, thrombocytopenia, neutropenia	fungal culture
Cryptosporidium	watery diarrhea, abdominal cramping	stool examinations
Oral or esophageal candidiasis	dysphagia; odynophagia; characteristic white, cheesy plaques	visual examination; definitive diagnosis: fungal culture
Kaposi's sarcoma	macular, papular, or nodular purplish mucocutaneous lesions	visual examination; definitive diagnosis: biopsy
Herpes zoster (HZV)	painful erythematous, vesicular lesions along a dermatome	visual examination; definitive diagnosis: HZV culture
Cytomegalovirus (CMV) retinitis	visual changes including floaters, scotomata, decreased visual acuity, or blindness	ophthalmoscopic examination demonstrating hemorrhages and perivascular exudates
AIDS wasting	weight loss, anorexia	diagnosis of exclusion; no pathology identified other than HIV infection
Lymphoma	weight loss, night sweats, fever, mass may or may not be noted	biopsy, fine-needle aspiration
Mycobacterium avium complex (MAC)	weight loss, diarrhea, fevers, night sweats	AFB cultures of stool, blood, sputum, and bone marrow; lymph node biopsy
Mycobacterium tuberculosis (MTb)	fever, chills, night sweats, weight loss, cough	AFB cultures of sputum, urine, stool, blood, and bone marrow; chest x-ray may demonstrate cavitary disease or infiltrate; ± PPD

AFB, Acid fast bacillus; PPD, purified protein derivative test.

TABLE 16–5. OPPORTUNISTIC INFECTIONS THAT AFFECT THE CENTRAL NERVOUS SYSTEM

Infection	Presenting Symptoms	Diagnosis
CNS toxoplasmosis	fever, headache, seizures, neurologic deficits	Head CT or MRI demonstrating single or multiple ring enhancing lesions; reactive serum toxoplasmosis titer may or may not be present
Cryptococcal meningitis	fever, headache, meningeal signs may or may not be present	Lumbar puncture with CSF fungal culture; reactive cryptococcal antigen
Progressive multifocal leukoencephalopathy (PML)	mental status changes, neurologic focal deficits	Head MRI demonstrating deep white matter lesions is suggestive; definitive diagnosis requires brain biopsy
AIDS dementia complex (ADC)	cognitive, motor, or behavioral dysfunction	EEG demonstrating diffuse slowing; physical exam: altered mental status exam or abnormal neurologic exam without other pathology
Primary brain lymphoma	focal neurologic deficits, headache, seizures	Definitive diagnosis requires brain biopsy; radiographic findings are variable and may be indistinguishable from toxoplasmosis

CNS, central nervous system, CSF, cerebrospinal fluid; CT, computed tomography; EEG, electroencephalogram; MRI, magnetic resonance imaging.

are obtained fairly close together. If these values are numerically close (within 100 points of each other), they are considered accurate. Studies are currently underway to determine other markers for disease progression. These include p24 antigen and beta$_2$-microglobulin. These markers may prove to be more useful and may in future be used more often than the CD4 levels.

Regardless of the stage of the HIV infection, early intervention is the key to the best management. When a patient's CD4 $\geq$ 500 cells/mm^3, no treatment is needed and the patient need only be seen at 3- to 6-month intervals for determination of CD4 levels and for progression of symptoms. When levels fall below 500 cells/mm^3, the clinician should discuss the treatment options that are available to the patient.

Nucleoside analogues have been studied the most extensively. The nucleoside analogues inhibit reverse transcriptase, the enzyme needed to convert RNA to DNA. Zidovudine, or ZDV, (Retrovir) was the first nucleoside analogue that was approved for the treatment of HIV and AIDS. Zidovudine (ZDV) is also known as azidothymidine, or AZT (Table 16–6). Zidovudine is the drug of choice for initial therapy and is currently offered to asymptomatic or symptomatic patients with CD4 levels $\leq$ 500 cells/mm^3 (Table 16–7). Didanosine (ddi) is considered second-line therapy by most and should be initiated if the patient is failing or intolerant of AZT. Failure means that a patient's CD4 levels decrease by 50% after beginning the therapy or the patient develops an opportunistic infection. Some experts feel that zalcitabine (ddC) is an equally good alternative for second-line therapy. Combinations are used clinically and in treatment trials. Stavudine (D4T) is another nucleoside analogue that has been recently approved. It is also available to patients who are intolerant of conventional therapy. There are a number of other medications and vaccines undergoing clinical trials, although at present none have been approved by the Food and Drug Administration (FDA).

TABLE 16–6. CURRENT ANTIRETROVIRAL THERAPIES

Name	Other Names	Common Dosages	Common Side Effects
Zidovudine	AZT, ZDV, azidothymidine, Retrovir	100 mg PO 5 × daily or 200 mg PO tid	headache, nausea, fatigue, anemia, neutropenia
Didanosine	ddI, dideoxyinosine, Videx	200 mg PO bid (weight-dependent)	pancreatitis, peripheral neuropathy
Zalcitabine	ddC, dideoxycytidine, Hivid	0.75 mg PO tid	pancreatitis, peripheral neuropathy, stomatitis
Stavudine	D4T, Zerit	40 mg PO q 12 hr	Peripheral neuropathy, elevated liver enzymes

bid, twice a day; PO, by mouth; tid, three times a day.

TABLE 16–7. PRIMARY TREATMENT RECOMMENDATIONS DERIVED FROM 1993 CONFERENCE OF THE NATIONAL INSTITUTE OF ALLERGY AND INFECTIOUS DISEASES

Patient Status	CD4 Levels	Recommended Treatment
PATIENTS WITH NO PRIOR AZT THERAPY		
Asymptomatic	≥500 cells/mm^3	continued observation
Asymptomatic	200–500 cells/mm^3	continued observation or AZT 600 mg/d in 3 divided doses
Symptomatic	200–500 cells/mm^3	AZT 600 mg/d in 3 divided doses
Asymptomatic or symptomatic	≤200 cells/mm^3	AZT 600 mg/d in 3 divided doses
PATIENTS TOLERATING AZT MONOTHERAPY		
Clinically stable	≥300 cells/mm^3	continue monotherapy with AZT 600 mg/d in 3 divided doses
Clinically stable	≤300 cells/mm^3	continue monotherapy with AZT 600 mg/d in 3 divided doses or change to ddl 125 mg–300 mg q 12 h depending on weight
PATIENTS FAILING OR INTOLERANT OF AZT		
Symptomatic with clinical failure	50–500 cells/mm^3	change to alternative therapy with either ddl, ddC, or D4T
Clinical failure	≤50 cells/mm^3	change to ddl, ddC, or D4T monotherapy*
Asymptomatic with clinical failure	≥500 cells/mm^3	discontinue AZT and continue observation (no antiretroviral therapy)
Asymptomatic, intolerant of AZT	50–500 cells/mm^3	Alternative monotherapy†
Intolerant to AZT	≤50 cells/mm^3	change to ddl or ddC monotherapy† or observation with no antiretroviral therapy

AZT, zidovudine; ddCyd, dideoxycytidine; DDI, dideoxyinosine.
*Monotherapy is preferred to combination therapy because of increased serious toxicities.
†National Institute of Allergy and Infections Diseases.
Adapted from Sande MA, Carpenter CCJ, Cobbs CG, et al. Antiretroviral Therapy for Adult HIV-Infected Patients: recommendations from a state-of-the-art conference. JAMA. 1993;270:2583-2589.

Prevention and management of opportunistic infections are both important factors in the evaluation of HIV-infected individuals. Prophylaxis for certain opportunistic infections should be initiated at various CD4 levels (Table 16–8). The management of opportunistic infections can be a difficult task for both clinician and patient. Table 16–9 shows current recommended treatment modalities for the most common opportunistic infections and alternative treatment regimens for patients unable to tolerate the treatments of choice.

Life-style Changes

Prevention and control of HIV infection must begin with thorough education. Since more than 93% of all HIV transmission in adults occurs as a result of sexual intercourse and sharing needles for injection of intravenous drugs, education remains the cornerstone of prevention.[7] Individuals should be aware of high-risk behaviors and comply with preventive measures to reduce the risk of transmission. Condoms can be an effective measure in reducing the risk of HIV transmission when used

TABLE 16–8. RECOMMENDED PROPHYLAXIS REGIMENS FOR FIRST EPISODE OF OPPURTUNISTIC DISEASE IN ADULTS AND ADOLESCENTS

Opportunistic Infection	Prophylaxis		Indication
	Treatment of Choice	*Other Choices*	
Pneumocystis carinii pneumonia (PCP)	TMP-SMX DS PO qd	Aerosolized pentamidine monthly or dapsone daily	CD4 < 200 or unexplained fever for > 2 wks, or oropharyngeal candidiasis
Mycobacterium avium complex (MAC)	Rifabutin 300 mg qd	Clarithromycin, azithromycin	CD4 < 75
Toxoplasmosis	TMP-SMX DS PO daily	Pyrimethamine plus dapsone	CD4 < 100 and seropositive for toxoplasmosis
Oral and esophageal candidiasis	*Fluconazole 100–200 mg daily	Ketoconazole	CD4 < 50

bid, twice a day; PO, by mouth; TMP-SMX, trimethoprim-sulfamethoxazole; DS, double strength.
*Fungal prophylaxis is still undergoing clinical trials; may lead to drug resistance in some cases.
Adapted from Centers for Disease Control and Prevention. USPHS/IDSA Guidelines for the Prevention of Opportunistic Infections in Persons Infected with Human Immunodeficiency Virus: A Summary. MMWR, 1995;44:24

TABLE 16–9. RECOMMENDED THERAPY FOR COMMON OPPORTUNISTIC INFECTIONS

Opportunistic Infection	Treatment of Choice	Other Choices
Pneumocystis carinii pneumonia	Po$_2$ < 60: Prednisone taper plus TMP-SMX IV × 21 d Po$_2$ > 60: TMP-SMX DS PO qid × 21 d or atovaquone tid × 21 d	Prednisone taper plus pentamidine IV × 21 d Clindamycin PO q 6 h plus primaquine base PO q d 21 × d
Histoplasmosis	Amphotericin B IV, then maintenance therapy with itraconazole PO	Itraconazole PO bid
Cryptosporidium	No standard therapy is available. Paromomycin PO tid–qid, length of treatment not yet determined Symptomatic therapy with diphenoxylate with atropine (Lomotil), loperamide (Imodium), or paregoric	No alternative therapy
Toxoplasmosis	Sulfadiazine or clindamycin plus pyrimethamine plus leukovorin lifelong all PO	TMP/SMX DS plus pyrimethamine plus leukovorin all PO
Cryptococcal meningitis	Amphotericin B IV × 2 wk then lifelong maintenance therapy with fluconazole PO	Amphotericin B IV × 2 wk then lifelong maintenance therapy with itraconazole†
Mycobacterium avium complex (MAC)	Clarithromycin PO bid plus ciprofloxacin PO bid or ethambutol PO qd	Amikacin IV or azithromycin PO
Oral/esophageal candidiasis	Fluconazole PO	Itraconazole or ketoconazole PO
Cytomegalovirus (CMV) retinitis	Ganciclovir (DHPG) IV bid × 2 wk then daily for lifelong maintenance	Foscarnet IV
Kaposi's sarcoma	Observation; local radiation or chemotherapy (depending on location and severity)	Excision of lesions for cosmetic purposes

bid, twice a day; IV, intravenously; PO, by mouth; qid, four times a day; tid, three times a day; TMP-SMX, trimethoprim-sulfamethoxazole.

†Itraconazole used for maintenance therapy of cryptococcal meningitis is associated with a greater number of relapses.

correctly. Condoms should be stored away from extreme temperatures and sunlight. When opening or handling the condom, care should be taken to avoid puncturing it. The tip of the condom should be free from trapped air and the penis erect prior to placement of the condom. Lubrication, when necessary, should be water-based rather than oil-based to preserve the integrity of the condom. Latex condoms used in combination with a spermicide containing nonoxynol-9 have been proven to be more effective at reducing the risk of HIV transmission.[8] It should be noted that abstinence is the most effective measure of prevention.

Women who have had a hysterectomy or tubal ligation are not at risk for pregnancy, but they are at risk for acquiring an STD or HIV infection if a condom is not used. Any HIV-infected woman of child-bearing potential should be educated on the risk of HIV transmission to the fetus. Recent findings on the use of AZT early in pregnancy revealed a decrease in the risk of perinatal transmission; therefore, all pregnant women should be encouraged to have an HIV test performed.

Adolescents are becoming sexually active at an earlier age; education and prevention must begin before sexual activity begins.

If a patient is using intravenous drugs, education is essential for understanding and preventing transmission. The patient should be encouraged to participate in a drug rehabilitation program. If the patient is not willing to seek help for his or her addiction, he or she needs to be informed of the danger in sharing needles and how to properly dispose of used needles. Cleaning the equipment with bleach should reduce the risk of transmission but it does not guarantee that HIV is inactivated.[8]

If an individual is in a high-risk group, routine HIV testing should be recommended. This will ensure early intervention and allow the patient to prevent transmission to others. Once infected with HIV, the patient should attempt to ensure proper nutrition, adequate rest, and moderation of unhealthy behavior, such as use of alcohol, tobacco, and recreational drugs.

Patients infected with HIV do not need to be isolated from family members or friends; however, personal hygiene items such as razors and toothbrushes should be separated so that they are not inadvertently used by someone else. There is no evidence that HIV can be transmitted by casual contact such as holding hands and hugging. Special precautions should be taken when handling body fluids such as vomitus and diarrhea, however. Bleach and water in equal proportions should be used to clean spilled body fluids to inactivate the virus once it's outside the body. Gloves should always be worn when handling any body fluids.

Once HIV infection occurs, the immune system is no longer capable of fighting certain infections. Two that are of particular interest are toxoplasmosis, which is carried in cat feces, and histoplasmosis, which is carried by domestic and wild birds. Care should be taken when changing litter boxes and when cleaning birdcages. When possible, it is best to let someone else take care of these tasks. Outside the United States, bottled water should be used whenever possible to prevent parasitic intestinal infections. When bottled water is not available, antibiotic prophylaxis can be helpful in preventing certain infections. Proper food storage and preparation will prevent certain intestinal infections as well.

There are many life-style changes associated with HIV infection. Prevention is the most important aspect of this disease. Once a person is infected with HIV, early intervention, good nutritional status, and certain precautions should be taken to live longer with a better quality of life.

References

1. Gorbach SL, Bartlett JG, Blacklow NR, et al. *Infections Diseases*. Philadelphia, Pa: WB Saunders Co; 1992:812–817, 1633–1639.
2. Holmes KK, Mardh PA, Sparling PF, et al. *Sexually Transmitted Diseases*. New York, NY: McGraw-Hill Inc; 1990:821–840, 804–806, 817–818, 872–873.
3. Centers for Disease Control. Recommendations for the treatment of sexually transmitted diseases. *MMWR*. 1993;42(RR-14):23–66.
4. Fitzpatrick TB, Johnson RA, Polano MK, et al. *Color Atlas and Synopsis of Clinical Dermatology*. New York, NY: McGraw-Hill Inc; 1992:379,402–404, 410.
5. Muma RD, Lyons BA, Borucki MJ, et al. *HIV Manual for Health Care Professionals*. Norwalk, Conn: Appleton & Lange; 1994:94.
6. Havens CS, Sullivan ND, Tilton P. *Manual of Outpatient Gynecology*. Boston, Mass: Little Brown & Co Inc; 1986.
7. Muma RD, Lyons BA, Borucki MJ, et al. *HIV Manual for Health Care Professionals*. Norwalk, Conn: Appleton & Lange; 1994:8.
8. Centers for Disease Control. 1993 Sexually Transmitted Diseases Treatment Guidelines. *MMWR*. 1993;42(RR-14):5–6.

17

Musculoskeletal Disorders

Debra D. Davis
J. Dennis Blessing

■ BONE FRACTURE

General Characteristics

The purpose of this discussion is to provide information to be given patients who have sustained a fracture (Fig. 17–1) and are to be followed up after intervention. Outpatient management of fractures is usually done by splint or cast immobilization. Even when properly applied and maintained, casts and splints can pose a threat to the integrity of nerves, arteries, veins, skin, and soft tissues. The problems are usually due to compression from edema or hematoma, the cast or splint, or both. Patient education should be directed toward reducing the risk of complications and identifying complications before irreversible damage occurs.

Signs, Symptoms, and Diagnosis

The signs and symptoms of fracture are pain, deformity, and disability usually secondary to trauma. Vascular and neurologic complications may be present. Diagnosis is by radiologic study.

Management

Edema and hematomas are common developments after injuries. The degree of their development can be limited by proper use of elevation, support, avoidance of weight bearing, and ice. Device compression can occur as casts and splints harden or from inelasticity of supporting and padding materials. Complications can be due to multiple factors.

If aids to ambulation, such as crutches or walkers, are used, instruction in their use will have to be part of patient education. Referral to a physical therapist may be the preferable course. Improper use of crutches or walkers may complicate existing conditions or create new ones.

Life-style Changes

Instructions to patients will vary, depending on the fracture type, the bone fractured, type of intervention, type of immobilization, etc. Consideration is given to patient resources and support systems. Outcome will be improved if complications are limited. The patient instructions provided are general in nature. They will need to be modified to fit the needs of the patient depending on the particular injury, and the type of intervention. See patient information and instructions in Part 3.

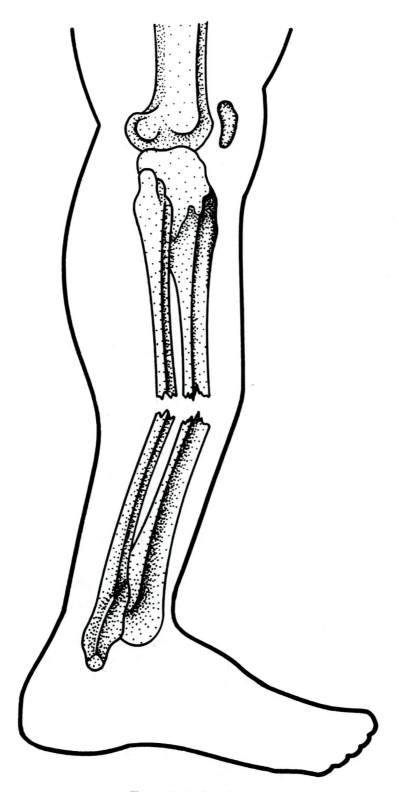

Figure 17–1. Bone fracture

■ SPRAINS AND STRAINS

General Characteristics

Strains and sprains are some of the most common types of injuries. They can occur during exercise, athletic competition, and routine acts of daily living. Though the terms "sprain" and "strain" are used by some as interchangeable and the injuries in some ways are similar, it is important for the health care provider to have in mind very distinct definitions for these types of injuries:

- Strain: A soft-tissue injury that results from the stretching of a muscle, tendon, or ligament other than those involving a joint.
- Sprain: A joint injury that involves the soft-tissue structures of the joint. The soft tissues involved are usually tendons and ligaments but not cartilage (Fig. 17–2).

■ *Sprains*

Any joint can suffer a sprain. It is beyond the scope of this chapter to cover every possible joint sprain. The most common type of sprain is ankle sprain. The principles of treatment and patient education for ankle sprain can be extrapolated to most other joint sprains with some modifications.

Signs, Symptoms, and Diagnosis

The most common type of ankle sprain occurs when the foot is inverted and there is an injury to the ligaments of the lateral side of the ankle. This injury can involve a single ligament or multiple ligaments. The range of injury can be from brief, mild discomfort to severe pain and disability.

Regardless of the degree of injury, the initial evaluation and treatment of ankle sprain are similar. Most individuals with very mild sprains and very transient discomfort or limitation will not seek medical evaluation. Those who do usually have a higher level of pain, edema, deformity, develop interruption of daily activities, such as walking. Observation and x-rays to determine whether fracture has occurred form the basis of diagnosis.

Management

The following plan should be followed as part of the initial treatment plan. A helpful acronym to remember is RICE:

- R = Rest
- I = Ice
- C = Compression
- E = Elevation

1. Rest: The patient must not bear weight on the foot.
2. Ice: This should be applied over the injured area for 20 minutes every 4 hours.
3. Compression: Compression dressings and splints should be left in place. The toes should be moved every hour. The toes should be examined for color changes such as turning blue or black. Sensation in the toes should be normal. If there is a loss of sensation, a "pins-and-needles" sensation, or a change in color, the patient should notify his or her health care provider immediately.
4. Elevation: The patient should keep the injured ankle elevated above the level of the heart as much as possible. Ambulation with crutches or other non–weight-bearing modalities will result in slowing the resolution of edema, and dependent edema may result.
5. Non-narcotic analgesia may be used, eg, non-steroidal anti-inflammatory drugs. (NSAIDs).
6. Follow-up should be arranged in 3 to 7 days for reevaluation.
7. At follow-up, further treatment depends on the ability of the patient to walk without pain.

Life-style Changes

Patients without pain and edema may return to nonstrenuous activity and can increase their level of activity slowly. Patients should be advised that activity may cause some discomfort and swelling. This should be treated with ice and elevation. Patients with significant pain and edema may need continued rest, compression, elevation, and no weight bearing. Heat should be substituted for ice after 3 days. Selected patients will benefit from physical therapy. Individuals with unstable ankles should be referred to an orthopedist. Patients should be warned that a slow, progressive return to activity is best. Some patients will have some discomfort and edema for a long period of time. Patients with chronic problems should be referred to an orthopedist.

■ *Strains*

Almost any soft-tissue structure can suffer a "strain." The term *strain* has been used to describe a number of musculoskeletal problems from well defined to poorly defined and very mild to

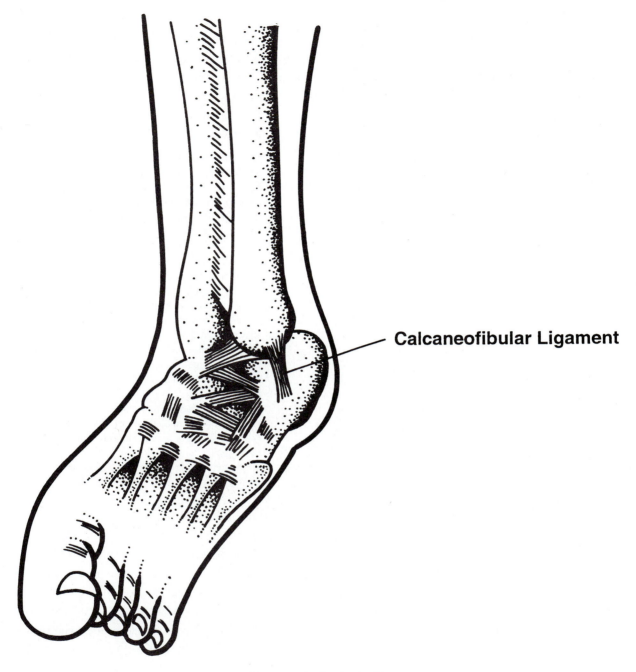

Calcaneofibular Ligament

Figure 17–2. Sprained ankle

very serious. In most instances the term *strain* is used to describe musculoskeletal injuries resulting from exertion or overuse that produce limited discomfort and short-term disability. Careful evaluation for more serious injuries and problems must be completed in individuals with severe pain, disability, radiculopathy, slow improvement, etc.

Treatment is usually of short duration, with patient education centering on gradual increase in exertional activity and conditioning. Nonnarcotic analgesia may help. Physical therapy will help in more serious and prolonged problems. Most patients with strains will not be seen immediately but at some time after the precipitating event. Treatment should include rest, heat, nonnarcotic analgesia, and a slow return to normal activities. Immobilization may or may not help or be practical. For sedentary patients, some exercise program should be recommended. This can include specific exercises, such as for the back, or general exercise, such as walking. For individuals in higher-level exertional activities or athletic competitions, a conditioning program is necessary.

■ HERNIAS

General Characteristics

Hernia is a general term that must be used with a descriptive term added to have meaning. The general definition is "the protrusion of a structure through the wall that normally contains it." Thus the adding of a qualifying term such as *inguinal, femoral, ventral*, etc. provides definition and meaning. Hernias can be congenital or acquired. Most hernias are not life-threatening, but they can become so if structures become incarcerated and ischemic.

Signs, Symptoms, and Diagnosis

Although almost any structure can herniate (Fig. 17–3), 75% of hernias occur in the inguinal region. Inguinal hernias are more common in men than women. Inguinal hernias are of two types: direct and indirect. Indirect inguinal hernias are a type of congenital hernia and occur when the processus vaginalis does not close and abdominal structures protrude into the inguinal regions, the inguinal canal, and scrotum. Direct inguinal hernias result from a weakness in the abdominal wall.

Femoral hernias occur in the groin and upper inner thigh in the region of the inguinal crease. Umbilical hernias are commonly present at birth and close without intervention. Umbilical hernias that do require intervention are those that are very large, remain after age 4, or pose a risk of incarceration. Incisional hernias occur at sites of previous surgical procedures. A number of factors can contribute to incisional hernia: poor healing, infection, and wound strain.

Management

It is generally recommended that hernias be surgically corrected. This decision is weighted by a number of factors such as age, general health, risk to benefit, expectations, and quality of life. Certainly all individuals with a hernia should have a surgical consultation as part of the evaluation process.

Life-style changes

The *two most important aspects* of patient education for hernias are to provide patients with information on (1) reducing their hernia and what to do if it cannot be reduced and (2) what to do if they think their hernia is incarcerated.

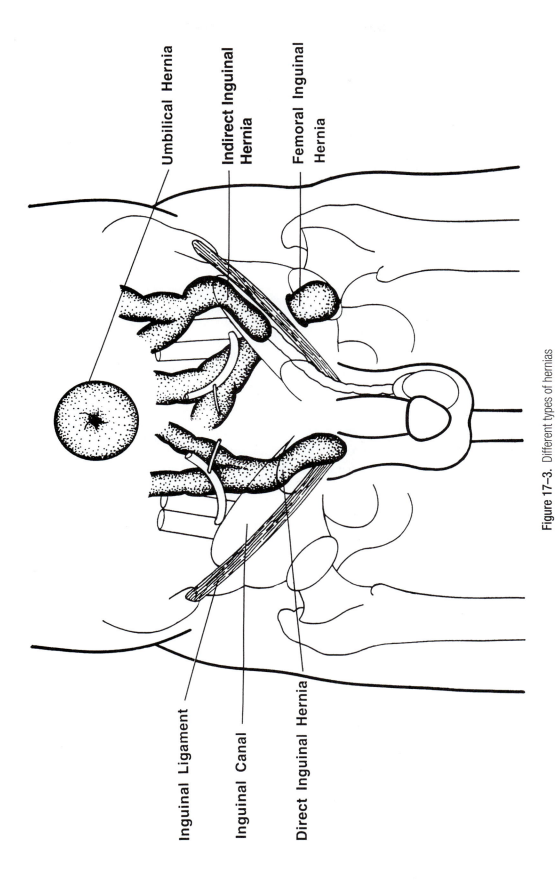

Umbilical Hernia

Indirect Inguinal Hernia

Femoral Inguinal Hernia

Inguinal Ligament

Inguinal Canal

Direct Inguinal Hernia

Figure 17–3. Different types of hernias

OSTEOPOROSIS

General Characteristics

Osteoporosis is a condition of decreased bone mass that results in thin, fragile bone that fractures easily. Osteoporosis affects more than 20 million people in the United States and is currently the most common disorder of bone metabolism. The incidence of osteoporosis is increasing because of a proportional increase in the population that is over the age of 65. Although osteoporosis is a clinically preventable disease, its silent progression is often overlooked until a clinically relevant incident such as a fracture brings the condition to the health care provider's attention.

Osteoporosis is associated with a number of factors (Table 17–1). The most common, however, relate to increasing age and the postmenopausal state. There is a "normal" age-related bone loss (type II osteoporosis) as a result of decreasing osteoblastic activity that begins around age 40 to 50 in both men and women. In women around the age of menopause, this age-related bone loss is coupled with increased activity of osteoclasts induced by falling estrogen concentrations (type I osteoporosis). Decreased bone replacement together with the increased resorption results in profound bone loss that may amount to as much as 50% in some women. Any condition that results in decreased estrogen levels essentially produces the same effects as does menopause. Oophorectomy, early menopause, or prolonged amenorrhea for any reason all lead to low estrogen states resulting in osteoporosis. Exercise-induced amenorrhea in young women has been shown to produce osteoporosis similar to that of postmenopausal women. Furthermore, it is unknown as to whether osteoporosis in these women is completely reversible.

Genetics plays a role in the predisposition to osteoporosis as well. White or Asian ethnicity, positive family history, and small body frame are all recognized as risk factors (Table 17–2).

Inadequate intake of calcium over many years results in an overall decrease in peak bone mass. This means that less bone is available when age-related bone loss and increased bone reabsorption begin to occur later in life. Smoking and immobilization are also known predisposing risk factors. Conversely, weight-bearing exercise can increase bone density and is believed to slow the rate of bone loss.

TABLE 17–1. ETIOLOGY OF OSTEOPOROSIS

Primary Osteoporosis	Secondary Osteoporosis
Hormonal and Age-Related	Disease states
Type I osteoporosis (post-menopausal)	Diabetes
Type II osteoporosis (age-related, begins around age 40–50, clinical manifestations seen after age 75)	Thyrotoxicosis
	Hyperadrenocorticism
	Hyperparathyroidism
	Rheumatoid arthritis
	Alcoholism
Early menopause	Liver disease
Oophorectomy	Epilepsy
Amenorrhea (anorexia nervosa)	Chronic obstructive pulmonary disease
Exercise-induced amenorrhea	Malignancy (multiple myeloma)
Idiopathic	
Juvenile and adult osteoporosis	Inheritable Connective Tissue Disorders
	Osteogenesis imperfecta
	Ehlers-Danlos syndrome
	Marfan's syndrome
	Homocystinuria
	Iatrogenic
	Excessive vitamin D administration
	Glucocorticoid administration
	Heparin therapy
	Methotrexate
	Excessive thyroid replacement
	Anticonvulsants
	Nutritional
	Malabsorption
	Vitamin C deficiency
	Malnutrition
	Calcium deficiency
	Vitamin D deficiency

All skeletal areas are affected by osteoporosis, but because trabecular bone is less compact than cortical bone (Fig. 17–4), the structure of trabecular bone is weakened to a much greater degree, making it more susceptible to fracture. Primary sites that are affected include the spine, hip, and distal radius.[1–6]

Signs, Symptoms, and Diagnosis

Early in the disease, patients are most likely to be asymptomatic. If signs and symptoms are present, they may consist of gradual loss in height resulting from vertebral compression

TABLE 17–2. RISK FACTORS FOR THE DEVELOPMENT
OF OSTEOPOROSIS

Genetic
  Family history of osteoporosis
  Asian or white ethnicity
  Small habitus
Other
  Smoking
  Alcohol use
  Caffeine intake
  Inadequate dietary calcium intake
  Immobilization

fractures, mild thoracic kyphosis, or complaints of vague discomfort in the thoracic cage. Late in the disease, patients more commonly present with symptoms of spinal compression fractures and fractures of the distal radius and femoral neck.

The trauma that induces the fracture may be very mild and may occur with routine activity. With vertebral fractures, the patient typically reports an acute onset of back pain, that is intensified with standing, sitting, or even slight movement. Coughing, sneezing, or defecation may increase the pain. Often the pain will radiate anteriorly around the flank and into the abdomen. The pain is improved with bed rest in the recumbent position and patients are treated with bed rest and analgesics until they are able to resume sitting or standing comfortably.

Vertebral fractures usually occur anteriorly, creating a wedge-shaped deformity (Fig. 17–5). Multiple vertebral fractures produce a kyphotic deformity (Fig. 17–6). Thoracic kyphosis has also been referred to as "widow's hump" or "dowager's hump."

Unfortunately, the diagnosis of osteoporosis is often made late in the disease when deformity or fracture is already present. Spinal radiographs will demonstrate wedge-shaped deformities and loss of horizontal trabeculae, but they cannot provide an accurate assessment of bone density.

Currently there are several ways to measure bone density to determine if disease is present. These include dual-photon absorptiometry (DPA), quantitative computed tomography (QCT), and dual-energy x-ray absorptiometry (DEXA). Of the three, DEXA is the most cost-effective and exposes the patient to the least amount of radiation. It is considered to be very accurate and can be done in the office setting. Although noninvasive bone-density absorptiometric techniques are becoming more readily available, most experts agree that it is not yet economically feasible to do routine screening at this time.

Transiliac bone biopsy is done only when bone loss occurs premenopausally in women or in men younger than age 65, or when another type of metabolic bone disease is suspected. Appropriate laboratory tests should be done as directed by the history in order to rule out osteoporosis resulting from secondary causes.[4]

Management

While the management of osteoporosis must include treatment of acute pain and fractures, the primary focus should be directed toward prevention of bone loss before the development of symptoms and prevention of further bone loss once disease is present.

Estrogen-replacement therapy has been shown to be effective in preventing loss of bone density. Estrogen therapy is recommended for the prevention of osteoporosis in perimenopausal, postmenopausal, and surgically menopausal women. There is still some concern over the possible association between hormone replacement therapy (HRT) and endometrial cancer, as well as the possible increased risk of breast cancer. Estrogen therapy reduces the rate of fracture by 50% or more, and most experts agree that the benefits outweigh the risks. Estrogen can be given either orally or transdermally through one of several regimens (Table 17–3). The contraindications to estrogen therapy are few but do include the following: a history of breast cancer or other estrogen-dependent neoplasia, a history of thrombophlebitis or thrombosis, undiagnosed abnormal genital bleeding, and known or suspected pregnancy. If a woman has not had a hysterectomy, it is recommended that she also receive progesterone to reduce the risk of endometrial hyperplasia and endometrial cancer. Yearly gynecologic examinations and regular breast examination followed by mammography are also recommended.

Calcitonin inhibits bone resorption through the antagonism of parathyroid hormone (PTH), resulting in increased bone mass; however, the efficacy begins to decline after 18 to 24 months of treatment, at which time bone loss resumes. Calcitonin is useful in treating postmenopausal women in whom estrogen replacement therapy is refused or contraindicated. Calcitonin therapy is administered parenterally either on a daily basis or three times a week, depending upon the preparation used (Table 17–3). Treatment is expensive when com-

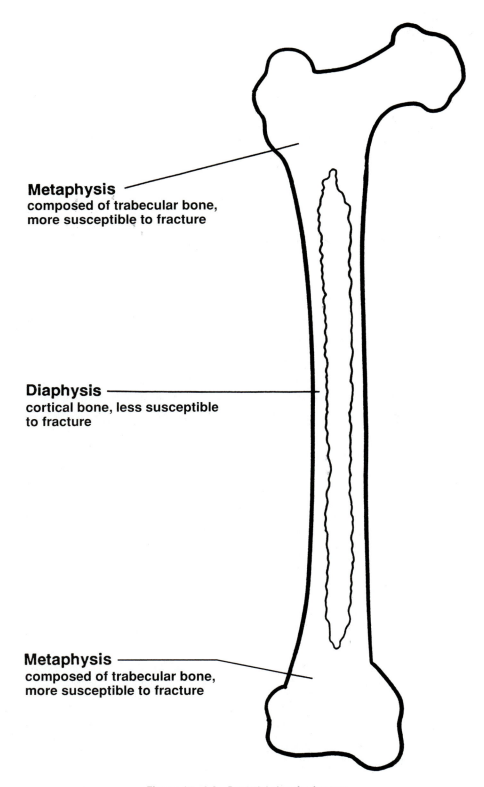

Metaphysis
composed of trabecular bone,
more susceptible to fracture

Diaphysis
cortical bone, less susceptible
to fracture

Metaphysis
composed of trabecular bone,
more susceptible to fracture

Figure 17–4.A. Potential sites for fracture

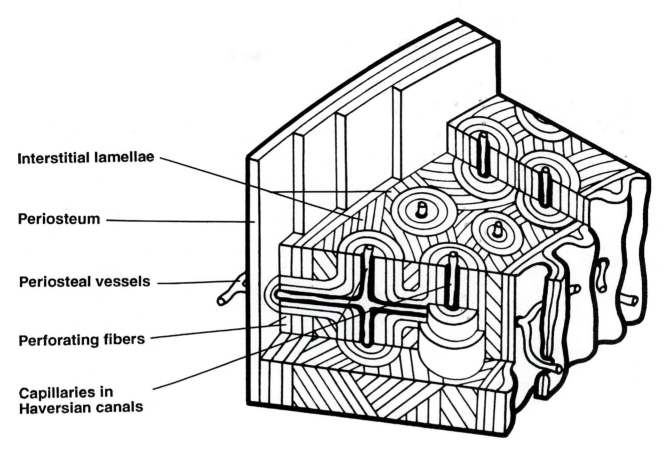

Figure 17–4.B. Structure of cortical bone

pared with estrogen replacement therapy. Calcitonin is associated with nausea (which can be reduced by administering the drug at bedtime) and skin hypersensitivities. Skin testing should be done prior to initiation of treatment. An added benefit of calcitonin is its analgesic property, which occurs as a result of endorphin stimulation.

Etidronate (Didronel) is a biophosphonate that effectively increases vertebral bone mass. Etidronate must be administered cyclically, since continuous therapy interferes with bone mineralization. The drug is poorly absorbed and so should be given daily on an empty stomach (Table 17–3). Studies concerning the true efficacy of this drug are still under investigation.

Vitamin D is indicated for the treatment of osteoporosis only when vitamin D deficiency has been established. True vitamin D deficiency is rather rare, since the vitamin is produced in sufficient quantities either through sunlight exposure or in a balanced diet that includes vitamin D-fortified foods.

Fluoride treatment has been shown to decrease vertebral fractures; however, there is a corresponding increase in the incidence of hip fractures. Fluoride is not generally recommended for the treatment of osteoporosis.[7–8]

Life-style Changes

Life-style changes include ensuring adequate amounts of calcium either through diet or calcium supplementation, regular weight-bearing exercise, and elimination of risk factors such as smoking, alcohol intake, and medications that are associated with osteoporosis.

While it is thought that calcium does not prevent bone loss, there is a consensus that adequate calcium intake is important in achieving a satisfactory peak bone mass. Dietary sources of calcium include certain types of fish and shellfish, nuts and grains, green vegetables, and dairy products (Table 17–4). Dairy products have the greatest calcium content. Lac-

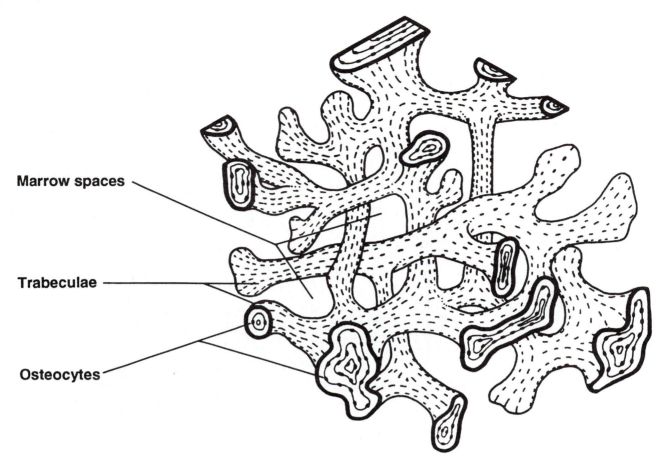

Marrow spaces

Trabeculae

Osteocytes

Figure 17–4.C. Structure of trabecular bone (schematic). On cut section (as in sections), trabeculae may appear as discontinuous spicules.

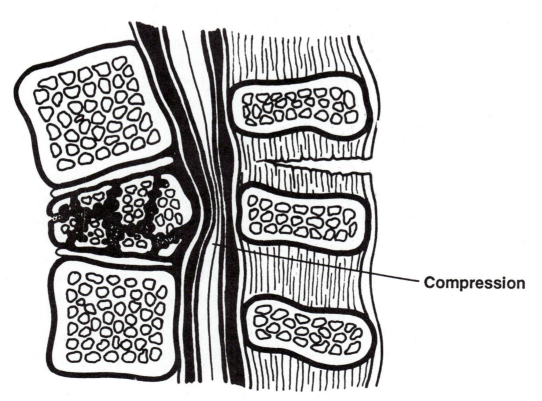

Compression

Figure 17–5. Wedge-shaped deformity

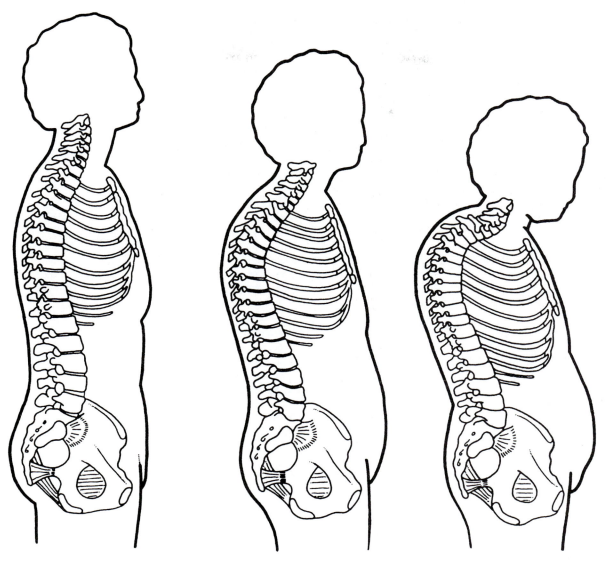

Figure 17–6. Progressive kyphotic deformity

tose intolerance may contribute to inadequate dietary calcium intake, resulting in increased risk of osteoporosis.

Most people are unable to meet the minimum daily requirements for calcium through dietary sources alone (Table 17–5). The lack of calcium in an individual's diet can be replaced through calcium supplementation. Numerous over-the-counter supplements are available (Table 17–6).

Patients should be encouraged to read the labels carefully to determine the amount of elemental calcium present in each tablet of the supplement they will be taking. They should also be advised to choose a supplement that will dissolve easily within the stomach. This can be tested by placing a tablet in 6

oz of vinegar at room temperature, stirring occasionally for 30 minutes. If the tablet dissolves within this time, it is probably a reasonable choice.

Calcium carbonate has the highest calcium content by weight, which means that patients have to take fewer tablets thereby improving the likelihood of patient adherence. It is also the least expensive. Calcium gluconate, citrate, or lactate preparations are also frequently recommended. Calcium dolomite or bone-meal preparations should not be used, since they may contain trace amounts of lead or other metals and result in heavy-metal poisoning. The recommended daily requirement for calcium can be found in Table 17–5.

TABLE 17–3. DOSING REGIMENS FOR THE PREVENTION AND TREATMENT OF OSTEOPOROSIS

Estrogen-Replacement Therapy

Conjugated estrogen (Premarin) or estropipate (Ogen) 0.625 mg/d PO or estradiol (Estrace) 0.5 mg/d PO days 1–25 of each month

Plus medroxyprogesterone (Amen, Cycrin, Provera)* 5–10 mg/d PO, days 13–25 or days 16–25 each month

Calcium 1500 mg/d

Alternative Regimen #1

Conjugated estrogen (Premarin) or estropipate (Ogen) 0.625 mg/d PO or estradiol (Estrace) 0.5 mg/d PO, continuously throughout month

plus medroxyprogesterone (Amen, Cycrin, Provera)* 2.5–5.0 mg/d PO on continual basis

Calcium 1500 mg/d

Alternative Regimen #2

Estradiol transdermal estrogen (Estraderm) 0.05 mg/d by transdermal patch; patches are replaced twice per wk

Plus medroxyprogesterone (Amen, Cycrin, Provera)* 5–10 mg/d PO, days 13–25 or 16–25; or 2.5–5.0 mg/d PO on a continual basis

Calcium 1500 mg/d

Calcitonin

Calcitonin-salmon (Calcimar, Miacalcin) 100 IU, SQ or IM daily or qid for 3–7 wk

Calcitonin, Synthetic (Cibacalcin) 0.5 mg/d SQ (some patients may have clinical improvement with 0.5 mg, 2–3 times per wk or 0.25 mg/d)

Continue for 3–7 wk

Calcium 1500 mg/d and vitamin D 400 U/d

Diphosphonates

Etidronate disodium (Didronel) two 200 mg tablets (400 mg) PO daily for 2 wk, q 12 wk

Calcium 500 mg/d

*Note: For women who have undergone hysterectomy, medroxyprogesterone is not necessary. IM, intramuscularly; PO, by mouth; qid, four times a day; SQ, subcutaneously.

TABLE 17–4. CALCIUM CONTENT OF COMMONLY USED FOOD ITEMS

Food Type	Serving	Calcium Content (mg)
PROTEIN		
Fish & Shellfish		
Oysters	1 C	226
Sardines (with bones)	3 oz	372
Shrimp	3 oz	99
Beef	3 oz	11
Chicken	3 oz	12
Almonds	1 oz	75
VEGETABLES		
Broccoli	1 C	136
Collard greens	1 C	357
Turnip greens	1 C	268
Green beans	1 C	62
Lima beans	1 C	80
Tofu (bean curd) (varies depending on processing method)	1/2 C	(100–300)
BREADS & GRAINS		
Bread, white	1 slice	19
Bread, wheat	1 slice	22
Tortilla, corn	6-in diameter	60
DAIRY PRODUCTS		
Milk		
Whole	8 oz	291
2%	8 oz	297
Skim	8 oz	302
Cheese		
American	1 oz	174
Cheddar	1 oz	204
Mozzarella (Part skim)	1 oz	207
Cottage	4 oz	78
Yogurt		
Plain (low fat)	8 oz	415
Fruit (low fat)	8 oz	343
Frozen	8 oz	200
Ice Cream		
Hard	8 oz	185
Soft serve	8 oz	274

Exercise is believed to slow the rate of bone loss and to improve coordination and strength, which can prevent falls and fractures. The optimal frequency, duration, or type has not been determined up to this point; however, weight-bearing exercise such as walking, aerobics, cross-country skiing, or dancing for 30 to 60 minutes three, four, or five times a week is generally recommended. It should be mentioned that exercise should be undertaken in moderation. Exercise that produces amenorrhea in premenopausal women is associated with producing osteoporosis.

While the acute fractures and complications associated with osteoporosis must be adequately managed, the best management for this disease lies in prevention.

TABLE 17–5. RECOMMENDED DAILY REQUIREMENT OF CALCIUM

Category	Elemental Calcium
Children	
Ages 1–10	800 mg
Adolescents/young adults	
Ages 11–24	1200 mg
Adults	
Men and premenopausal women	1000 mg
Pregnant and lactating women	1200 mg
Postmenopausal women	1500 mg

TABLE 17–6. CALCIUM CONTENT OF VARIOUS CALCIUM PREPARATIONS

Preparation	Percentage of Elemental Calcium
Calcium carbonate	40
Tribasic calcium phosphate	39
Dibasic calcium phosphate	23–30
Calcium citrate	21
Calcium lactate	13
Calcium gluconate	9

References

1. Dempster D, Lindsay R. Pathogenesis of osteoporosis. *Lancet*. 1993;341:801–804.
2. Female athlete triad, risk for women. *JAMA*. 1993;270:921–923.
3. Fitzgerald P. Endocrine disorders. In: Tierney L, McPhee S, Papadakis M, eds. *Current Medical Diagnosis and Treatment*. 33rd ed. Norwalk, Conn: Appleton & Lange; 1994:949–951.
4. Krane S, Holick M. Osteoporosis. In: Wilson J, Braunwald E, Isselbacher K, et al, eds. *Harrison's Principles of Internal Medicine*. 12th ed. New York, NY: McGraw Hill Inc; 1991:1921–1933.
5. Longitudinal study pursues questions of calcium, hormones and metabolism in life of skeleton. *JAMA*. 1992;268:2357–2358.
6. Zilkoski M. Osteoporosis. In: Mengel M, Schwiebert L, eds. *Ambulatory Medicine: The Primary Care of Families*. Norwalk, Conn: Appleton & Lange; 1993:452–458.
7. Allen S. Primary osteoporosis: methods to combat bone loss that accompanies aging. *Postgrad Med*. 1993;93(8):43–55.
8. Lindsay R. Prevention and treatment of osteoporosis. *Lancet*. 1993;341:801–804.
9. Barrett-Connor E, Chang J, Edelstein S. Coffee-associated osteoporosis offset by daily milk consumption: the Rancho Bernardo study. *JAMA*. 1994;271:280–283.
10. Prince R, Smith M, Dick I, et al. Prevention of postmenopausal osteoporosis. *N Engl J Med*. 1991; 325:1189–1195.
11. Trachtenbarg D. Treatment of osteoporosis: what is the role of calcium? *Postgrad Med*. 1990;87(4):263–270.

18

Psychiatric Disorders

Barbara A. Carnes

■ DEPRESSION

General Characteristics

Depression is an emotion characterized by feelings of sadness, low spirits, gloom, disappointment, frustration, and dejection.[1] Many individuals experience these feelings in response to the disappointments, frustrations, and losses in life. Clinical depression, a prevalent medical disorder, is often referred to as the "common cold" of psychiatry. The symptoms are seen frequently in a general medical clinic but often the diagnosis is missed. While the onset of depression can occur at any age, onset during the mid-twenties is the average.[2]

Depression can be associated with the normal grief process,[3] the climacteric period of middle-aged women,[4] and poor health in elderly women.[5] Socioenvironmental factors such as economic deprivation and single parenthood can contribute to the development of depression in young women.[6] Depression has been identified as one of the feelings associated with unemployment in white male hourly-wage workers.[7] The increased rate of suicide in older white men has been associated with depression.[8]

Most commonly seen alone, the symptoms of depression can be associated with other primary physical disorders such as multiple sclerosis, encephalitis, systemic lupus erythematosus, and chronic Epstein-Barr virus syndrome. Organic disorders such as cerebral ischemia, Meniere's disease, tuberculosis, endocrinopathies, electrolyte imbalance, and vitamin deficiencies can also produce symptoms of depression and anxiety. In addition, pharmacologic agents such as rauwolfia alkaloids, beta blockers, trichomonacides, antiarrhythmics, and estrogens can lead to the development of these symptoms.[9]

Clinically, *mood* is the term used to describe a prolonged emotion such as depression that impacts the whole self. A *depressive disorder* is a condition characterized by one or more periods of depressed mood, which persists for a minimum period of time, is associated with a distinct cluster of symptoms with no known organic factor or psychotic disorder, and is not associated with any abnormal elevation of mood (hypomania, mania).[2]

There are a variety of theories that try to explain the etiology of depression. Evidence such as the increased risk for depression in first-degree relatives, recurrent episodes, and the response of symptoms to antidepressant medication suggests a biochemical disturbance in monoamine neurotransmitter systems (norepinephrine and serotonin), an imbalance of acetylcholine-adrenergic balance, or decreased dopamine.[1,10]

Psychodynamic theory suggests that depression is associated with a perceived difference between the ideal self and the actual self, which results in low self-esteem and self-recrimination. There is a loss of a sense of well-being. Anger associated with loss is directed inward. Depression can be a signal to alter psychologic behavior; failure to work through the associated feelings of frustration and loss, if left unchecked, can overwhelm the individual as the more intense feelings of a deeper depression.[11]

Beck proposes that negative cognitive distortions of self, the world, and the future are the foundation for depression.[12] According to this theory, depressed individuals view themselves as the source of psychologic, physical, or moral problems; they presume that any personal deficits make them worthless and undesirable. These individuals view the present and their world in a negative way. Furthermore, they believe that the environment makes exorbitant demands and erects insurmountable obstacles that interfere with their accomplishment of goals. Finally, depressed individuals have a negative view of the future. They expect the frustrations, hardships, and deprivation of the present to continue forever. Based on these cognitions, individuals expect to fail, believe that recovery will never come, and believe that they will always be sad. Depressed individuals view themselves as losers.[13–15]

Seligman's theory of learned helplessness proposes that individuals who initially expect that their actions will produce desired effects may come to learn through experience that their efforts are, in reality, ineffective.[16] As a result of this learning, they may cease to offer voluntary responses. The deficits that could develop as a result of this learned helplessness can lead to anxiety, depression, and hopelessness. Seligman and his associates suggest that depressed individuals have a negative view of themselves as a result of an internal attribution of uncontrollable outcomes.[17,18] The individual's negative view of the present is based on the perception that responses and outcomes are independent. The individual's negative view of the future reflects the expectation that negative events will continue to occur and that these events will be uncontrollable. While this sequence of events may occur in any situation, it is likely to lead to motivational, cognitive, and emotional deficits only when it occurs in those situations that individuals perceive to be important.

In the depression stage of the grief process, Kubler-Ross has described two forms of depression associated with the sense of deep loss surrounding terminal illness.[3] She suggests that reactive depression is a response to past losses (financial security, job, life-style, and missed opportunities) and that preparatory depression is a time of quiet reflection in the face of losing all loved objects.

Signs, Symptoms and Diagnosis

Bereavement.   The loss of a loved one can trigger bereavement, which is characterized by feelings of depression and related symptoms of decreased appetite, weight loss, and periods of insomnia. Bereavement is a normal process and can be accompanied by feelings of guilt associated with thoughts about what might have helped or not helped the loved one. Major depression is a potential complication of normal be-

reavement and can be accompanied by prolonged feelings of worthlessness and intense functional impairment.[19]

Adjustment Disorder with Depressed Mood.

Adjustment disorder with depressed mood is a common disorder and one that is likely to be seen in general practice. An adjustment disorder signals a disruption of an individual's normal process of adaptation; in other words, the level of the stressor exceeds the individual's ability to cope effectively. The depressed mood is associated with recent difficult life experiences such as physical illness, marital discord, financial worries, or work-related concerns. While the symptoms are less severe and disabling than those associated with dysthymia or major depression, the individual's response to the experience seems greater than the degree of dysfunction generally associated with the experience. Symptoms displayed do not meet the specific criteria for other psychiatric disorders including dysthymia and major depressive disorder.[20]

To make the diagnosis of adjustment disorder with depressed mood, the individual or others will suggest a time relationship (within 3 months) between the onset of symptoms and psychosocial stressor(s). The duration of the symptoms is less than 6 months. There will be evidence of impaired functioning such as misconduct, withdrawal, inhibition in work, school, relationships, or social functioning. The level of impairment is more severe (stronger or lasts longer) than expected but not severe enough to warrant other diagnoses.[20]

Dysthymic Disorder.   Dysthymic disorder is a persistent mood state that is less severe but more chronic than major depression. The prevalence of dysthymia is unknown; it occurs more frequently in women than in men. The biologic and psychosocial theories of causes are similar to those of major depression. Dysthymic disorder is characterized by long-standing mild or moderate feelings of depression that are not as severe as those associated with major depression. Individuals often complain that they have felt depressed their whole life and that they have lost interest or pleasure in things that they had once found pleasurable. Affected individuals report unrealistic, idealistic expectations of themselves and an exaggerated reaction to normal stressors. In addition, they describe chronic, unremitting feelings of inadequacy, self-denigration, low self-confidence, and hopelessness. These thoughts and feelings are often expressed in a dramatic manner characterized by behaviors

such as demanding, complaining, and blaming themselves and others; obsessional traits can also be observed. The abuse of alcohol and other drugs is common in this group. These behaviors contribute to the individual's limited social life and troubled relationships.[10]

The diagnosis is made on the basis of severity and chronicity of the symptoms. Symptoms of dysthymic disorder contribute to a mild to moderate interference with the individual's personal and social functioning, resulting in an inability to sustain adequate performance.[10]

Major Depressive Disorder. It is estimated that major depressive illness affects millions of people a year. Approximately twice as many women (10% to 25%) as men (5% to 12%) are diagnosed with this disorder during their lifetime.[2,10]

There is great variation in the clinical characteristics of major depression. The symptoms can be confused with dementia in the elderly and can occur as a complication of normal bereavement; it can be associated with seasonal change ("seasonal mood disorder"). Symptoms can occur concurrently with dysthymia and cyclothymia. While initial symptoms can occur at any age, the average age of onset is approximately 40 years. When the onset is earlier, more frequent recurrence of the condition is expected. Symptoms can develop gradually, or there can be a dramatic development of symptoms following a significant loss or stress. It is possible that symptoms will subside spontaneously in weeks or months or they can become chronic and exist over a period of years. Approximately 50% of individuals with this disorder are completely recovered 1 year after the onset of symptoms. The risk of relapse is high during the period immediately following recovery (25% of individuals relapse within 12 weeks).[10]

A major depressive episode is characterized by at least a 2-week history of depressed mood or loss of interest in or pleasure from things that were enjoyed in the past. In addition, patients report at least five of the following symptoms: 1) a significant weight loss or gain, 2) insomnia or hypersomnia, 3) psychomotor agitation or retardation, 4) fatigue or loss of energy, 5) feelings of worthlessness or excessive guilt, 6) decreased ability to think or concentrate, and 7) recurrent thoughts of death or suicide.[2,10] Recurrent episodes of suicidal preoccupation or profound delusional content generally suggest that the prognosis for recovery is poor.[10]

At major depression's most severe level, symptoms also include extensive paranoid or nihilistic delusional systems, hallucinations, more psychomotor disturbance, and a poor response to antidepressant medication.[10]

Management

Depression is a common emotional disorder that exists on a variety of levels and affects both men and women. Because of the stigma associated with mental illness, patients are often reluctant to report symptoms that they consider a sign of weakness. Teaching patients about the importance of mental health and reassuring them that depression and anxiety are signals alerting the self to get help will be a great service to the individual.

It is important that health care workers explore their own thoughts and feelings about grief and depression. Finding and utilizing resources to promote one's own well-being will facilitate the ability to work effectively with others who are experiencing these emotions.[1]

Use therapeutic communication skills to assist the individual in exploring and expressing feelings. Assess coping methods and, if necessary, teach more effective coping strategies. Encourage the development and use of support systems, including community resources.

It is important to note that individuals often self-medicate through the use of caffeine, alcohol, over-the-counter medications, or street drugs in an attempt to alleviate symptoms. These approaches can have harmful sequelae, including dependence on the substance. In addition, use of these substances can ease the emotional discomfort, thereby removing the motivation to identify the cause of the feelings and to initiate positive steps toward self-awareness and change.[10]

Individuals who are experiencing sleep interruption can be helped to restore sleep. Caffeine and caffeine-containing products should be avoided as they can increase the number of times an individual wakes during the night. Encourage patients to manage their anxiety by engaging in activities such as reading a book or listening to music that they find relaxing and by avoiding evening activities they find stimulating or that increase tension. While exercise can be an effective method to induce fatigue, caution the individual to complete an exercise at least 2 to 3 hours before bedtime. Suggest that the individual develop a routine pattern of preparation for sleep (consistent time, warm bath, warm milk, light snack) and create a dark and quiet environment for sleep. If the individual experiences difficulty falling asleep, suggest staying out of bed until he or she feels sleepy or getting out of bed if unable to fall asleep and resuming relaxing activity until sleepy. If insomnia continues, explore the use of sedative-hypnotic medication.[6,21]

Maintaining adequate nutrition and elimination are important aspects of care. Encourage individuals to eat appropriate amounts of calories while avoiding excess sugar, fat, salt, and caffeine. Individuals who are taking monoamine oxidase (MAO) inhibitors must follow prescribed dietary restrictions. Encourage the individual to drink adequate amounts of fluids, including water. Adequate exercise promotes proper elimination, and the use of large muscle groups during exercise contributes to feelings of well-being.[6]

Management of the symptoms of depressive disorders is guided by the extent and duration of the symptoms. The goal is to assist the patient with adjustment, to relieve symptoms, and to foster positive change. Approaches to achieve these goals include individual or family therapy, self-help groups, and biomedical interventions including medication (Table 18–1) or electroconvulsive therapy (ECT). Medications can be used to control biologic symptoms and facilitate the use of other therapies to explore the issues associated with the experience.[10]

Suicide Prevention. Some people see suicide as the only way to end the pain associated with deep depression. It is a permanent solution to a temporary condition. Actively listen to hear what the individual is saying and not saying. Be alert for signs such as hopelessness, ambivalence, inability to see a future for her- or himself, giving away possessions, and the sudden lifting of mood. Assess specificity and lethality of the individual's plan, as well as the individual's ability to carry out the plan. Remain with the person and explore alternative ways of coping. If necessary, refer the patient for evaluation and treatment by the psychiatric team. Arrange accompanied transportation to the team if an attempt at suicide during transfer is suspected.[22]

Life-style Changes

Depression can interrupt the life of the individual and family. Decreased libido can interfere with relationships as can the decreased pleasure of previously enjoyed activities. Depression can be a signal to identify stressors and to mobilize defenses by identifying and changing unrealistic expectations and negative thoughts.

TABLE 18–1. COMMON ANTIDEPRESSANTS

Medication	Dosage	Side Effects
Trazodone hydrochloride (Desyrel)	150 mg/d in divided doses to start, followed by an increase of 50 mg/d every 3–4 d, as needed and tolerated, up to 400 mg/d in divided doses for most outpatients	Priapism; mental or physical impairment; neutropenia
Amitriptyline hydrochloride (Elavil)	75 mg/d in divided doses to start, followed by an increase in late afternoon or bedtime dose, up to a total of 150 mg/d in divided doses	Arrhythmias; sinus tachycardia; prolongation of cardiac conduction time; mental or physical impairment; withdrawal symptoms
Desipramine hydrochloride (Norpramin)	100–200 mg/d in one or more doses	Cardiac conduction defects; arrhythmias; tachycardias; stroke; acute myocardial infarction
Nortriptyline hydrochloride (Pamelor)	25 mg tid or qid or 75–100 mg/d in a single daily dose	Arrhythmias; sinus tachycardia; prolonged cardiac conduction time; myocardial infarction; stroke; mental or physical impairment; withdrawal symptoms
Paroxetine hydrochloride (Paxil)	20 mg/d q AM to start; increase dosage, if needed, in increments of 10 mg/d at intervals of at least 1 wk, up to 50 mg/d	Mental impairment; mania or hypomania; seizures; hyponatremia; weight loss; dry mouth
Fluoxetine hydrochloride (Prozac)	20 mg q AM to start; if no clinical improvement is observed after several weeks, increase up to 80 mg/d in divided doses	Rash; urticaria; anaphylaxis; CNS stimulation; appetite depression; dry mouth; weight loss; mania; hypomania; seizures; hyponatremia; mental or physical impairment; abnormal platelet function; drug dependence
Sertraline hydrochloride (Zoloft)	50 mg once daily (AM or PM) to start; if no clinical improvement, dosage may be increased at intervals of no less than 1 wk, up to 200 mg/d	Mental impairment; mania; hypomania; weight loss; uricosuria; hyponatremia; drug dependence

CNS, central nervous system; qid, four times a day; tid, three times a day.

■ ANXIETY

General Characteristics

Fear and *anxiety* are terms that are often used interchangeably to describe a common response to a perceived threat. More specific is the use of the term *fear* to name the physical and emotional response to a recognized threat that is external to the individual and the term *anxiety* to name the physical and emotional response to a threat that is elusive and difficult to identify.[23]

Beck suggests that *fear* is a cognitive function and that *anxiety* is an unpleasant, subjective emotional experience in response to fear.[24] Peplau purports that anxiety is energy that is felt as tension or excitement and its presence is inferred from observation of the individual's behavior.[25] This energy can be channeled to enhance learning and personal growth, or it can grow and overwhelm the individual.

Garber, Miller, and Abramson define *anxiety* in terms of helplessness and uncertainty.[26] They propose that "a kind of helplessness" develops when an event "cannot be interpreted or given meaning, and it cannot be dealt with."[26] They suggest that while for some individuals this time of uncertainty can be used to prepare for an event and thereby increase personal control, for others it can trigger a time of increased uncertainty and apprehension. In the latter case, this increased uncertainty and apprehension might lead to helplessness when the individual is unable to use coping alternatives effectively.

According to Spielberger, anxiety that exists at a given moment is labeled "state."[27] State anxiety is characterized by "subjective feelings of tension, apprehension, nervousness, and worry, and by activation or arousal of the autonomic nervous system."[27] Trait anxiety, on the other hand, is a more enduring quality and a function of personality.

Although the exact etiology of anxiety is elusive, there are a variety of theories that attempt to explain its origins. Peplau proposes that at any given time, when individuals become aware of their "expectations or prestige or status needs"[25] and the fact that these expectations or needs are not met, there is a vague sense of discomfort and feelings of powerlessness. The energy (anxiety) associated with these feelings is transformed into behaviors that provide relief from the uneasiness. Since these behaviors produce relief, if repeated often enough they can become automatic. The behaviors can contribute to growth, creativity, and self-development (gardening, studying, resolving conflict), or they can simply bring relief (pacing, hand-wringing, deep-breathing), or they can be destructive and interfere with relationships (blaming, arguing).[25]

The increased incidence of anxiety in female first-degree relatives of individuals with anxiety disorders and in identical twins suggests a genetic, biologic root for anxiety. While there is evidence of increased adrenergic activity (increased epinephrine release) in anxious patients, it is unclear whether this is an existing condition or a response to a given situation. At the level of beta-adrenergic receptors, beta blockers tend to decrease anxiety, whereas beta stimulators have the opposite affect.[28]

In addition, anxiety has been associated with medical conditions that affect various organ systems. Angina, acute myocardial infarction, cardiac arrhythmias, congestive heart failure, asthma, emphysema, pulmonary embolism, seizure disorders, vertigo, anaphylactic shock, hypo- and hyperthyroidism are associated with feelings of anxiety. Furthermore, medications including thyroid supplements, digitalis, cold medications, and antispasmodics can produce feelings of anxiety. Withdrawal from medications such as sleep medications, some antihypertensives, and antianxiety drugs can trigger symptoms of anxiety as can paradoxical reactions to antianxiety and antidepressive medications. Caffeine, alcohol, and marijuana are known to produce symptoms similar to anxiety.[28]

Beck views fear as the source of anxiety.[24] When individuals intellectually assess a given situation and conclude that there is actual or potential danger (fear), this can trigger an emotional response (anxiety). Fear can be either realistic or unrealistic that is, either based on "sensible assumption, logic and reasoning, and objective observation" or founded in "fallacious assumptions and faulty reasoning"[24] or on an appraisal that is contrary to observation. Whichever the case, the degree of anxiety will depend on the individual's assessment and not on the accuracy of that assessment. Beck suggests that anxiety attacks result from fear of internal physical, mental, or social catastrophe. These catastrophes include heart attacks, cancer, "going crazy," and public disgrace. It is often difficult for the individual to specifically identify the catastrophe, but the expectation is that it is occurring or is about to occur. Beck equates anxiety with pain in that both provide a warning to the individual to reduce the factors that are causing the discomfort.

According to Garber, Miller, and Abramson, "when individuals are uncertain about the symbolic meaning of events, as well as what to do about them, they become anxious."[26] They state further that it is not uncontrollability per se that is the defining feature of anxiety, but rather, it is the individual's *uncertainty* about the outcome that triggers the anxiety. Helplessness contributes to the intensity of anxiety to the extent that it contributes to the uncertainty of that outcome.

Spielberger suggests that anxiety can be a function of personality.[27] He proposes that *trait anxiety* "refers to relatively stable individual differences in anxiety-proneness, that is, to differences between people in the tendency to perceive stressful situations with elevations in the intensity of their state anxiety (S-Anxiety) reactions."[27] *State anxiety* is a response to a particular situation. These observations provided the foundation for State-Trait Anxiety Inventory (STAI) published in 1970 and revised (Form Y) in 1980.

Signs, Symptoms, and Diagnosis

Anxiety exists at a variety of levels from mild to severe. Individuals experiencing mild anxiety are alert; their ability to attend to themselves and the environment and to focus broadly enables individuals with mild anxiety to learn and to make decisions. Individuals can learn to tolerate this level of anxiety. In moderate anxiety, the individual continues to be alert but there is a narrowing of the breadth of focus. Individuals at this level are able to focus on relevant details and are capable of learning. Anxiety at these levels can be experienced as a challenging and motivating force; it can spark creativity. In severe anxiety, individuals are not able to get the "big picture." Disorganized thinking and a focus on small details hinder the individual's ability to collect all the information needed to accurately assess a situation. Individuals at this level of anxiety cannot learn. Panic, the highest level of anxiety, precludes learning. Personality is disorganized and communication is not effective. Attention is narrowed and focus is on a minute detail, which can be blown out of proportion. Events become distorted. This is a time of "terror." Obtaining relief is the main intent.[25]

It is difficult to differentiate the point at which anxiety as a normal response to a given situation becomes an anxiety disorder. Based on community surveys, of the individuals reporting symptoms of anxiety, those who report mild anxiety (approximately 33%) do not seek assistance; about the same number report intermediate anxiety and seek assistance from their family physician. The rest, who suffer from intense anxiety, seek the services of the psychiatric treatment team.[28]

The characteristic features of the anxiety disorders are symptoms of anxiety and avoidance. The anxiety disorders identified by the American Psychological Association (APA) include panic disorder (with or without agoraphobia), agoraphobia, social phobia, specific phobia, obsessive compulsive disorder, and generalized anxiety.[29] Posttraumatic stress disorder is included in the category, but the Association notes that it is the reexperiencing of the trauma rather than anxiety or avoidance that is the major concern in this case. The APA asserts that anxiety disorders, particularly specific phobia, are the most frequently found disorders in the general population. Panic disorder is the disorder that usually leads people to seek help from mental health professionals.[29]

Panic Disorders.   Panic disorder is diagnosed more frequently in women than in men; symptoms usually begin between adolescence and the mid-30s and can occur for several months or for many years. It is characterized by panic attacks that are sudden and brief, usually lasting about 10 minutes and no longer than 30 minutes. Attacks are characterized by at least four symptoms of anxiety such as dyspnea, tachycardia, chills, and complaints of dizziness, hot flashes, chest pain, and fears of dying or of "going crazy." The diagnosis is made if these attacks are not the result of the individual's being the focus of attention from others (social phobia) and if there is no physical disorder contributing to the development of the symptoms. Criteria for panic disorder include a history of either four panic attacks within a 4-week period, or a panic attack followed by the fear of having another panic attack that has lasted for at least 1 month. Panic disorder is a common condition that can occur alone or can be associated with agoraphobia. It causes limited impairment of work and social functioning; complications can include abuse of anxiolytics and alcohol.[23,29]

Agoraphobia.   Agoraphobia commonly exists with and rarely exists without panic disorder. It is anxiety about being in places or situations from which escape might be difficult (or embarrassing) or in which help might not be available in the event of having a panic attack or panic-like symptoms.[29] The anxiety-provoking symptoms can include fainting, losing control of bowel or bladder function, and having cardiac distress. Usually beginning between 20 and 40 years of age, the symptoms of agoraphobia are more common in women than men. In its mild form and with adjustments being made to manage working and traveling, it causes little disturbance of life-style. In its most severe form, when individuals are homebound, lifestyles can be disturbed greatly. Complications can include abuse of anxiolytics and alcohol.[23,29]

Social Phobia. This disorder is characterized by an irrational fear of humiliation or embarrassment associated with situations in which the individual is the subject of public attention. Fears of public speaking and interacting in social situations are common. This disorder often coexists with panic disorder and specific phobia and is more common in women than men. Symptoms can first appear in childhood and early adolescence and these are usually chronic. This anticipatory anxiety can impact life-style when the avoidance of the feared situation impairs social or occupational activities, or relationships; generally this occurs only in severe cases. Complications can include substance abuse (alcohol, barbiturates, anxiolytics); and if there is severe impairment, a depressive disorder can develop.[23,29]

Specific Phobia. Specific phobias are persistent, unreasonable or excessive fears related to a particular thing or situation. When individuals approach the feared object, anxiety increases; it decreases when they remove themselves from the object. When individuals persist in contact, the anxiety becomes intense. Feared objects or situations include dirt, animals, closed spaces, and heights. Individuals recognize that this fear is excessive or unreasonable. In its mild form, this condition is very common in the general population and usually treatment is not sought. The disorder occurs more frequently in women than men. The age at onset of symptoms varies; usually the phobias of childhood disappear but those that continue into adulthood rarely diminish without treatment. Usually there is little interference with daily life if the feared object or situation is rare or can be avoided.[23,29]

Obsessive Compulsive Disorder. Symptoms of obsessive compulsive disorder can begin in adolescence or the early adult years and are almost equally common in men and women. The mild form of this disorder is common and rarely causes a great deal of distress or disruption in daily life. This disorder is characterized by recurrent *obsessions*, which are "persistent ideas, thoughts, impulses, or images"[29] and by *compulsions*, which are "repetitive behaviors performed in response to an obsession, and according to certain rules." Common obsessions are fear of hurting others, contaminating self or others, and questioning whether or not routine tasks have been performed. Repetitive hand washing, touching, counting, and checking are common examples of compulsive behavior. Initially, individuals feel increasing tension as they attempt to resist obsessions. There is a release of tension as the activity is carried out. When compulsive behavior is blocked, anxiety rises. Compulsive behavior is recognized as unreasonable by the individual and at moderate to severe levels of the disorder, the behavior can be very disruptive and time-consuming. In addition to substance abuse (anxiolytics and alcohol), major depression can be a complication of obsessive compulsive disorder.[23,29]

Posttraumatic Stress Disorder (PTSD). The diagnosis of PTSD is made if symptoms associated with reliving a past, psychologically traumatic experience continue for 1 month or more. The traumatic experience must be unexpected and out of the realm of probable experience for most people. These experiences are characterized by a significant threat to life, self, or property and can be experienced alone or with others. Traumatic experiences can include natural disasters (hurricanes, tornadoes, earthquakes, and floods), major accidents leading to injury and loss of life (mass transportation accidents, multivehicle accidents), violence or the threat of violence to self or loved ones (rape, kidnapping), and situations that have the potential for serious injury or death to self or others resulting from acts of violence (mass homicide, war). The traumatic event triggers intense fear, terror, and feelings of helplessness. Recurrent and intrusive memories of the event continue despite the individual's avoidance of reminders of the event and attempts to stop thinking about the situation. Depending on symptoms, impairment can range from mild to severe. Affected individuals can report difficulty sleeping, recurrent nightmares, hypervigilance, difficulty concentrating, decreased memory, headache, emotional lability, irritability, survivor guilt, and fear of losing control. None of these responses were characteristic of the individual prior to the experience. Individuals experience a dissociative state in which they relive the traumatic experience; this causes intense psychologic distress.[23,29]

Individuals with PTSD often have symptoms of depression, anxiety, and cognitive impairment. These symptoms could be severe enough to meet the requirements for a formal diagnosis of a psychiatric disorder. Self-defeating behaviors, including substance abuse, are common and can be the individual's attempt to alleviate the pain of the situation. There is also a potential for suicidal actions.[23,29]

Generalized Anxiety Disorder.

A diagnosis of generalized anxiety disorder is uncommon. This disorder is characterized by excessive worry about two or more life circumstances for a period of at least 6 months. The usual age at onset of the symptoms is during the 20s to 30s; the disorder occurs about equally in men and women. In its pure form, it contributes mild impairment. Symptoms of motor tension, autonomic hyperactivity, vigilance, and scanning are associated with this disorder. It is not uncommon for signs of mild depression to be associated with this disorder. Depressive disorder and panic disorder can occur simultaneously but are unrelated to the generalized anxiety disorder.[23,29]

Management

Anxiety is ubiquitous. It is important that health care providers be aware of their own level of anxiety and the relief behaviors that they use. Since anxiety is contagious, the health care worker needs to approach the patient in a calm manner and talk with a calm tone of voice. Remember that anxiety can distort the message heard. Clear, concise, direct communication is important.

The uncertainty surrounding illness and feelings of powerlessness in dealing with the health care system are additional stressors that can trigger increased levels of anxiety in health care seekers. Anxiety in the mild and moderate levels can be an asset to healing as it can provide the motivation for healthy adaptation. Severe and panic levels of anxiety can compound the problems of the health care seeker. Health care professionals need to monitor the manifestation of anxiety in health care seekers, help the individual maintain a healthy level, and refer for further diagnosis and treatment when needed.

While monitoring behaviors for signs of increasing anxiety, it is important to address the behavior and assist the indi-

vidual to maintain an effective level of anxiety. This process in itself can be educational and health-producing. First, the anxiety must be identified. When anxiety behaviors are observed, asking the individual questions such as "Are you anxious?" "Are you nervous?" "Are you uncomfortable?" helps the individual to focus on the present. This question, in various forms, might have to be asked several times, especially if denial is one of the individual's anxiety relief behaviors. Once the individual affirms the anxiety, ascertain the usual way the individual relieves the anxiety. Questions such as "What helps you?" and "What usually relieves it?" encourage the individual to connect feelings and behaviors while they afford the health care provider the opportunity to assess the appropriateness of relief measures. Next, establish the patient's expectations prior to the anxiety-triggering situation, and then the patient's perception of what actually happened in the situation. Connect the unmet expectations to the anxiety and the anxiety to the relief behavior. This provides the health care worker with the individual's picture of the situation and allows the patient to make the connection between feelings of anxiety and relief behaviors. It is at this point that there is an opportunity to facilitate change. If relief behaviors have been ineffective, the anxiety can provide the motivation for the client to learn alternative coping methods such as problem solving, relaxation techniques and assertiveness skills.[23,25,30–33]

Once an organic basis for the symptoms has been ruled out, various approaches are available for the treatment of anxiety disorders. It is often difficult for people to take advantage of the assistance available, as psychiatric disorders are often viewed as a sign of weakness and people are much more comfortable with the diagnosis and treatment of a physical illness. While a variety of treatment modalities are available for symptoms of anxiety, medications such as benzodiazepines, tricyclic antidepressants, MAO inhibitors, and beta-adrenergic antagonists are often the most acceptable to the patient[23,28,33] (Table 18–2).

Individual, group, and family therapy can be used to increase insight and to provide reassurance and support for the individual and those impacted by the behavior. Within these approaches, theoretical underpinnings will direct the specific approach. Behavior therapy techniques include thought stopping, substituting positive for negative behavior, systematic de-

TABLE 18–2. ANTIANXIETY AGENTS

Medication	Dosage	Side Effects
Lorazepam (Ativan)	2–3 mg bid or tid to start, followed by 1–10 mg/d, as needed, in divided doses, with largest taken before bedtime; usual maintenance dosage: 2–6 mg/d in divided doses	Drug dependence; withdrawal reactions; mental impairment; slowed reflexes
Chlordiazepoxide hydro-chloride (Librium)	Adult: 5–10 mg tid or qid Child (>6 yr): 5 mg bid to qid, or up to 10 mg bid or tid, if needed	Mental impairment; slowed reflexes; drug dependence; withdrawal reactions; increased activity with poten-tiating compounds
Oxazepam (Serax)	10–15 mg tid or qid	Drug dependence; drowsiness; dizziness
Clorazepate dipotassium (Tranxene)	15 mg/d to start, followed by 15–60 mg/d, in a single daily dose at bedtime or in divided doses	Drug dependence; mental impairment; slowed reflexes; barbituratelike withdrawal symptoms; dry mouth
Diazepam (Valium)	2–10 mg bid to qid, depending on severity	Mental impairment; slowed reflexes; drug dependence; withdrawal reactions; seizure activity
Hydroxyzine pamoate (Vistaril)	50–100 mg qid	Drowsiness; dry mouth
Alprazolam (Xanax)	0.25–0.50 mg tid to start, followed by increases at intervals of 3–4 d, up to 4 mg/d in divided doses, if needed, or if adverse reactions occur, by a reduction in dosage	Physical dependence; psychologic dependence; seizure activity; drug tolerance; suicide; mental impairment; mania; hypomania; increased stimula-tion; muscle spasms; sleep disturbances; dry mouth

bid, twice a day; qid, four times a day; tid; three times a day.

sensitization, flooding, and aversive conditioning. The aim of cognitive therapy is to modify faulty thoughts that contribute to the anxiety. This is accomplished through the use of planned exercises and homework assignments. These approaches require the patient's commitment to practice and to use these techniques.[23,28,33]

PSYCHOACTIVE SUBSTANCE USE AND ABUSE

General Characteristics

The complexity that surrounds the understanding, diagnosis, and treatment of problems associated with substance use and abuse can lead the health care worker to avoid addressing the issue with patients. Hughes proposes that the numerous terms such as "alcoholism, alcohol problem, alcohol abuse, drug misuse, drug abuse, drug dependency, chemical dependency"[34] and others that are found in the literature related to this topic can contribute to this complexity. The fact that the definition of the same term can differ from one author to another also challenges understanding. Finally, the fact that individuals often use more than one substance further compounds the difficulty of addressing this topic.[34]

The APA defines *substance* as "a drug of abuse, a medication, or a toxin."[35] At any given time, problems associated with abuse of or dependence on legal and illegal substances exist across all levels of society. A variety of cultural factors influence the use of substances. These factors include "attitude toward substance consumption, patterns of substance use, accessibility of substances, physiological reactions to substances, and prevalence of Substance-Related Disorders."[35] The cyclical pattern of psychoactive substance use and abuse throughout history has been summarized by various authors.[34,36,37]

In addition to affecting the person who abuses the substance, drug and alcohol abuse affect the family,[38] the community, and society. In the United States, it is estimated that the current levels of substance abuse contribute to at least 75,000 deaths and costs approximately 152 billion dollars a year.[37] In the workplace, productivity, quality, and job efficiency are compromised when employees with substance use disorders are late or absent or when they make errors as a result of poor concentration. These behaviors can contribute to poor relationships with coworkers and can increase the potential for accidents.[39]

Affected individuals also experience serious health problems and can put themselves and others in danger from life-threatening accidents. Alcohol has been cited in 45% of violent crimes, 45% of marital violence, 20% of nonfatal industrial accidents, 15% of nonfatal and approximately 50% of fatal traffic accidents.[35,40] It is reported that 40% of suicide attempts involve alcohol[40] and that substance-induced mood disorders could contribute to the fact that approximately 10% of those with substance dependence commit suicide.[35]

Substance use disorders impact personal health as evidenced by their association with ineffective personal hygiene, malnutrition, cirrhosis, cerebrovascular accidents, cardiac arrhythmias, respiratory arrest, and death. Depending on the route of administration, consequences can include the erosion of the nasal septum, septicemia, subacute bacterial endocarditis, hepatitis, or infection with human immunodeficiency virus (HIV). In addition, the use of substances by pregnant women can adversely affect the development of the fetus; in some cases, substance use leads to physiologic dependence in the fetus and withdrawal symptoms in the neonate.[35]

The APA addresses disorders associated with and resulting from the abuse of a drug, the development of side effects of medication, and the exposure to toxins.[35] Some of the abused drugs cited in the discussion of substance-related disorders are alcohol, anxiolytics, sedatives, hypnotics, amphetamines, cannabis, cocaine, inhalants, and hallucinogens. Side effects of medications such as anesthetics, analgesics, anticonvulsants, antidepressants, muscle relaxants as well as nonsteroidal anti-inflammatory, antimicrobial, antihypertensive, and cardiovascular agents can contribute to the development of symptoms. In addition, some of the toxic substances of concern are heavy metals such as lead, poisons containing strychnine, some pesticides, antifreeze, carbon dioxide and carbon monoxide, and inhalants such as fumes from fuels and paints.[35]

Individuals use substances in variable patterns and for a variety of reasons. *Experimental* use is based in curiosity or a desire for the anticipated short-term effects; there is no identifiable pattern of use. *Social-recreational* use of a substance is voluntary and usually occurs as a shared experience with others who find the practice acceptable and pleasurable. *Circumstantial* or *situational* use is use of the substance to cope with a perceived need related to a specific situation. This use is limited to the situation, and patterns of use differ in frequency, intensity, and duration. *Intensified* use is long-term, and use of the substance occurs at least once each day in response to a perceived need related to a persistent problem or situation. *Compulsive* use is frequent, intense, and of long duration.

Psychologic dependence occurs and leads to physical or psychologic discomfort when the substance is not used.[41]

Generally, the route of administration, speed of onset of intoxication, and duration of effects influence the development of abuse or dependence. Use of those substances that can be administered by routes that quickly and efficiently produce desired results such as more intense intoxication, those that have a rapid onset such as immediate intoxication, and those substances that are short-acting tend to increase the chance that abuse will escalate and that dependence and possibly toxic effects will result.[35]

While there are several theories related to the causes of substance abuse, "no single theory or perspective has yet proved sufficiently broad or flexible to explain the varied and highly complex phenomena of addiction."[34] Coleman suggests that the development of substance abuse disorders is due to the interplay among biologic, psychologic, and environmental factors and supports continuing research to gain a better understanding of the problems that can lead to the development of optimum treatment approaches.[37]

Hughes has described several perspectives that currently determine perception of substance use disorders. In American society, the moral perspective predominates and maintains that substance misuse problems are signs of "weak will and immorality."[34] Individuals in this situation are labeled as "drunks" and "alcoholics." From this perspective, affected individuals are viewed as being totally responsible for their situations. In order to gain sobriety and thereby respectability, they must "exercise willpower and gain control of themselves."[34]

The perspective from which treatment is most often viewed is the medical or disease perspective, which proposes that the susceptibility to addiction is a function of body chemistry. Alcoholism is viewed as a progressive disease that the individual cannot control; complete abstinence is seen as the ultimate goal.[34] This perspective suggests that either the physical trait or a predisposition to substance abuse is inherited. Evidence supporting the biologic component of alcoholism consists of a variety of observations related to the differences between those who abuse alcohol and those who do not. These observations include electroencephalogram (EEG) changes, decreased sensitivity to alcohol, decreased levels of the enzyme MAO, and the presence of the dopamine D_2 receptor. Factors contributing to the abuse of substances other than alcohol have not been studied as extensively.[37]

Another perspective suggests that there is an "addictive personality," but Hughes and Coleman found little evidence in their reviews of the research that supports this contention.[34,37] Some practitioners also base treatment on the belief that individuals learn addictive behaviors in their attempts to cope with life's problems and that these ways of coping can be unlearned or modified.[34]

Signs, Symptoms, and Diagnosis

This section contains a general overview of the categories of substance-related disorders. Criteria for the diagnosis of specific substance disorders within each category are too extensive for inclusion here. Several excellent sources are available.[35,42] The APA divides the pathologic problems of psychoactive substance use into the categories of abuse, dependence, and substance-induced disorders (substance intoxication and substance withdrawal).[35]

Beginning in the teen years, substance intoxication is generally an individual's initial substance-related disorder. While there is a high prevalence rate for use of substances for individuals between 18 and 24 years, the onset of substance dependence disorders is generally during the 20s, 30s, and 40s. Generally, these disorders are more prevalent in men than in women.[35]

Substance Intoxication. Substance intoxication is characterized by the development of a reversible, clinically significant syndrome that is substance-specific and results from the effects of the substance on the central nervous system. The syndrome is characterized by maladaptive behavioral or psychologic changes, including "disturbances of perception, wakefulness, attention, thinking, judgment, psychomotor behavior, and interpersonal behavior".[35] The symptoms vary among individuals based on the substance, "the dose, the duration or chronicity of dosing, the person's tolerance for the substance, the period of time since the last dose, the expectations of the person as to the substances' effects, and the environment or setting in which the substance is taken."[35] These symptoms can last for hours or days and must be differentiated from symptoms associated with withdrawal from a substance or from those associated with another physical or mental condition.

Substance Withdrawal. Substance withdrawal is characterized by a substance-specific syndrome that develops when heavy or prolonged use of a substance is reduced or stopped. Withdrawal can occur after the use of alcohol; amphetamines and or similar drugs; cocaine; opiates; or sedatives, hypnotics, or anxiolytics. These symptoms affect the individual's ability to carry out important social, occupational, and family responsibilities; and they cannot be explained by other conditions. Individuals often crave and use the substance in order to reduce the symptoms of withdrawal.[35]

Substance Abuse.   Substance abuse is a recurrently maladaptive pattern of use of a substance that leads to significant impairment or distress. This pattern of use is evident for at least a 12-month period and does not meet the criteria for substance dependence. The pattern is characterized by the individual's continued use of the substance despite knowing that its use contributes to or exacerbates occupational, psychologic, or physical problems. These problems are characterized by the failure to meet major obligations including those related to family, school, and work. The maladaptive pattern also includes use of the psychoactive substance in situations in which its use contributes to physical hazards, for example, driving a motor vehicle while under the influence of the substance. This pattern of use can lead to recurrent legal problems. While tolerance, withdrawal, and compulsive use are not characteristics of substance abuse, continued abuse of a class of substances can evolve into substance dependence for that class of substances.[35]

Substance Dependence Disorders.   Substance dependence disorders are characterized by cognitive, behavioral, and physiologic symptoms and continued use of a substance despite indications of serious problems that are substance-related. Individuals experiencing dependence are likely to experience *craving*, "a strong subjective drive to use the substance."[35] Depending on the substance used, this pattern of behavior usually results in tolerance, withdrawal, and compulsive substance-taking behavior. The diagnosis is made when at least three of the criteria for the disorder are met during the 12-month period of maladaptive substance use. In addition to tolerance and withdrawal there are five other criteria, all of which are characteristic of compulsive use, that define substance dependence.[35]

Tolerance exists when increased amounts of the substance must be used in order to achieve the desired effect, or the effect of the substance decreases with continued use of the

same amount of the substance. *Withdrawal* is a characteristic cluster of unpleasant physical or subjective symptoms that develop when use of the substance stops. Symptoms of withdrawal vary according to the substance used.[35]

Compulsive substance use is a pattern of characteristic behaviors. These behaviors can include the individual's:

- using larger or more frequent doses of the substance than intended,
- persistent desire or unsuccessful attempts to control substance use,
- spending large amounts of time to procure, use, and recover from effects of the substance to the detriment of other important activities,
- withdrawing from usual activities in order to associate with substance-using group, and
- continuing use of substances despite recognition that this use is contributing to the creation and maintenance of current problems.[35]

Management

In the practice arena, it is important for health care workers to examine their own perspective and its influence on their care and treatment of affected individuals. Unexamined thoughts and feelings can lead to ambivalence, which can then contribute to "therapeutic inconsistency and contraindication" on the part of caregivers.[34] As members of the public, health care workers are influenced by the attitudes of society. Hughes has identified factors that can influence the approach of health care workers toward individuals with substance-related problems. These factors include "religious background, familial influences, education and training, personal and professional experiences."[34] As members of society, health care workers are also impacted by "societal stereotypes of alcoholics and drug addicts as irresponsible, weak-willed, and immoral" and by beliefs that characterize addiction as a "chronic, progressive disease characterized by relapse."[34] These stereotypes and characterizations can contribute to health care workers' feelings of ineffectuality and hopelessness. In turn, this can lead to the belief that only a specialist can provide effective treatment with substance-abuse problems. There are not enough specialists to provide substance abuse treatment, and treatment facilities may be nonexistent or crowded, expensive, or unacceptable to clients. The interplay of these factors results in delayed or missed opportunities for intervention.[43]

On the other hand, when health care workers view substance abuse as a health care concern, it creates the potential for addressing the problem as a routine health care issue. Bien et al. have reviewed the research related to using brief interventions as an alternative approach to those with less-than-severe alcohol-related problems and conclude that brief intervention may initiate natural processes of change that would not take place in other circumstances.[43]

Brief intervention is focused on increasing persons' awareness of the problem and advising them about the need to change their behavior. The approach is cost-effective and can be useful in primary health care settings and in employee assistance programs. Common elements of this approach include providing feedback, advice, and information related to self-help options. The health care worker uses an empathic approach to enhance patient feelings of self-worth and self-control, to establish responsibility for the problem and the solution, and to provide ongoing follow-up. This approach has been cited consistently as a positive motivating factor in getting patients to address the issue.[43]

Using findings from the physical examination, the health care worker links identified symptoms to the effects of the substance used. This can challenge denial and can increase patients' awareness of some of the problems caused by their behavior. Patients are clearly advised to reduce or to stop drinking; this advice can be presented in either verbal or written form. Implicitly or explicitly advising patients "that their drinking is their own responsibility and choice,"[43] and that they need to decide what to do about it, can enhance patients' feeling of personal control. Providing patients with a range of self-help treatment resources is an effective way to provide the information needed for patients to explore their options and select the method that best fits their need. Bien and his associates report that health care workers' "warm, reflective, empathic, and understanding" approach to patients has contributed to a positive change in patient behavior.[43] In addition, sharing the belief with patients that they are capable of changing behavior has been beneficial. Follow-up visits can be seen as supportive and contribute to change and the maintenance of changed behavior.

The recidivism rate is high for individuals who abuse substances. Change is difficult. If individuals have used substances to cope with different situations, the challenge of their learning to cope without using substances is great. The health care worker is also challenged to help the individual to find alternative ways of coping and to support efforts to change.

There are a variety of supportive approaches available that need to be tailored to the individual situation. Obviously, the management of life-threatening physical or psychologic crises must take priority in treatment decisions. References addressing specific interventions for specific substances are available. Depending on the substance used, detoxification can be accomplished in a treatment facility or on an outpatient basis. Continuing treatment can include pharmaceutical interventions to manage withdrawal symptoms, individual, group, or family counseling. Transitional living arrangements (halfway houses) can support some individuals as they move from a structured treatment setting back to their chosen environment. Education is a major component of prevention and treatment.[44-46]

Alcoholics Anonymous (AA) is a worldwide system of self-help groups composed of individuals at all levels of sobriety and providing the opportunity for mutual group and individual support for those working toward the goal of total abstinence. The composition of individual AA groups can vary, and there are groups in which members share common characteristics such as occupation (eg, blue collar workers, physicians, lawyers, nurses), life-style, and age. Some groups have "open" (visitors are welcome) meetings while others are "closed" (open only to members).[45]

Groups that follow the philosophy and principles of AA are also available for those who are seeking abstinence from narcotics (Narcotics Anonymous), those whose lives are disrupted by individuals with substance problems (Alanon, Alateen), for those who are survivors of living with an alcoholic family member (Adult Children of Alcoholics [ACOA]), and for those whose codependent behaviors have enabled the substance user (Co-dependents Anonymous). The purpose of these groups is to foster the understanding of the fact that individuals are not responsible for and cannot control the behaviors of others. Individuals can and should be encouraged to join these groups, even if the person abusing substances has not chosen to join AA or NA.[45]

Because of the shame and guilt that is often associated with the abuse of substances, it can be very difficult for individuals to take the first step to getting help. It is important for the health care worker to be aware of the variety of groups available in the area and to share this information with the patient. It might be necessary for individuals to "shop around" for a group that matches them. It is also important for the person to learn that the philosophy of AA is "a way of life to be lived"[47] and not just a series of meetings to attend.

Education groups can be helpful in addressing some of the problems associated with or resulting from substance abuse. These groups have been successful in helping those individuals who have not developed the skills necessary to manage day-to-day living. Topics such as nutrition, child care, money management, job skills, and leisure activities as well as relaxation and assertiveness techniques have been addressed using this format. Individuals may also need education and emotional support related to emotional and physical abuse.[45–48]

When designing programs for individuals recovering from substance misuse, it is important to remember that cognitive ability varies and that many in our society are functionally illiterate. Cognitive ability can be impaired as a result of the substance misuse or as a function of the process of recovery. Individuals who are grieving for the losses resulting from their behavior (eg, the substance, job, family, financial security), those who fear legal sanctions, and those who are feeling shame and guilt are compromised in their ability to process information. These difficulties can be manifested in their decreased ability to reason abstractly and to remember recent events.[46]

Individuals may be reluctant to share their cognitive difficulties with others. The clear, concise presentation and repetition of information as well as the provision of notepads, writing implements, and visible reminders to reinforce information can be helpful. Encourage individuals to write down questions that facilitate their obtaining the information needed. Initially, it is very important to present only information that is essential and relevant at any given time. Simple informational pamphlets and brochures as well as inspirational material are available, some in a variety of languages. It is important to ascertain the reading level necessary to benefit from this material; remember to explore the possibility of audiotaped materials.[45–49]

Life-style Changes

Substance use disorders can impact all aspects of life. Physical and emotional health, family relationships, economic security, employment, and legal standing can all be affected. Because substance use disorders are a family disease, all are influenced by the illness and by recovery as well. Those affected can learn new, healthy ways of living and relating. They need to recognize and use the support available and necessary to assist them in reaching their goal.

References

1. Barile L. The client who is depressed. In: Lego S, ed. *The American Handbook of Psychiatric Nursing.* Philadelphia, Pa: JB Lippincott Co; 1984:391–397.
2. American Psychiatric Association. *Diagnostic and Statistical Manual.* 4th ed (rev) (DSM-IV). Washington, DC: American Psychiatric Association; 1995:317–27; 339–352.
3. Kubler-Ross, E. *On Death and Dying.* New York, NY: Macmillan Co; 1969:85–88.
4. Coleman PM. Depression during the female climacteric period. *J Adv Nurs.* 1993;18:1540–1546.
5. Heidrich SM. The relationship between physical health and psychological well-being in elderly women: a developmental perspective. *Res Nurs Health.* 1993;16(20):123–130.
6. Hauenstein EJ. Young women and depression: origin, outcome, and nursing care. *Nurs Clin North Am* 1991;26:601–612.
7. Carnes BA. (1985) *Attributional Style, Anxiety, Depression, and Hopelessness: A Study of Unemployed White, Male, Hourly-wage Workers in Southwest Arkansas.* Austin, Tex: University of Texas; 1985. Dissertation.
8. Mellick E, Buckwalter KC, Stolley JM. Suicide among elderly white men: development of a profile. *J Psychosoc Nurs Ment Health Serv.* 1992;30(2):29–34.
9. Ziemann KM, Dracup K. Patient-nurse contracts in critical care: a controlled trial. *Prog Cardiovasc Nurs.* 1992;5(3):98–103.
10. Reus VI. Mood disorders. In: Goldman HH. *Review of General Psychiatry.* 4th ed. Norwalk, CT: Appleton & Lange; 1995:246–265.
11. Bemporad JR. Long-term analytic treatment of depression. In: Ceckham EE, Leber WR, eds. *Handbook of Depression: Treatment, Assessment, and Research.* Homewood, Ill: Dorsey Press; 1985:82–99.
12. Beck AT. Thinking and depression I. idiosyncratic content and cognitive distortions. *Arch Gen Psychiatry.* 1963;9:324–333.
13. Beck AT. The phenomena of depression: a synthesis. In: Offer LD, Freedman DX, eds. *Modern Psychiatry and Clinical Research.* New York, NY: Basic Books. 1972.
14. Beck AT. The development of depression: a cognitive model. In: Friedman RJ, Katz MM, eds. *The Psychology of Depression: Contemporary Theory and Research.* Washington, DC: VH Winston & Sons; 1974.
15. Beck AT, Rush AJ, Shaw BF, et al. *Cognitive Therapy of Depression.* New York, NY: Guilford Press; 1979:1–22.
16. Seligman MEP. *Helplessness: On Depression, Development, and Death.* San Francisco, Calif: WH Freeman Co; 1975.
17. Seligman MEP. A learned helplessness point of view. In: Rehm L, ed. *Behavior Therapy for Depression.* New York, NY: Academic Press; 1980:123–139.

18. Abramson LY, Seligman MEP, Teasdale JD. Learned helplessness in humans: critique and reformulation. *J Abnorm Psych.* 1978;87(1):49–74.

19. American Psychiatric Association. *Diagnostic and Statistical Manual.* 4th ed (rev) (DSM-4). Washington, DC: American Psychiatric Association; 1995:684–685.

20. Weiss, DS, DeWitt KN. Adjustment disorders. In: Goldman HH, ed. *Review of General Psychiatry.* 4th ed. Norwalk, Conn: Appleton & Lange; 1995:302–308.

21. Swanson AR. The client who is experiencing sleep disorder. In: Lego S, ed. *The American Handbook of Psychiatric Nursing.* Philadelphia, Pa: JB Lippincott. Co; 1984:455–466.

22. Fortinash KM, Holoday-Worret PA. *Psychiatric Nursing Care Plans* 2nd ed. St Louis, Mo: Mosby Year Book; 1995:49,264–265.

23. Greist JH, Jefferson JW. Anxiety disorders. In: Goldman HH, ed. *Review of General Psychiatry* 4th ed. Norwalk, Conn: Appleton & Lange; 1995:266–282.

24. Beck AT. Turning anxiety on its head: an overview. In Beck AT, Emery G. *Anxiety Disorders and Phobias.* New York, NY: Basic Books Inc; 1985:3–18.

25. Field WE, Jr. *The Psychotherapy of Hildegard E. Peplau.* New Braunfels, Tex: PSF Productions; 1979:17–24.

26. Garber J, Miller SM, Abramson LY. On the distinction between anxiety and depression: perceived control, certainty, and probability of goal attainment. In: Garber J, Seligman MEP, eds. *Human Helplessness Theory and Applications.* New York, NY: Academic Press; 1980:131–169.

27. Spielberger, CD *Manual for the State-Trait Anxiety Inventory STAI (Form Y).* Palo Alto, CA: Consulting Psychologists Press; 1983.

28. Noyes R. Anxiety and phobic disorders. In: Winokur G, Clayton P, eds. *The Medical Basis of Psychiatry.* Philadelphia, Pa: WB Saunders Co; 1986:152–170.

29. American Psychiatric Association. Anxiety disorders (or anxiety and phobic neuroses). In: *Diagnostic and Statistical Manual.* 4th ed (rev) (DSM-4). Washington, DC: American Psychiatric Association; 1995:393–444.

30. Benson H. *The Relaxation Response.* New York, NY: William Morrow & Co; 1975.

31. Alberti R, Emmons M. *Your perfect right: a guide to assertive behavior.* 2nd ed. San Luis Obispo, Calif: Impact Publishers; 1974.

32. Smith MC. The client who is anxious. In: Lego S, ed. *The American Handbook of Psychiatric Nursing.* Philadelphia, Pa: JB Lippincott Co; 1984:387–390.

33. Fortinash KM, Holoday-Worret, PA *Psychiatric Nursing Care Plans* 2nd ed. St Louis, Mo: Mosby Year Book; 1995:19–22.

34. Hughes TL. Models and perspectives of addiction: implications for treatment. *Nurs Clin North Am.* 1989;24:1–12.

35. American Psychiatric Association. Substance-related disorders. In: *Diagnostic and Statistical Manual of Mental Disorders.* 4th ed. Washington, DC: American Psychiatric Association; 1994:175–272.

36. Baciewicz GJ. The process of addiction. *Clin Obstet Gynecol* 1993;36:223–231.

37. Coleman P. Overview of substance abuse. *Primary Care.* 1993;20(1):1–18.

38. Hagemaster, JN. Alcohol and other drug abuse. *AAOHN J.* 1991;39:456–460.

39. Conry PB. Drugs and alcohol in the workplace. *AAOHN J.* 1991;39:461–465.

40. Liskow B, Goodwin DW. Alcoholism. In: Winokur G, Clayton P, eds. *The Medical Basis of Psychiatry.* Philadelphia, Pa: WB Saunders Co; 1986:190–211.

41. Smith DE, Landry MJ. Psychoactive substance use disorders: drugs and alcohol. In: Goldman HH, ed. *Review of General Psychiatry.* 3rd ed. Norwalk, Conn: Appleton & Lange; 1992: 172–188.

42. Olson KR, ed. *Poisoning & Drug Overdose.* Norwalk, Conn: Appleton & Lange. 1994.

43. Bien TH, Miller WR, Tonigan JS. Brief interventions for alcohol problems: a review. *Addiction.* 1993;88:315–336.

44. Kanas N. Alcoholism. In: Goldman HH, ed. *Review of General Psychiatry.* 3rd ed. Norwalk, Conn: Appleton & Lange; 1992: 189–197.

45. Jefferson LV. Chemically mediated responses and substance-related disorders. In Stuart GW, Sundeen SJ, eds. *Principles and Practice of Psychiatric Nursing.* 5th ed. St. Louis, MO: Mosby Year Book: 1995;569–604.

46. La Salvia TA. Enhancing addiction treatment through psycho-educational groups. *J Subst Abuse Treat.* 1993.10:439–444.

47. Bollerud KA. Model for the treatment of trauma-related syndromes among chemically dependent inpatient women. *J Subst Abuse Treat.* 1990;7:83–87.

48. Chavkin W, Paone D, Friedmann P, et al. Psychiatric histories of drug-using mothers: treatment implications. *J Subst Abuse Treat.* 1993;10:445–448.

49. Friedrich RM, Kus RJ. Cognitive impairments in early sobriety: nursing interventions. *Arch Psychiatr Nurs.* 1991;5(2):105–112.

19

Pediatric Disorders

Karen S. Stephenson
Heather Walters Hull

■ ANEMIA

General Characteristics

Anemia in children is a very common condition that can frequently be treated with dietary changes and supplements. By definition, anemia refers to a condition of fewer red blood cells (RBCs) in circulation than is considered normal for a child based on the child's age. This is initially determined by comparing the child's hemoglobin and hematocrit to the normals established for his or her age as well as looking for any clinical symptoms of anemia. A child may become anemic because there is inadequate production of RBCs by the bone marrow, RBC destruction, or bleeding.

The most common cause of anemia in children is iron deficiency that is the result of inadequate ingestion of iron. This variety of anemia is so common that children are screened for it several times during childhood. Probably the most common scenario is that of the toddler who was taken off iron-fortified formula or has a diet largely composed of cow's milk. Lead ingestion is also a cause of iron deficiency and should be considered as part of the work-up if the family lives in a house built before 1970 or in older towns where lead-pipe plumbing may not have been updated. Children usually ingest lead by eating paint chips, which have a sweet taste that children like, or by inhaling dust that contains lead. The dust occurs during remodeling in older houses in which lead paint was used.

Iron-deficiency anemia is characterized by microcytosis with a low mean corpuscular volume (MCV) and a low red cell distribution width (RDW). If the reticulocyte count and RDW are both normal but the MCV is low, thalassemia minor is likely, especially if the child is of African, Asian, or Mediter-ranean descent. The genes for thalassemia can affect either the alpha or beta chains that produce hemoglobin. The alpha and beta chains are inherited as a pair with one half of the pair (one alpha and one beta chain) from each parent. Most of the time the beta chain is affected, and the pattern of inheritance determines whether someone has thalassemia major or thalassemia minor. Thalassemia major is produced by two abnormal beta chains (one from each parent) that leads to marked anemia. Thalassemia minor is heterozygous and many people with the one abnormal beta chain may not be anemic. Those who are anemic will have a hemoglobin that is 2 to 3 gm/dL lower than normal for the patient's age.

Thalassemia from abnormalities of the alpha chain is usually diagnosed by gene mapping. This abnormality results from abnormalities of 2 pairs of genes that control alpha chain production. Severity of anemia resulting from alpha chain abnormalities is based on the number of abnormal genes: one gene produces a carrier state to four abnormal genes that usually leads to death for the fetus or the newborn.

Distinguishing thalassemia minor from iron deficiency requires hemoglobin electrophoresis. In thalassemia minor, the abnormal gene will produce elevated A_2 hemoglobin. The A_2 hemoglobin is usually not elevated in iron deficiency unless the deficiency is chronic. Chronic iron deficiency may decrease hemoglobin A_2 levels and may make the A_2 levels falsely normal when both thalassemia and chronic iron deficiency co-exist. In addition, serum ferritin is normal in thalassemia and reduced in iron deficiency. Bone marrow iron stores are normal in thalassemia minor and absent in iron deficiency.

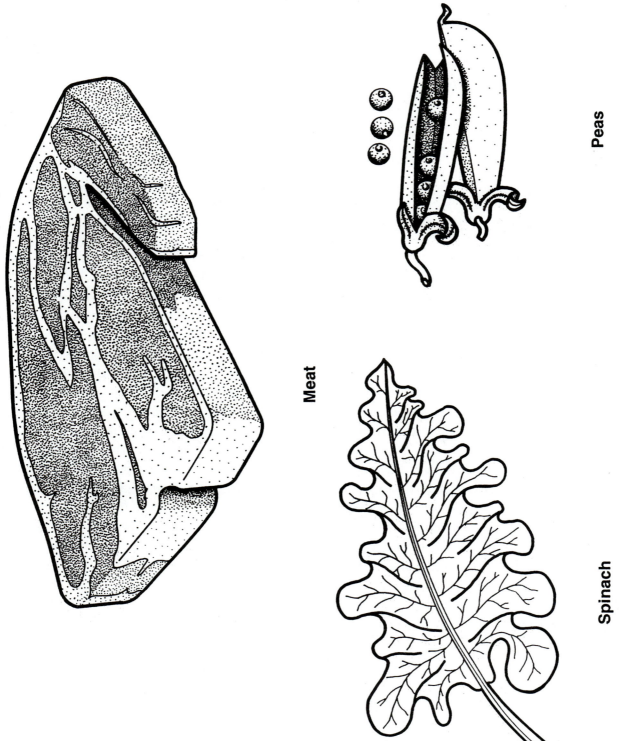

Peas

Meat

Spinach

Figure 19–1. Foods to treat iron deficiency anemia

The newer automated complete blood count (CBC) will provide both the MCV and the RDW as part of the initial CBC report. This saves money because further diagnosis may not be necessary; enough information to treat the patient is available initially.

If the MCV is normal and the child has a high reticulocyte count, hemolytic causes should be considered. Sickle cell anemia, hereditary spherocytosis, and autoimmune hemolytic anemia are possible diagnoses. In such a case, tests of the parents' blood, Coomb's test, tests of osmotic fragility, and a careful examination of the blood smear should be done. If the smear and reticulocyte count are normal, bleeding should be considered.

Children with a normal MCV and low reticulocyte count should be evaluated for a chronic disease with laboratory evaluation to include kidney, liver, and thyroid function studies in search of a chronic disease.

Causes of macrocytic anemia in children include folic acid and vitamin B_{12} deficiencies of childhood. Children who drink only goat's milk will not ingest enough folic acid. Children with malabsorption problems, those taking anticonvulsants, or those who have a concurrent hemolytic anemia will also have a folic acid deficiency. Vitamin B_{12} may not be absorbed for several reasons: lack of intrinsic factor, either congenital or acquired, lack of carrying molecule for B_{12}, or familial causes of malabsorption.

Management

Treatment of anemia depends on the cause. Dietary modifications may be needed (Fig. 19–1). Foods rich in iron include red meats, pinto beans and dried fruits, such as raisins, apricots, and prunes. Sources with lesser amounts of iron include spinach, peas, carrots, beans, sweet potatoes, and peaches.[1] Iron-deficiency anemia is the most common, for which oral iron is prescribed at the rate of 3 to 6 mg/kg/d of elemental iron for 3 to 6 months. About 2 weeks after the iron is begun, a reticulocyte count can be done to measure the response to iron. Iron therapy must be continued for 4 to 6 weeks after levels are back to normal to replenish iron stores. Thalassemia minor may appear similar to iron-deficiency anemia but does not respond to iron. Referral to a hematologist is recommended for management of thalassemia. If bleeding is suspected, a stool specimen for occult blood should be done. Children with hereditary spherocytosis usually have splenectomies performed around 5 years of age.

Children with sickle cell disease need to receive regular health care with special emphasis on eating well, watching closely for emerging illnesses, especially pneumococcal sepsis (due to autosplenectomy), and giving penicillin 125 mg orally twice daily for the first 5 to 6 years of life. These children should receive the 23-valent pneumococcal vaccine at age 2. This vaccine should be repeated 3 to 5 years later for those with either functional or anatomic asplenia. If the child originally was given the 14-valent vaccine, the 23-valent should be given. Parents must be cautioned to seek immediate treatment for the child with fever or other signs of sepsis, since the vaccine will not protect completely from pneumococcal infection, sepsis, or death.[2]

■ ASTHMA

General Characteristics

Asthma occurs frequently in children and is the most common cause of hospitalization for children (for additional information refer to Chapter 7). Events or conditions that may predispose children to asthma include exposure to tobacco smoke from parents and other caregivers, croup, bronchiolitis, atopic dermatitis, and exposure to inhalant allergens that may precipitate an episode of wheezing. Some of these include dust mites, pollens, molds, cold air, pollution, and animal dander. Exercise or emotional upset may also trigger an asthma attack.

Children may begin wheezing before age 2, and this is usually caused by a viral upper respiratory infection. Because asthma is a chronic disease, the diagnosis may become apparent over time with several episodes of wheezing. Forty percent of children who develop lower respiratory symptoms from bronchiolitis will later be diagnosed with asthma. Children do not outgrow asthma but their airways become larger and therefore they may not appear symptomatic. They may continue to have subclinical ventilation-perfusion deficits and may experience a recurrence during a viral illness.

There is usually a strong family history for IgE-mediated diseases (allergic rhinitis, atopic dermatitis, and asthma), and asthma is more common in boys until puberty, when the ratio of men to women becomes equal. Many people are unfamiliar with the term atopic dermatitis but will describe dry skin or eczema.

Signs, Symptoms, and Diagnosis

Increased mucus production, smooth muscle spasm, and inflammation in the airways are characteristic of asthma. Coughing, wheezing, tachycardia, tachypnea, and shortness of breath commonly occur during an acute asthmatic episode. Coughing may develop, with a smaller degree of bronchospasm than that required to produce audible wheezing. Coughing, especially at night and during physical activity or excitement, is the hallmark of asthma. These symptoms may be brought on by a viral upper respiratory infection, exercise, or exposure to inhalant allergens. Some children will cough after laughter or following other intense emotions. Some children will not wheeze but rather have coughing or profuse mucus production, with the cough worsening at night. Chil-

dren who seem to have had recurrent pneumonia may actually be asthmatic; on x-ray the infiltrate turns out to be atelectasis in the right middle lobe or lingula.

When a child is being evaluated for wheezing or cough, bronchiolitis, cystic fibrosis, aspiration of a foreign body, gastroesophageal reflux, and anatomic defects of the airway should be considered. The physical examination must include an assessment of the general condition of the child, especially signs of distress. The physical examination must include a thorough chest evaluation, including respiratory expansion, signs of respiratory distress, and auscultation for rales, rhonchi, or wheezing. Asking the child to fold his or her arms and hold them away from the chest increases the area available to evaluate both upper lobes. Asking the child to pretend to be blowing out a candle or actually blow on a paper towel to make it flutter will improve airway movement, especially in young children.

Pulmonary function testing is the most important diagnostic tool, and peak flow rates are easily measured in the outpatient setting. They are also used at home to evaluate the degree of bronchospasm as a basis for management decisions. Peak flow is commonly used, can be measured with portable equipment, and measured over time can establish norms for each child. Most importantly, it provides information that can allow the parent and the child to take more responsibility for the management of asthma. Peak flow measures the expiratory rate in liters per minute, but it requires that the child exhale with maximal effort. Children should exhale two to three times and then use the best measurement to determine the degree of bronchospasm. Normals for sex and height in centimeters have been established for children and adults; this information is included with the flow meter. Personal norms can be established over time for each child, and values should be within 5% to 10% of each other.

Management

Treatment of asthma includes: education of the patient and the parent, participation in childhood activities, minimal exposure to environmental irritants, and use of medications. The child should participate in the treatment of his or her illness as completely as possible, including daily measurement of peak flow readings, monitoring times for dosages, and identi-

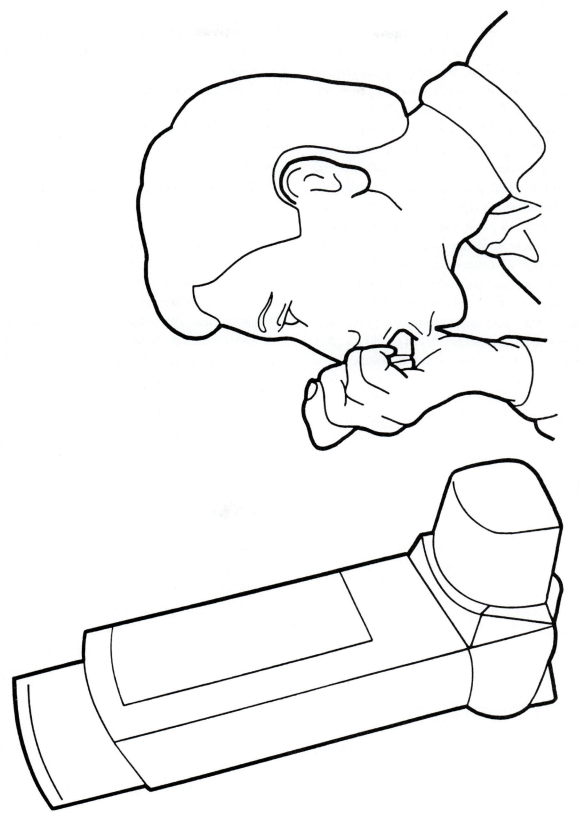

Figure 19–2. Asthma treatment using an inhaler

fying symptoms early. The child should also participate in activities as much as possible. Every effort should be taken to maintain the child's environment as irritant-free as possible. For instance, if the child is old enough to assume duties around the house, cleaning responsibilities (eg, dusting, sweeping, vacuuming) should not be given to him or her, but to someone else. The child can assume other duties where dust exposure is limited (eg, folding laundry, washing dishes).

Pharmacologic treatment of asthma includes the following: bronchodilatation with inhalatory medication (Fig. 19–2), addition of corticosteroids and systemic bronchodilators as warranted, and use of peak flow or arterial blood gases to monitor response to therapy. Sodium cromolyn can be used to prevent asthmatic episodes when wheezing can be predicted, as with exercise or allergen exposure. Sodium cromolyn is not used for acute asthma treatment. Albuterol, metaproterenol, or isoetharine in 2 mL of normal saline is recommended as initial therapy for asthmatic symptoms. In all categories of medicines, there are topical medications that can directly affect inflammation with fewer side effects than systemic drugs.

The best example is sodium cromolyn. Cromolyn works by destabilizing the mast cell membrane and reducing the amount of histamine released. Most children also receive a beta-adrenergic agonist; albuterol or metaproterenol are the preferred choices. Whether theophylline or steroids, either inhalatory or systemic, are then added is debatable. Both medications have serious side effects, but more recently, the trend is toward using steroids, because of the large role that inflammation plays in asthma, and away from using theophylline because of its narrow therapeutic window.

Home- or self-monitoring for the child with asthma provides objective data that can be used by the child, parent, and clinician to follow the clinical course of asthma. Peak flow is measured twice daily until the normal or best is established. On any given day, a reading that is 70% or greater is considered a good response to therapy. Values that fall between 70% and 50% require increasing treatment (for example, nebulization four times a day instead of three). A reading below 50% requires a call to the doctor, probably resulting in an additional dose of treatment or the addition of systemic steroids.

■ CARDIOVASCULAR RISK FACTORS

General Characteristics

Evaluating children and adolescents for cardiac risk factors is a relatively new emphasis in preventive pediatrics.[3] Adults have been screened for about 40 years for hypertension as a risk factor for myocardial infarction as well as other embolic events. The roles also played by premature disease in relatives, smoking, diabetes, sedentary life-styles, and hyperlipidemia have been added as a result of the Framingham studies, the Swedish lipid trials, and other studies. Out of those findings, coordinated screening programs for adults with emphasis on risk factors that are modifiable was begun in earnest in the United States and other developed countries.

Currently information about the significance of cholesterol to the care of children and adolescents has been studied. The efficacy of aggressive lowering of blood lipid levels in children has not been studied to the extent that it has in adults; therefore, guidelines for children are not as available as they are for adults. It also has not yet become a standard of care that each child be screened for elevated blood lipids.

Screening children for elevated lipid levels when they have a strong family history for coronary artery disease (CAD) does seem to be appropriate. Suggested guidelines include screening those who have male family members with CAD prior to age 50 and female family members with CAD prior to age 60. Adolescents whose parents have elevated lipid levels, hypertension, or other significant risk factors for CAD should also be screened. Directed questioning should provide the basis for screening. Other children with risk factors who also require screening include children who are obese (30% overweight for age-specific norms), who are hypertensive by age-specific criteria, are sedentary, have diabetes, or have begun smoking. A study by Becque et al demonstrated that 97% of obese teenagers were found to have four or more cardiac risk factors.[4] These include elevated triglycerides, decreased high-density lipoprotein (HDL) cholesterol, elevated blood pressure, diminished work capacity, and strong family history of coronary heart disease. Parents are responsible for the environment in which their children are raised. Activities on the part of parents that put parents at risk for CAD are more likely to be incorporated into the life-style activities of their children.

Management

Recommendations for reducing coronary risk factors in children include aerobic activity several days a week, a diet that is low in fat, and no smoking. Aerobic exercise should be one that the child or adolescent enjoys and should include 30 to 60 minutes of aerobic exercise with warm-up and cool-down periods before and after. The clinician should provide the patient with specific information; Rocchini recommends writing an exercise prescription that begins with 1 to 3 weeks of mild exercise, then beginning more strenuous exercise until the child or adolescent can do 30 to 60 minutes of activity.[3] Children should also be taught to calculate their target pulse, using the formula $(220 - age) \times 0.75 = target$. He also recommends that the clinician emphasize the improvement in well-being and encourage support from family and friends.

The most important dietary change is reducing the amount of fat to 30% or less of total calories for children three years of age or older. Fat provides the rich taste to many foods, and it requires commitment to reduce the fat intake (Fig. 19–3). Examples include red meats, pastries, and desserts. Most of the calories consumed should be from complex carbohydrates (50% to 60%) and protein should only be 10% to 20% of a child's or teenager's diet. If the parents are at risk also for CAD, these activities can be adopted by the whole family. Just as with the exercise regimen, the child or adolescent needs support of family or friends. Children should also watch a limited amount of television. Television watching is associated with sedentary life-styles, obesity, and high-fat diets.

Lipid-reducing medications have not been evaluated for children and at present are not recommended. Lipid levels for children based on sex and age have been documented, but the question of levels at which treatment should be initiated remains controversial. Suggested treatment goals for children and adolescents include reducing cholesterol levels to below 180 to 200 mg/dL, reducing low-density lipoprotein (LDL) cholesterol levels to 120/dL, and the LDL:HDL ratio to 3 or less. These suggestions are based on the 95th percentile levels established for children and adolescents between age 10 and 19 from data gathered by the National Heart, Lung, and Blood Institute and published in 1980.[5]

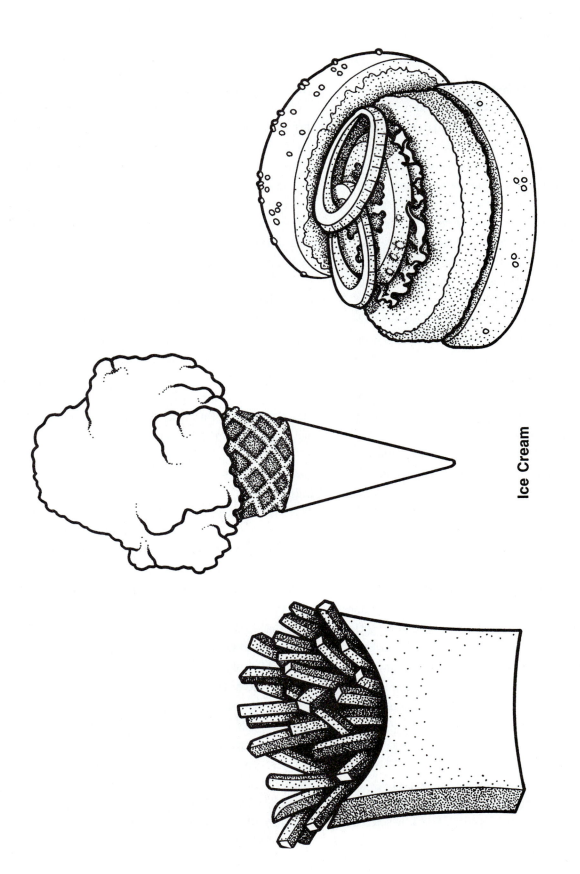

Hamburger

Ice Cream

French Fries

Figure 19–3. Foods high in fat

■ TAKING A TEMPERATURE

General Instructions

Taking a child's temperature is a skill parents need to take care of their sick children. There are several ways to take a child's temperature: by mouth (Fig. 19–4), under the arm, in the rectum, or by the ear. For the mouth, the child must hold the ther-mometer under the tongue with lips closed for 3 to 5 minutes. Generally a child should be 6 to 7 years of age before he or she can hold the thermometer under the tongue safely without breaking it. Taking an axillary temperature requires that the thermometer be held under the arm with the arm next to the

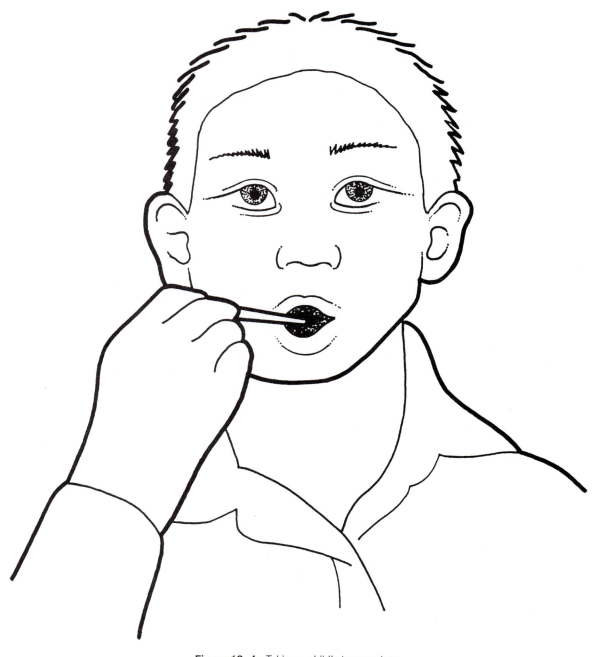

Figure 19–4. Taking a child's temperature

child's body for 3 to 5 minutes. For the rectum, the thermometer should be placed gently into the rectum for about 5 minutes. For the ear, there is a probe placed in the ear while the temperature is being taken. Measurement of temperature under the arm, in the rectum, or in the ear are suitable methods for children of all ages. Drinking liquids, eating, taking a bath, or smoking can change the temperature, so temperature should not be taken for about 15 minutes after any one of them.

Fever is an increase in the body temperature above what is considered normal. Most people consider 98.6°F as the normal body temperature. A fever is considered to be above 100.5° to 101°F. When the temperature is above 98.6°F and not at 100° to 101°F, it may be called a low-grade fever. It may or may not be an actual fever because body temperature varies during the day from waking to sleeping. The temperature is lowest just before we get out of bed and highest about 12 to 14 hours later. That first temperature may be about 97° or 97.5°F but may go up to 99.6° to 99.8°F toward the end of the day. The temperature starts to go down again with sleep. This is referred to as diurnal changes in the temperature and is the reason a temperature has to be above 100.5°F to be considered fever.

Different types of thermometers will give different temperature readings: a rectal temperature is 1 degree higher than an oral one. The axillary temperature is 1 degree lower. Thus a temperature is considered a fever when it is 101.5°F when taken in the rectum and when it is 99.5°F taken in the armpit.

It is important to ask how the temperature was taken when a child's temperature is reported.

The health care provider may want the parent to call when the child has a fever, especially if the child is a newborn (up to 2 months old) or when fever is really high, for example 103°F, before any treatment at home is given. The health care provider can then give instructions on treating the child. The child may need to be seen and given a checkup. Otherwise, the parent may want to give the child acetaminophen to help lower the temperature and help him or her to feel better. Acetaminophen should always be given rather than aspirin. When children have viral infections, like colds or the flu, aspirin can cause Reye's syndrome and may lead to coma and death. Unless the health care professional specifically tells the parent to give aspirin, it should not be given.

For children less than 2 years of age, the label informs the parent to contact the child's doctor about the dose of acetominophen for the child. Otherwise, the directions are on the box.

Some ways of treating fever at home may not be safe. In the past, an alcohol or cold water bath has been used to treat fever. It has been discovered that these baths cause the child to cease sweating which helps to remove excess body heat. Baths may be used, however, only water at a comfortable body temperature should be used. The child should not be left alone in the bathtub.

■ NEONATAL JAUNDICE

General Characteristics

Neonatal jaundice can occur from a multitude of conditions during the perinatal period. The clinician must distinguish the physiologic jaundice that commonly occurs in newborns from conditions that carry a more serious prognosis. Clues to the cause of jaundice are available from the laboratory evaluation of the infant as well as from the time in the newborn period in which the jaundice occurs.

Jaundice during the first 2 weeks of life is usually indirect hyperbilirubinemia, and physiologic jaundice is the most common type occurring during this period. This type of jaundice arises from the hemolysis of fetal RBCs no longer needed by the newborn, decreased bilirubin conjugation by UDPglucuronyl transferase, and abnormal bilirubin secretion from meconium. The blood-brain barrier also may allow bilirubin to be deposited in the brain; this can cause kernicterus resulting in motor impairment, mental retardation, or sensorineural hearing loss.

The second type of jaundice, direct hyperbilirubinemia or cholestasis, usually occurs after the first 2 weeks of life. The liver, spleen, and bone marrow process the fetal RBC cells and break them down into indirect or unconjugated bilirubin that, free in the circulation, can be a toxin to the newborn. The bilirubin is bound to albumin and carried to the liver, where it is converted to direct, or conjugated, bilirubin by the UDPglucuronyl transferase. This bilirubin is then water-soluble and can be excreted by the kidney.

Physiologic jaundice is the most common cause of jaundice during the first 2 weeks of life. It develops in the first 2 to 4 days of life and peaks on day 3 to day 4 at a level of 12.9 mg/dL but may rise to 15 mg/dL. If this type of jaundice develops in a premature infant, it peaks sooner, lasts longer, and doesn't exceed 15 mg/dL.

Hemolytic disease of the newborn may be secondary to ABO or Rh incompatibilities. When the incompatibility results from the Rh antigen, the condition is more serious and without treatment may result in erythroblastosis fetalis or death. ABO problems occur much more frequently but are less serious. Both result from RBCs from the fetus passing into the mother's circulation and, when different from the mother's, maternal production of antibodies against the fetal RBCs.

ABO incompatibility occurs in about 20% of pregnancies. Almost half the American population has O+ blood, which contains both anti-A and anti-B antibodies. The manner in which these antibodies are produced from RBCs without A and B antigens is unknown. The second most common blood type, A, occurs in 40% of the population and contains antibodies to B. Blood type B occurs in 11% of the population and has anti-A antibodies; the least common blood type, AB, occurs in only 4 % of the population and is without either antibody. It is thought that these antibodies are weaker than the Rh ones and, therefore, may be better tolerated.[6]

After the first 2 weeks of life, the most common cause of jaundice from indirect bilirubin is breast milk jaundice. This may persist for as long as 3 months, but it does not usually cause kernicterus. The bilirubin generally stays below 15 mg/dL, except in a rare condition, the Lucey-Driscoll syndrome, which may occur in the first few days and is associated with high levels of indirect bilirubinemia and kernicterus.

Two other types of hyperbilirubinemia result from a deficiency of or total lack of UDPglucuronyl transferase (Crigler-Najjar types I and II, respectively). Newborns may also be jaundiced because of congenital hypothyroidism.

Direct hyperbilirubinemia usually develops in newborns 2 weeks of age or older. This type of jaundice may result from problems within the liver as well as extrahepatic ones. The most common intrahepatic causes include neonatal hepatitis or viral hepatitis. Most of the cases of neonatal hepatitis (50% to 60%) are unrecognized, and the second most common cause are the pathogens responsible for infections in newborns: TORCH (toxoplasmosis, rubella, cytomegalovirus, herpes) hepatitis B virus varicella, adenovirus, *Listeria*, and other infectious agents.

Other cholestatic causes of neonatal jaundice may include toxic etiologies; parenteral nutrition, galactosemia, fructosemia, alpha$_1$-antitrypsin deficiency, and tyrosinemia. Further etiologies to consider include inspissated bile syndrome, hypoplastic bile ducts (Alagille syndrome), or cystic fibrosis. Causes that necessitate surgical intervention include biliary atresia and choledochal cyst.

Signs, Symptoms, and Diagnosis

The most important information about jaundice involves the prenatal history and the perinatal events. For example, did the mother acquire an intrauterine infection? Was the baby born prematurely? Was there an Rh incompatibility? Others to remember: diabetes, preeclampsia, hypothyroidism, type of feedings, or stress of any type at delivery.

The physical examination must be complete to look for clues about the cause of the jaundice. Does the infant have any evidence of congenital problems? Are there signs of chronic liver disease? Does the skin or sclera look yellow or green? What size and shape is the liver? Can the gallbladder be palpated? Are there abdominal signs of liver disease? Is the spleen enlarged? Is there a heart murmur, such as pulmonary artery hypoplasia, which is accompanied by bile duct problems? Is there clubbing of the extremities, which may be associated with cirrhosis?

Laboratory evaluation includes particular attention to the bilirubin level as well as finding the relative amounts of indirect and direct bilirubin. The following work-ups address the two different types of jaundice. If the problem is in the indirect portion, additional laboratory tests should be performed: CBC; reticulocyte count; RBC smear; platelet count; direct and indirect Coombs' tests, serum haptoglobin, cold agglutinins, antinuclear antibodies (ANA) and, glucose-6-phosphate dehydrogenase (G6PD) levels; thyroid function tests; and urine culture.

Direct jaundice requires a different evaluation. This work-up includes serum cholesterol, blood and urine culture, VDRL, TORCH antibodies, hepatitis B surface antigen, reducing substance in urine, $5'$ nucleotidase, serum alpha$_1$-antitrypsin, Pi typing of alpha$_1$-antitrypsin, galactose-1-uridyl-transferase activity in RBCs, amino acid screen of urine and blood, and sweat chloride test.

Management

The etiology directs the management of the condition. If the problem is thought to be from breast feeding, a 2- to 3-day hiatus with formula in the interim will correct the problem. Physiologic jaundice can be treated with increased fluids or, if the bilirubin is high enough, by phototherapy. Graphs are available in most neonatology books for the exact levels at which phototherapy should be begun. There are now fiberoptic blankets that can provide the phototherapy portion of the treatment of the jaundice. Children must remain well-hydrated during phototherapy. This increases urine output and elimination of conjugated bilirubin. Exchange transfusion may also be warranted in cases in which the hemolytic process produces high levels of bilirubin that would place the newborn at risk for brain damage.

Metabolic disorders can also be treated with special formula, in particular, formula that contains medium-chain triglycerides (Portagen) can be used for prolonged cholestasis. Several drugs, including phenobarbital or cholestyramine promote bile secretion, diminish pruritus, and alleviate cholestasis. Surgery is indicated for problems that interrupt bile flow.

■ OTITIS MEDIA AND SINUSITIS

General Characteristics

Otitis media and sinusitis share many of the same characteristics, are frequently precipitated by the same factors, and are treated similarly. The conditions arise in similar structures in the skull: small bony cavities with a minute opening, lined with mucosa that is continuous with the mucosa of the throat. Under normal conditions, these cavities are air-filled, but when infected, they are colonized by normal flora from the oral cavity.

Both conditions are most frequently caused by: *Streptococcus pneumoniae,* nontypable *Haemophilus influenzae,* and *Moraxella catarrhalis. Moraxella* was previously known as *Branhamella.* Beta-hemolytic (group A) streptococcus occurs much less frequently unless there is some contributing circumstance, such as premature birth, lengthy stays in the hospital, or immunodeficient states. These three most common organisms have significant numbers of strains that are beta-lactamase producers.

Otitis media and sinusitis are usually precipitated by viral upper respiratory tract infections or inhalant allergies. Both cause swelling of the mucosal lining of the oral cavity, which causes the minute openings of both sets of cavities to swell shut. In the case of the ear (Figure 19–5) the eustachian tube is no longer able to equalize the air pressure in the middle ear. In young children, this process is exacerbated by a tube that is still shorter, more horizontal, and flimsier than that of older children and adults. Once the openings are swollen shut, it may take several weeks or months for the ears and sinuses to recover from the acute infection. Swollen adenoids (likely in chronic allergic rhinitis) or nasopharyngeal tumors may also

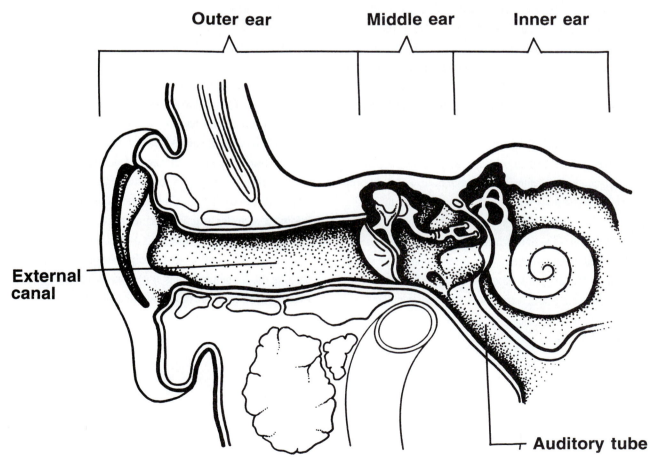

Outer ear   **Middle ear**   **Inner ear**

External canal

Auditory tube

Figure 19–5. Anatomy of the ear

block the eustachian tube. As the infection becomes chronic, the organisms that infect both cavities may change. It becomes more likely that the common three organisms may be resistant to amoxicillin or that other bacteria, such as gram-negative enteric bacilli and group A beta-hemolytic streptococcus are infecting the middle ear and sinuses.

Signs, Symptoms, and Diagnosis

Acute otitis media presents with ear pain or pulling on the ear, fever, or irritability. There may also be an antecedent viral upper respiratory infection or allergic rhinitis. Examination of the ear may reveal impaired or absent mobility, loss of landmarks, and bulging or full tympanum. Erythema may accompany these signs but is not diagnostic of acute otitis media. It is imperative that each examination include pneumatic otoscopy, especially because a return of mobility signals a resolution of the acute infection and implies that hearing may be returning to normal if the hearing loss was a conductive one. Performing an adequate otoscopic examination requires distraction or restraint of the child. Once that is accomplished, pneumatic otoscopy does not significantly lengthen the examination.

Sinusitis in children may have a subtle presentation. This may include rhinitis that is profuse and purulent, fever, and periorbital swelling, or the cold symptoms may not be acute but may linger for longer than 7 to 10 days. The quality of the discharge is not diagnostic; the cough may occur both during the day and at night, but frequently the cough worsens at night. Parents may also notice halitosis. The physical examination is directed toward the nasal mucosa, the presence of purulent drainage around turbinates, and evaluation of the tonsils and cervical lymph nodes. Some examiners find transillumination of the sinuses helpful.

Additional laboratory examination may be needed to confirm the diagnosis of otitis media or sinusitis. Tympanograms have been used recently to provide additional data that includes the degree of compliance of the tympanum and the pressure. Flat tympanograms imply middle ear effusion; peaked waves with normal compliance imply normal tympanic movement; and increased negative pressure with normal compliance is consistent with serous otitis.

Sinus films can be used to confirm a diagnosis of infection by looking for thickened mucosa in the sinuses, air–fluid levels, and opacification of the sinuses. Air–fluid levels are rarely seen in children less than 5 years of age, and the sinus cavities in children less than 1 year of age are only outpouches rather than closed cavities. For children, the mucosal thickening must be 4 mm or greater, whereas in adults it should be 5 mm or greater. Cultures of the nasal mucosa have not proved effective in identifying the cause of sinusitis because the nasal and oral mucosa have many normal flora, but many or all are not identified by routine culture techniques. It is more appropriate to gauge the proper antibiotic coverage on the basis of known research and each patient's response to therapy.

Management

Antibiotic choices are based on information of the causative organisms, percentage of beta-lactamase producers in a community, and the degree of efficacy versus cost to the patient. Because both gram-negative and gram-positive organisms cause these infections, broad-spectrum antibiotics must be prescribed. Amoxicillin has been the drug of first choice because of its broad spectrum and low cost. Because many bacteria are resistant, many health care providers have made erythromycin ethylsuccinate and acetyl sulfisoxazole (Pediazole) a first drug choice. Trimethoprim-sulfamethoxazole has been used successfully for treating otitis media but has been shown to increase bacterial resistance. This drug is not only not suitable for treating group A beta-hemolytic streptococcus (only 5% have this bacterium) but is also a long-acting sulfa drug with the risk of erythema multiforme and allergy.

■ ALLERGIC RHINITIS

General Characteristics

Allergic rhinitis is a common condition among children and adults. The rhinitis may occur seasonally or perennially. When and under what conditions it occurs usually implies what the causative agent is. Typical allergens for seasonal allergies include pollens from trees, grasses, and weeds. Nonseasonal causes are air pollution, cigarette smoking, mold spores, animal dander, perfumes, chemicals, dust mites, feathers, and some insects (roaches). Foods may also precipitate allergic symptoms. Children develop symptoms to these conditions secondary to an allergic response triggered by exposure to allergens. The allergens are identified by IgE antibodies, which present the mast cells and basophils with the allergens. Several substances (histamines, leukotrienes, D_2 prostaglandin, and chemotaxic agents) are released from mast cells and basophils. This in turn produces the symptoms commonly associated with allergic rhinitis. Allergic rhinitis is frequently associated with asthma and atopic dermatitis because all three are IgE-mediated; there is also a strong genetic predisposition to all three.

Signs, Symptoms, and Diagnosis

Symptoms and signs of allergic rhinitis include sneezing, itching of the nose, ear, palate, and pharynx, clear rhinorrhea, nasal stuffiness, postnasal drip that leads to coughing, especially at night and upon arising, and constant sniffing and clearing of the throat to handle the secretions. Because of this, the child may be unable to breathe through his or her nose and may breathe through the mouth. Children may be observed repeatedly pushing upward on the tip of the nose, demonstrating the "allergic salute," or be heard using their tongue to scratch their throat. Parents may key in on these auditory noises and bring the child in for those reasons rather than the sneezing or postnasal drip symptoms. The allergy irritability syndrome has recently been described as a sense of lethargy and fatigue associated with allergic rhinitis. Other symptoms include anorexia, poor self-image, frequent school absences, and poor school performance. The preschool child is irritable and not contented to play.

History taking should address the symptoms and try to identify the precipitant of the symptoms. Information about similar symptoms as well as asthma and atopic dermatitis (dry skin) in other family members should be elicited. Other diagnoses to consider while taking a history include sinusitis (purulent drainage, fever, and cough), abuse of nasal sprays, and vasomotor rhinitis. Other causes of nasal obstruction include nasal polyps, foreign body, malignancy (especially if discharge is bloody), deviated septum, hypertrophy of the adenoids, encephalocele, rhinitis of pregnancy, benign nasopharyngeal fibroma, and hypothyroidism.

Physical examination should concentrate on nose, throat, ears, conjunctivae, and lungs. A nasal speculum should be used to evaluate the nasal turbinates. Pale or purplish boggy turbinates, mucosa with clear rhinorrhea, conjunctival injection and edema, and a crease across the nose from the "allergic salute" are commonly found in children with allergic rhinitis.

Microscopic evaluation of the nasal mucus may reveal eosinophils or segmented neutrophils indicative of allergies or sinusitis, respectively. The color alone of the nasal discharge is not diagnostic of the condition, though clear drainage is most likely allergic and green or yellow drainage may indicate sinusitis. For sinusitis, other signs and symptoms must suggest the diagnosis (eg, lasting longer than 7 to 10 days, fever, facial or dental pain). Sinus films can then be done to confirm the diagnosis. Sinus films can be abnormal in small children, even though there may be no clinical symptoms. Sinus films in children less than 1 year old are not usually indicated. The sinuses have not completely closed and are more like anterooms rather than closed chambers.

Management

Avoidance is the most effective means of managing allergic rhinitis, but it is not always practical. There are now vacuum cleaners and air filters that have electrostatic features that are much better at removing the offending allergens. The child's room should be made as allergy-free as possible including removing carpet, drapes, stuffed animals, feather pillows, plants, and animals. Bedding should be washed regularly and dried on high heat to kill the dust mites.

Medications for allergic rhinitis include antihistamines, sodium cromolyn, and steroids. There are quite a few antihistamines available by prescription and over the counter. Sometimes several may have to be used before an effective one is found. Sodium cromolyn works by destablizing the mast cell membrane, and topical corticosteroids work by alleviating the inflammatory response to the allergen. Which of the two is used depends on the experience and personal preference of the patient and the clinician. Both work well and have complementary roles in the treatment of allergic rhinitis.

■ SEIZURE DISORDERS

General Characteristics

Seizure disorders in children include several classifications of seizures. The term seizure is used to describe several different neurologic events or conditions that may occur: febrile seizures, epilepsy, single seizures (isolated instance), and seizures from metabolic, infectious, or other causes.

Febrile seizures usually occur in children in early childhood (6 months to 5 years of age) with a febrile illness and without evidence of intracranial or other cause. Ninety percent of febrile seizures occur in children less than 3 years of age.

Single seizures do not have a pattern of recurrence and seizures secondary to another process have a identifiable cause. Epilepsy is used to refer to a chronic disorder characterized by seizures without any identifiable cause. Epilepsy is characterized by one or more seizure types, specific findings on electroencephalogram (EEG), specific age of onset, and predictable clinical course.

Seizures are classified as either partial or generalized and as either simple or complex (Table 19–1). Partial seizures begin in a portion of the cerebral hemisphere, and this is supported by history and EEG findings. Generalized seizures, on the other hand, are located in both hemispheres by history and EEG findings. Simple seizures are those in which there is no impairment of consciousness, whereas in complex seizures there is. An aura, a premonitory sensory or motor phenomenon, is considered a simple partial seizure.

TABLE 19–1. CLASSIFICATION OF CHILDHOOD SEIZURES

Types	Symptoms	EEG Findings	Treatment
Generalized Seizures			
Childhood absence epilepsy or petit mal epilepsy	blank stare with unresponsiveness; changes in tone; automatisms	3-Hz spike slow-wave discharges	Valproic acid or ethosuximide
Tonic-clonic or grand mal epilepsy	short cry; stiffness; falling down; clonic jerks with relaxation; may bite tongue; may be incontinent	bilateral synchronous 2-6-Hz spike and slow-wave discharges	Valproic acid, carbamazepine, phenytoin
Juvenile myoclonic epilepsy	myoclonic jerks of neck and shoulder; tonic-clonic-tonic; seizure shortly on waking; photic stimulant	4-6-Hz multiple-spike slow-wave discharges	Valproic acid, clonazepam, nitrazepam
Infantile spasms, salaam seizures, flexor spasms (West's syndrome)	onset at age 2 mo–1 y; flexion of extremities, head, trunk for seconds to 1 min; may cry, laugh; autonomic dysfunction; caused by prenatal events*	high-voltage, arrhythmic slow waves with multifocal spikes while awake (beta seizures)	Corticotropin (ACTH), prednisone
Lennox-Gastaut syndrome, minor motor seizure syndrome	atypical absence; myoclonic; tonic; atonic seizures; caused by prenatal events*	1.5-2.5-Hz spike wave with slow background	Tonic: phenytoin Others: valproic acid, ethosuximide
Partial Seizures			
Sylvian seizures syndrome (benign Rolandic epilepsy)	during sleep; may become aphonic; salivate; tonic or clonic jerks of face or limbs	spikes over central (Sylvian) and midtemporal (Rolandic) area	Treatment not needed
Simple partial seizures syndrome (focal seizure or jacksonian seizure)	one side of body, without loss of consciousness; numerous motor or sensory findings; caused by CNS problem (CVA, tumors, AV problems, etc)	focal spikes or slow waves in appropriate cortical regions	Carbamazepine, phenytoin, valproic acid, phenobarbital, primidone, clonazepam
Partial complex seizure syndrome (temporal or psychomotor seizures	may have motor or psychic findings; impaired consciousness	focal spikes and sharp waves	Valproic acid, carbamazepine, phenytoin

AV, atrioventricular; CNS, central nervous system; CVA, cerebrovascular accident.

*Causes include prenatal infections, cerebral malformations, chromosomal abnormalities, neonatal hypoglycemia or hypoxia, kernicterus, aminoacidopathies, organic acidurias, meningitis, encephalitis, hemorrhages, phakomatoses, lysosomal disorders, neuronal ceroid lipofuscinosis, mitochondrial disorders, and Aicardi's syndrome.

Signs, Symptoms, and Diagnosis

Possible seizures should be evaluated by getting answers about the following: age at onset; possible developmental delays; the particulars of the seizure, any loss of consciousness, causes, or aura, body parts involved, any loss of continence or postictal phase, length of time it lasts; and history of central nervous system (CNS) insult.

The physical examination should be complete, with attention to an age-appropriate neurologic examination. Examination for bruits, hemiparesis, and papilledema is necessary.

A laboratory examination that includes blood chemistries and an EEG also must be done. Instructing the patient to hyperventilate during the EEG to facilitate the occurrence of seizures is also helpful. Screening blood chemistries recommended are fasting glucose, calcium, magnesium, and electrolytes. A lumbar puncture can be done to rule out an infectious process (encephalitis or meningitis), subarachnoid hemorrhage, or degenerative storage disease. A computed tomographic (CT) scan or magnetic resonance imaging (MRI) may also be necessary; the MRI is more expensive, more difficult, and may require sedation. The MRI scan is preferred for tumors or anatomic malformations. Unless the EEG demonstrates a seizure disorder that is straight-forward (eg, absence seizures with typical EEG findings) the need for imaging must be considered to rule out an intracranial cause for other types of recurrent seizures.

Management

There are several drugs available to the health professional in treating children with epilepsy. These include phenobarbital, phenytoin, valproic acid, carbamazepine, and ethosuximide. Ethosuximide is the drug of choice for petit mal seizures and works well in most patients. Carbamazepine, phenytoin, valproic acid, and primidone are appropriate for partial, primary, and secondary generalized tonic-clonic seizures. Phenobarbital has been the most common drug used for these types of children 1 year of age or younger. Carbamazepine has not been approved for use in children under 6 years of age. Care must be used in prescribing each drug because they all have significant side effects that require frequent monitoring of liver, kidney, and bone marrow function.

Drug levels should be monitored periodically depending on the clinical course; noncompliance or difficulty maintaining control warrants frequent follow-up visits. When drug levels are ordered, it should be remembered that these drugs have long half-lives and that it may take at least five half-lives or 21 days to establish a steady state. Only one drug should be used at the beginning, and if a second drug is added, time should be allowed to taper off the first drug. EEGs can be used to follow the clinical course. A child must be seizure-free for 2 to 5 years before the medications are tapered to see if the child can tolerate being off the drug.

Because seizure disorders are chronic conditions, the psychosocial aspects of treatment are very important. Both child and parent need support and encouragement to successfully care for the disorder. Both need support in taking the medicine on a regular basis; children may stop their drug when they are seizure-free and then restart if a seizure occurs. If this happens close to their medical visit, the drug level may not reflect levels that exist when they are taking their medicine correctly. The child and parent should be referred to a support group in the area and time be set aside to answer questions and discuss the psychosocial aspects of this condition, especially with teenagers.

■ TONSILLITIS AND PHARYNGITIS

General Characteristics

Tonsillitis and pharyngitis are common problems in children, and most are caused by viruses. The role of group A beta-hemolytic *Streptococcus* has complicated the treatment of these conditions. Even though a minority of sore throats are caused by streptococci, missing the diagnosis can have serious consequences for the child. Pharyngitis from any cause usually occurs during the school year and is most common among children who are 5 to 8 years of age. Tonsillar tissue is largest in children at these ages and gradually reduces in size during the teenage years.

Streptococcal pharyngitis occurs in 15% to 40% of cases of pharyngitis. The classical symptoms are a sore throat, fever, erythema of the pharynx and tonsils, and exudate (Fig. 19–6). The tonsillar lymph nodes are usually enlarged and tender. There may also be petechiae of the soft palate, as well as signs of scarlet fever: sandpaper rash, most intense in the axillas and groin, and strawberry tongue. Headache, abdominal pain, and vomiting support the diagnosis of streptococcal infection, whereas symptoms of cough, rhinorrhea, and conjunctivitis support a viral or allergic cause. Streptococcal pharyngitis

does not commonly occur in children under age 3, and it may be mistaken for a viral infection because of rhinorrhea, cough, and pharyngitis. Acute rheumatic fever remains a rare complication in acute streptococcal pharyngitis; in the 1980s, the rate was 0.5 to 2.0 cases per 100,000 Americans.

Other bacterial causes to consider include groups C and G beta-hemolytic *Streptococcus, Corynebacterium diphtheriae*, gonococcal pharyngitis, *Francisella tularensis* and *Mycoplasma*. Diphtheria is not common among adequately immunized children, but this disease is escalating in this country. Tularemia is associated with eating improperly cooked rabbit meat or contact with an infected animal.

Mycoplasma pneumoniae infections can also frequently cause sore throats, but the lung is the primary site of infection. Other symptoms such as headache, malaise, fever, and cough are frequent in this illness. Mycoplasmal infections may cause pneumonia, bronchitis, croup, otitis media, bronchiolitis, and bullous myringitis.

Viral pharyngitis may be caused by adenovirus, Epstein-Barr virus (EBV), echovirus, and Coxsackie virus. Adenoviral pharyngitis occurs in winter and spring, is common in children

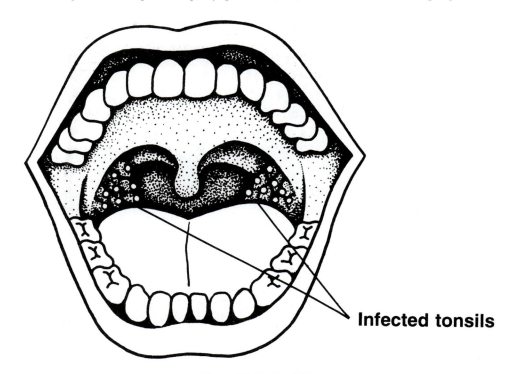

Infected tonsils

Figure 19–6. Tonsillitis

under 3 years of age, and presents with fever, nasal discharge, congestion, and cough. Adenovirus is also a cause of laryngotracheobronchitis or pneumonia. During the summer months, the presentation may be somewhat different, with high fever, conjunctivitis, and tonsillitis.

One point to remember is that infectious mononucleosis, caused by EBV, may present with cervical adenitis; exudative tonsillitis; or pharyngitis, fever, and malaise. Each child with these symptoms should have his or her liver and spleen palpated. These children may also have petechiae on their palate or generalized lymphadenopathy. A streptococcal culture may not be as helpful as anticipated because of the carrier state. Treating exudative tonsillitis caused by mononucleosis with penicillin may cause an idiopathic rash that will resemble a penicillin allergy.

Echovirus and Coxsackie virus commonly cause pharyngitis, but fever is the predominant symptom.

The evaluation must also rule out peritonsillar or retropharnygeal abscesses. The clinician should look for medially displaced tonsils, palpate them for fluctuance, and palpate the lymph nodes. Peritonsillar abscesses usually occur in adolescents, whereas retropharyngeal ones occur in young children. Younger children may have inspiratory stridor, drooling, fever, and problems swallowing. In this situation, the clinician should remember to consider epiglottitis, especially caused by *H. influenzae*, and proceed with caution during the examination to prevent laryngospasm after producing the gag reflex.

Signs, Symptoms, and Diagnosis

The factors described above will help identify the causes of the sore throat and other associated symptoms based on the etiology. A complete examination is necessary, with attention to head, ears, eyes, nose, throat, lungs, and abdominal organs.

Management

The most difficult part of managing tonsillitis or pharyngitis is the decision to evaluate for a streptococcal infection and how to manage the illness in light of those studies. Because many of the symptoms of viral and streptococcal pharyngitis overlap, the decision to look for streptococcal infection cannot be based on clinical findings alone. Rapid streptococcal antigen screens are available and are very specific, but have a 10% to 15% false-negative rate. If children do have symptoms that may imply streptococcal infection, those children with negative rapid test results should have cultures done. The cultures will take 24 to 48 hours to produce results. Penicillin should not be given as a precaution measure, but only when streptococcal infection is documented. Monospot testing can be done to rule out infectious mononucleosis. If the child does have a streptococcal infection, he or she remains contagious for 36 to 48 hours after the medication is started.

■ WHEN A CHILD HAS A VIRUS

Many of the illnesses that children have are viruses, and most of these last 7 to 10 days. Symptoms may include runny nose, coughing that is dry or productive, fever, sore throat, sneezing, vomiting, diarrhea, crankiness, or decreased appetite.

There are no medications that can cure viral illnesses except for influenza (the "flu"). The child may need antibiotics, however, if an ear infection develops. There are medicines that are available at the drugstore for treating the runny nose and cough. Some of them contain antihistamines or decongestants. These medicines can help dry the runny nose and decrease the cough. Some suggest that these not be used for children under 1 year of age. A bulb syringe can be used to remove mucus from the child's nose. Taking the child into the bathroom and turning on the shower with warm water will help the child cough and clear the airways.

A cool-mist humidifier rather than a steam humidifier can also be used. Both kinds of water will make the air moister, but steam humidifiers can be pulled over by small children and can cause burns. Cool-mist humidifiers must be cleaned frequently, every day or so, to prevent mold and fungus from growing in the bowl holding the water and then being sprayed into the room.

During this time, the child may not be hungry but should be offered plenty of fluids to prevent dehydration. The urine may darken in color when not enough fluid is given. Light color indicates that enough fluids are being taken. The best fluids for keeping urine flow normal are water, breast milk, or formula. Many times children who are ill will not take any of those fluids but will take juice or soda. If the child is not vomiting or having diarrhea, these are acceptable until the child's appetite gets better. If the child wants to eat or drink, small amounts should be offered in the beginning. Small amounts of soft foods that do not contain meat or milk, such as crackers, dry cereal, bananas, toast, or rice, will be tolerated best.

If the child has diarrhea, he or she should be given an over-the-counter oral electrolyte replacement solution such as Pedialyte, Ricelyte, or Hytren (Fig. 19–7). These help replace the water and salts lost in diarrhea and vomiting. Drinks such as apple juice, chicken broth, or soda contain too much salt or sugar and take the place of the water that is needed. When a child is vomiting, monitoring the color of urine can determine whether he or she is taking in enough fluids. If the child feels like it, he or she can take small amounts of solids (a few bites in the beginning) as tolerated. The soft foods suggested above are good choices. This is also known as the BRAT diet, for bananas, rice, applesauce, and toast.

Acetaminophen can be used to bring down fever. Fever is a frequent part of childhood illness, and even fairly high temperatures, such as 102°F, will not hurt a child, although it may frighten the parent. It needs to be explained that the fever is part of the body's defense against the virus. Some health care providers recommend not giving medicine for fever because it may prolong the illness an extra day. The child is sick until the fever has been gone for 24 hours.

A child may continue to have symptoms for a week or so, especially not eating well or a cough that continues for a couple of weeks. It also may be common for the child's bowels to move immediately after eating for a while after diarrhea stops.

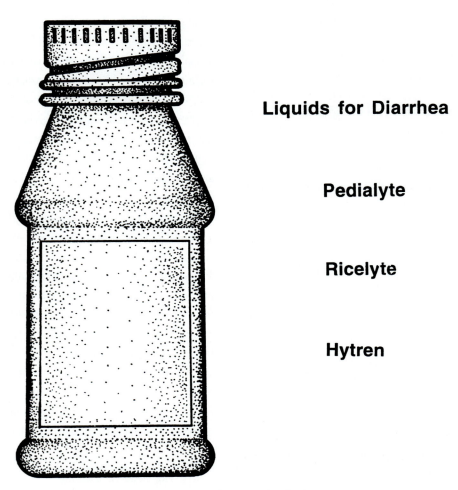

Liquids for Diarrhea

Pedialyte

Ricelyte

Hytren

Figure 19–7. Treatment for diarrhea

■ GASTROENTERITIS IN CHILDREN

General Characteristics

Acute gastroenteritis, a common pediatric illness, is characterized by diarrhea, which may be accompanied by varying degrees of vomiting, anorexia, abdominal pain and cramping, or fever. Diarrhea is a *change* in frequency, consistency, and volume of stools. Stool frequency normally varies from one stool every other day to 3–4 stools per day in children. With mild diarrhea, stools are loose or mushy, while severe diarrhea produces more frequent, watery stools. Green stools indicate rapid passage through the gastrointestinal tract and indicate moderate to severe diarrhea. More than 10 stools per 24 hours indicates severe diarrhea. Breast fed infants normally have watery yellow stools which are "seedy" in consistency, and occur after feedings, every 2–4 hours.[7,8]

Acute diarrhea is most often self-limiting and infectious, caused by viral, bacterial and parasitic pathogens. Rotovirus is the most common viral diarrhea, producing watery stools without blood or heavy mucus. Bacterial diarrhea produces more acute illness with higher fevers and blood or mucus in the stool. Parasitic diarrhea produces more variable symptoms with history of exposure to contaminated water supplies, day care epidemics, or specific animal sources. Food poisoning due to bacterial enterotoxins is abrupt in onset with vomiting greater than diarrhea and a history of exposure to contaminated foods. Diarrhea may also accompany respiratory and urinary tract infections or antibiotic therapy. Chronic diarrhea suggests other etiologies such as malabsorption, inflammatory bowel, immune deficiency, allergy, lactose intolerance or inadequate treatment of acute diarrhea (Table 19–2).

The most serious risk for infants and young children with gastroenteritis is dehydration, a total body fluid deficit resulting primarily from fluid loss through watery stools, but also from vomiting or fever, or from reduced fluid intake. Other risk factors include:

1. electrolyte imbalance due to sodium, chloride, potassium, and bicarbonate losses or inadequate fluid and electrolyte replacement, and
2. metabolic acidosis due to loss of bicarbonate in the stools or tissue hypoxia from hypovolemia.[9]

Signs, Symptoms, and Diagnosis

Evaluation includes a history, physical exam, and laboratory tests. The potential for dehydration exists in each patient and can be assessed by determining weight loss from the pre-illness state and clinical signs (Tables 19–3 to 19–5). Infants and children under 3 years can dehydrate rapidly due to high metabolism and greater intestinal fluid losses.

Laboratory Tests

Routine laboratory tests are usually considered unnecessary for most mild to moderate cases of diarrhea. However, serum electrolytes are helpful in evaluating the degree of dehydration. Urinalysis may indicate dehydration or urinary tract infection. An elevated complete blood count with a left shift usually indicates a bacterial etiology. Stool may be tested for occult blood and leukocytes, and if positive for either, culture for enteric bacterial pathogens should be done. Stool culture and examination for ova and parasites is indicated for the patient with high fever, blood and mucus in stool, or diarrhea longer than one week. Stool may be tested for rotovirus antigen if diagnosis is needed for isolation or other public health requirements.[11]

Management

Expert consultation is recommended for patients with severe dehydration; infants with dehydration, bloody stools, and fever; septic or toxic appearing patients; persistent diarrhea despite appropriate care; and failure to rehydrate.

Patients with mild to moderate dehydration are treated with oral rehydration therapy, close follow-up and education for home management. Fluid replacement and slow return to regular diet are key to effective treatment. Antidiarrheal medications are not effective, and can dangerously decrease gastrointestinal motility in children.

Oral rehydration therapy begins with a rehydration phase of 4 hours, in which clear liquid electrolyte solutions are offered (50 ml/kg for mild and 100 ml/kg for moderate diarrhea). For the vomiting infant, small volumes (5–15 ml) are offered frequently, and large volumes are avoided. Recommended electrolyte fluids which offer balanced sodium, potassium, glucose, base and osmolality are: Pedialyte, Rehydralyte, Infalyte, Ricelyte, and WHO (World Health Organization) solution.[9,12]

Clear liquids alone offer no caloric replacement and have limited use. Liquids high in sodium, such as boiled skim milk or broth, should be avoided due to danger of hypernatremia.

TABLE 19–2. MAJOR CHARACTERISTICS OF COMMON ACUTE DIARRHEA

Etiology	Stool	Characteristics	Medication
Viral *Rotovirus* 　*Incubation* 1–3 days 　*Source*—Person to Person 　　　　　Water 　　　　　Food 　*Other*—Norwalk, entero, 　　　　adrenovirus, 　　　　enterovirus	Watery Few WBC	Onset abrupt Low grade fever Vomiting, nausea, abdominal 　pain May have URI 80% occurrence in winter Less than 2 yrs of age	None
Bacterial *E. Coli* (Pathogenic) 　*Incubation*—Variable 　*Source*—food, water	Small watery, green, 　explosive, blood, 　mucus & +WBC	Onset abrupt or gradual High fever—appear toxic Vomiting Abdominal distention/pain Tenesmus Incidence higher in summer History of travel or epidemic	TMP/SMZ* Ampicillin Gentamycin
Salmonella 　*Incubation*: 6–72 hours 　*Source*—Food, drink (poultry, 　　　　eggs, dairy) 　　　　—Animals (poultry, rep- 　　　　tiles, livestock, pets)	Watery, green, foul 　+Gross/Occult 　blood, 　mucus, 　+WBC	Onset abrupt High fever Vomiting, nausea Colicky abdominal pain Possible life-threatening 　septicemia & meningitis Higher incidence in summer History of exposure to turtles	None unless extraintestinal 　infection or sepsis Ampicillin Amoxicillin TMP/SMZ* Third generation cephalosporin
Shigella 　*Incubation*: 1–7 days or >24 　　　　hours 　*Source*—Food, drink (salads)	Small, watery, 　frequent, 　gross blood, 　mucus	Onset variable, usually abrupt High fever Abdominal pain, cramping Tenesmus Possible meningeal signs— 　headaches, nuchal rigidity, 　delirum, seizures Higher incidence in summer	TMP/SMZ* Ampicillin
Helicobacter Jejuni 　*Incubation*: 1–7 days 　*Source*: 　　Water 　　Animals (birds, pets, 　　　livestock) 　　Food (chicken, salads, 　　　unpasturized milk) 　　Sporadic	Watery, foul smelling, 　gross blood, mucus	Fever Abdominal pain—cramping, 　periumbilical, can mimic 　appendicitis	None or erythromycin
Parasitic *Giardia lamblia* 　*Incubation*: 1–4 weeks 　*Source*: Water (lakes, streams) 　　Humans (day care epidemics) 　　Animals (puppies)	Watery, foul smelling Flatulence No blood No WBC Infectious cysts- 　present 30–60%	Onset variable—acute or 　chronic malabsorptive No fever Abdominal distension Flatulence Nausea, vomiting	Furazolidone Metronidazole

(continued)

TABLE 19–2. MAJOR CHARACTERISTICS OF COMMON ACUTE DIARRHEA (*Continued*)

Etiology	Stool	Characteristics	Medication

Cryptosporidium
  Incubation: 2–14 days
  Source:
    Animals (birds, reptiles, live-
      stock, pets)
    Water supply—resistant to
      chlorination; appropriate
      water filtration systems
      critical
	Watery or bloody	Low grade fever
		Abdominal cramping
		Anorexia
		Weight Loss
		Subclinical illness
		Day care outbreaks
		Highest incidence in very young
		History of animal exposure
			Metronidazole
			Spiramycin
			Clarithromycin
			
			Paromomycin or Azithromycin
			  may be tried

Food Poisoning & Other (Enterotoxin) *As Above*: E. Coli			

Staphlococcus aureus
  Incubation: 4–6 Hrs
  Source: Food (poultry, pork,
    salads, eggs, pastries)
	Explosive
	Watery
	+WBC
		Vomiting worse than diarrhea
		Severe abdominal cramping
		History of food ingestion &/or
		  group outbreaks	

Clostridium perfringens &/or
Bacillus cereus
Incubation: short 1–16 hours
Sources: Food (meat, poultry, grains,
  rice, vegetables—mexican style
  food)
	Explosive
	Watery
	+WBC
		Abdominal pain & cramping
		Vomiting
		Fever uncommon	

Other: Clostridium difficile *Incubation*: Unknown *Source*: Antimicrobial—associated	Blood Mucus Pus +WBC Cytotoxin in stool	Abdominal pain Fever Systemic toxicity History of prior antibiotic use	Vancomycin Metronidazole Oral bacitracin

* TMP/SMZ, Trimethoprim-sulfamethoxazole.

Fluids with high sugar and high osmolar loads, such as soft drinks, full strength fruit juices or Kool-Aids, should be avoided.[7,8,12]

If an infant is breast-feeding, this method of feeding should continue. Offering extra oral rehydration solutions between breast-feedings can be used to replace ongoing fluid losses.

After rehydration (8–12 hours), reintroduce easily digested food from a regular diet, such as bananas, rice, rice cereal, carrots, toast, crackers, and lean meats. Cow's milk formulas should be used with caution, due to maldigestion of lactose that can occur during infectious diarrhea. After 24 hours of improvement, cow's milk can be introduced in half-strength, or a soy formula at half-strength. If diarrhea increases, regress the diet and increase as tolerated.[7–11]

Diaper rash from diarrhea is best treated by frequent diaper changing and keeping the skin clean and dry. Use of protective ointments, such as zinc oxide paste or petroleum jelly are helpful in reducing irritation. Education in terms of reducing spread of infection should be directed toward careful handwashing, especially after diapering or toilet activities and before feeding.

Parents should be instructed to notify a health professionals if the child becomes worse, a fever develops, abdominal pain occurs, blood is found in the stools, and further dehydration develops.

TABLE 19–3. DEGREE OF DEHYDRATION[10]

Mild (5% weight loss)
Increased thirst, dry mucus membranes, decreased urination
Moderate (6–10% weight loss)
Very dry mucus membranes, reduced skin turgor, decreased tears, sunken eyes or fontanelle, oliguria, irritable, lethargic
Severe (>10% weight loss)
Parched mucus membranes, poor skin turgor, tenting of skin, no tears, very sunken eyes or fontanelle, anuria, tachycardia, decreased blood pressure, poor perfusion, hyperpnea (metabolic acidosis)

TABLE 19–4. HISTORY

Question	Comment
Type and frequency of stools	Determines severity
Blood and/or mucus in stool	May indicate *Shigella, Salmonella,* or *Helicobacter*
Signs of dehydration	Determining number of diaperings, urine color, and stool consistency is helpful
Vomiting, nausea, type and amount of feedings, decreased intake, duration	Helpful questions to determine amount of dehydration
Fever	May indicate bacterial etiology
Abdominal pain	May indicate bacterial etiology or appendicitis
Rashes	May indicate viral etiology
Exposure to illness or contaminated foods	May indicate *Shigella* or *Salmonella*
Source of water, day care attendance, animal contact, travel	Helpful to identify pathogen
Fast or heavy breathing	May indicate metabolic acidosis
Recent antibiotic therapy	Should consider *Clostridium difficile*

TABLE 19–5. IMPORTANT ASPECTS OF THE PHYSICAL EXAMINATION

Vital signs
Activity level
Capillary refill
Degree of dehydration
Abdominal tenderness or masses
Postural changes
Associated rashes

■ CROUP SYNDROMES IN CHILDREN

General Characteristics

Croup refers to acute inflammatory diseases of the larynx, which are characterized by varying degrees of "brassy" or "barking" cough, inspiratory stridor, hoarseness and respiratory distress. Croup syndromes can be described by etiology or anatomic areas affected (Table 19–6):

- Epiglottitis (supraglottis above the opening to the larynx)
- Laryngotracheobronchitis (LTD) (viral croup, which affects larynx, trachea, and bronchi)
- Tracheitis (bacterial laryngotracheitis)
- Spasmodic croup (sudden onset, non-infectious spasmodic laryngitis).

Viral croup, which is usually a self-limiting mild disease, is the most common type of croup. Croup primarily affects children in the 6 month to 3 year age range, affects boys more than girls, and occurs more often in the fall and winter months. Patients usually present with a history of low grade fever and mild upper respiratory symptoms for several days prior to onset of stridor and croupy cough, and then may progress to severe respiratory distress.[13,14] Inflammation of the small-diameter larynx of young children renders them susceptible to airway obstruction. It is, therefore, important to assess the degree of respiratory distress and to distinguish benign croup from severe croup and life-threatening conditions such as:[13,14,15]

- Acute epiglottitis (true medical emergency)
- Retropharyngeal abscess
- Bacterial tracheitis
- Foreign body aspiration
- Angioedema

Acute epiglottitis is a true medical emergency, with the potential for airway obstruction in the first 6 to 12 hours, due to an edematous, "cherry red" epiglottis. The patient presents with abrupt onset of high fever, toxic appearance, inspiratory stridor, drooling, difficulty in swallowing or vocalizing, and extreme restlessness. Cough is rare. *Retropharyngeal abscess* presents with a more gradual onset of similar symptoms, plus stiffness or hyperextension of the neck. *Acute bacterial tracheitis* also presents with the above symptoms in a patient with history of croup that has suddenly worsened. Purulent, thick secretions begin to obstruct the airway and the patient becomes more croupy, toxic and febrile. *Foreign body aspiration* and *angioedema* present abruptly with histories of choking or drug/toxic exposures, respectively. *Spasmodic croup*, although generally benign, can be very frightening. A healthy, afebrile child, who may or may not have a mild URI, abruptly begins with inspiratory stridor and a loud "barking," "brassy" and "seal-like" cough. The onset is frequently at night.[14,16]

Signs, Symptoms, and Diagnosis

Evaluation primarily includes listening to the child (via telephone if necessary) and the history and physical examination. Laboratory tests and x-rays are of limited value in mild croup. The use of throat culture, CBC, and neck x-rays are helpful for differential diagnosis. Due to the risk of airway obstruction, the severity of respiratory distress remains the most significant assessment (Tables 19–7 to 19–9), with degree of fever and toxicity also being important considerations.[16,17]

Management

The majority of childhood croup is mild, viral croup and can be managed at home with supportive therapy, which includes mist therapy for humidification, antipyretics for mild temperature elevation, oral hydration and rest with minimal handling. Parents should be educated about at-home treatment and the usual 5 to 10 day progress of viral croup. They should be instructed to report signs of increasing respiratory distress and toxicity. Hospitalized patients may benefit from racemic epinephrine and corticosteroids.[13,19,20]

Spasmodic croup often improves with either warm or cool mist and reassurance. Warm steam from a shower in a closed bathroom often relieves symptoms. If there is no improvement after several minutes, the child should be examined. An aerosol treatment of racemic epinephrine, in the emergency room, often produces improvement.[14]

Moderate and severe croup usually require physician referral and hospitalization. Emergency transportation may be needed. If acute epiglottitis is suspected, examination of the

TABLE 19–6. CROUP SYNDROMES[13,14,19,21]

	Acute Epiglottis	Retropharyngeal Abscess	Acute Laryngotracheo-bronchitis	Acute Bacterial Tracheitis	Acute Spasmodic Laryngitis
Synonyms	Supraglottitis	None	Viral Croup Subglottic laryngitis	Membranous Croup	Spasmodic Croup "Midnight" Croup "Twilight" Croup "Allergic" Croup
Age	1–8 years Usually >2 years	1–3 years: variable	3 months–3 years Peak 6 months–2 years	1 month–6 years	1–4 years
Etiology	Bacteria H. Influenze B S. Pneumococci	Bacteria Strep. A S. aureus Anaerobics	Virus Parainfluenza Influenza Respiratory Syncycial Virus	Bacteria S. aureus H. Influenzae Strep. A	Unknown Virus–Allergy
Onset	Rapid	Gradual	Gradual	LTB worsens despite therapy	Sudden, usually at night
Signs & Symptoms *	High fever Toxic Inspiratory stridor Cough rare Drooling Dysphagia Dysphonia Agitation MEDICAL EMERGENCY —potential airway obstruction in first 6–12 hours: "Cherry Red," edematous epiglottis	High fever Toxic Acute pharyngitis Drooling Respiratory distress Dysphonia Neck hyperextension	Mild fever Non-toxic URI Inspiratory stridor "Barking," "Brassy," "Seal-like cough Hoarseness Dyspnea	High fever Toxic Stridor Croupy cough Purulent, thick secretions obstruct airway	No or low fever Inspiratory stridor "Barking," "Brassy," "Seal-like" cough May have history of mild URI
Treatment ** ***	Protect Airway— endotracheal tube or tracheostomy IV antibiotics Cephalosporins: Ceftriaxone Cefotaxime IV fluids Monitoring Humidity & O$_2$ Hospitalization–ICU	Protect Airway— IV antibiotics— Penicillin, Oxacillin Cefuroxime Surgical incision & drainage Hospitalization Otolaryngology consult	At-home therapy: Mist humidity Antipyretics Oral hydration Observation In-hospital therapy: Mist humidity Racemic epinephrine O$_2$ Steroids (short course) Intubation if severe	Protect Airway— Intubation & frequent suctioning IV antibiotics Penicillin Cephalosporins Hospitalization–ICU	Warm or cool mist (Warm steam from hot shower in closed bathroom) Reassurance If no improvement, Racemic epinephrine aerosol may help

* Examination of posterior pharynx can be dangerous and may precipitate airway obstruction in the toxic patient with stridor, especially if acute epiglottis is suspected. Throat inspection should be attempted only when immediate intubation can be performed if needed.

** Refer to physician if significant fever is associated with stridor, airway obstruction is threatened, if the clinical condition is worsening despite treatment, if croup is a recurrent problem or if infant is under 6 months of age.

*** Do not leave patient unattended. Do not agitate. Avoid invasive procedures if possible. Allow patient to sit upright on parent's lap. Do provide a quiet reassuring atmosphere.

TABLE 19–7. RESPIRATORY DISTRESS AND CROUP[13,18]

Sign/Symptom	Mild	Moderate	Severe
Stridor with croupy cough and hoarseness	When disturbed	Intermittent	Continuous, even at rest
Breath sounds	Normal	Slightly diminished	Markedly diminished
Respirations	Mild rate increase Can lie supine without distress	Moderate rate increase Prefer sitting up Labored breathing	Rapid rate Tripod & "sniff" position Labored breathing
Retractions	None	Mild	Marked
Color	Normal	Normal to pallor	Cyanotic hypoxia
Mental status	Normal to fussy or fearful	Anxious/restless	Frantic/unable to sleep
Drooling	None	None	Yes
Dysphagia	None	None	Yes
Dysphonia	None	None	Yes

TABLE 19–8. INDICATORS OF THE DEGREE OF RESPIRATORY DISTRESS[21]

Question	Comment
Croup or "crowing" sound/stridor constantly (even when relaxed) or intermittent > 3 times/day	Severe croup or moderate croup
Croupy cough	Absent in acute epiglottitis
Difficulty breathing	Degree of hypoxia and respiratory insufficiency
• Retractions	Indicate severity
• "tugging" between ribs	Indicate severity
• Respirations fast or labored	Tachypnea indicates severe case
• Lips bluish or dusky	Cyanosis indicates severe case
• Agitated, constantly uncomfortable	Increases with severity
• Unable to sleep more than 1 hour	Severe case
Drooling or trouble swallowing, sitting with chin forward to breath	May indicate epiglottitis especially if no cough
Unable to bend neck forward, stiff neck	May indicate retropharyngeal abscess
	Child may hyperextend neck
Condition worsened, fever spike	May indicate bacterial tracheitis
Choking on toy, food, or other foreign body	May be unrelated to URI, indicates foreign body aspiration
Sudden onset after medication or insect bite	May indicate laryngeal angioedema
Age < 6–12 months	Unstable infants may need referral
Poor fluid intake	May indicate dehydration
Temperature > 103 degrees	May indicate bacterial infection
Hoarseness	More common with viral croup

TABLE 19–9. LABORATORY TESTS [14,16,17]

Test	Comment
CBC	Elevated, left shift, with bacterial infection
Throat Culture	Rule for streptococcal pharyngitis
RSV nasopharyngeal rapid tests	Identification of Respiratory Syncytial Virus: • IFA (rapid immunofluorescent antibody) or • ELISA (enzyme-linked immunosorbent assay)
Lateral neck X-ray	Shows swollen epiglottis "thumb print sign," or widening of retropharyngeal space (abscess)
Anteroposterior neck X-ray	Shows subglottal narrowing "steeple sign" (LTB) or irregular tracheal margins (tracheitis)

pharynx may precipitate airway obstruction, and should only be attempted when immediate intubation can be performed. Guidelines for initial management of moderate and severe croup are found in Table 19–10.

TABLE 19–10. GUIDELINES FOR IMMEDIATE MANAGEMENT OF DIFFICULT CROUP[13,14,19]

* If acute epiglottitis is suspected:
* Do not examine pharynx
* Refer to physician specialist
* Do not leave patient unattended
* Do not agitate patient
* Avoid invasive procedures if possible
* Allow patient to sit upright on parent's lap
* Provide a quiet, reassuring atmosphere
* Refer to physician if significant fever is associated with stridor
* Refer to physician if condition is worsening despite treatment
* Refer to physician if infant is under 6 months of age
* Refer to physician if croup is a recurrent problem

References

1. Hays, T. Hematologic Disorders. In Merenstein GB, Kaplan DW, and Rosenberg AA, eds. *Handbook of Pediatrics*, 17th ed. Norwalk, Conn: Appleton and Lange, 1994:638.
2. 1994 Red Book Report of the Committee on Infectious Diseases. 23rd ed. Elk Grove, Ill: American Academy of Pediatrics; 1994: 374–375.
3. Rocchini AP. Cardiovascular risk factors and prevention. In: McAnarney ER, Kreipe RE, Orr DP, et al. *Textbook of Adolescent Medicine*. Philadelphia, Pa: WB Saunders Co; 1992.
4. Becque MD, Katch VL, Rocchini AP, et al. Coronary risk incidence of obese adolescents: reduction by exercise plus diet intervention. *Pediatrics*. 1988;81:605.
5. National Heart, Lung, and Blood Institute. *The Lipid Research Clinic's Population Studies Data Book, vol. l. The Prevalence Study*. Washington, DC: Government Printing Office; 1980. US Dept of Health and Human Services, NIH 80-1527.
6. Ravel, R. *Clinical Laboratory Medicine: Clinical Application of Laboratory Data*. 5th. ed. St. Louis, MO: Mosby Year Book, 1989;49–51, 121.
7. Schmitt B. *Instructions for Pediatric Patients*. Philadelphia, Pa: W. B. Saunders Co; 1992:61–62.
8. Schmitt B. *Pediatric Telephone Advice*. Boston, Mass: Little Brown & Company; 1980:43–51.
9. Wong D. *Whaley and Wong's Nursing Care of Infants and children*. 5th ed. St. Louis, Mo: Mosby; 1995:1207–1243.
10. Green M, Haggerty R. *Ambulatory Pediatrics*. Philadelphia, Pa: W.B. Saunders Co; 1990:189–194.
11. Hay W, Groothuis J, Hayward A, Leven M, eds. *Current Pediatric Diagnosis and Treatment*. 12 ed. Appleton and Lange: Norwalk CT; 1995:624–626, 1184–1185.
12. Graef JW, ed. *Manual of Pediatric Therapeutics*. Boston, Mass: Little Brown & Co; 1994:204–206, 274–275.
13. Wong D. *Whaley and Wong's Nursing Care of Infants and Children*. 5th ed. St. Louis, Mo: Mosby; 1995:1391–1395.
14. Green M, Haggerty R. *Ambulatory Pediatrics*. Philadelphia, Pa: W. B. Saunders Co; 1990:175–181.
15. Steele R. *The Clinical Handbook of Pediatric Infectious Disease*. New York, NY: The Parthenon Publishing Group; 1994: 159–161.
16. Hay W, Groothuis J, Hayward A, Leven M, eds. *Current Pediatric Diagnosis and Treatment*. 12th ed. Appleton & Lange: Norwalk, Conn; 1995:501–503.
17. Graef JW, ed. *Manual of Pediatric Therapeutics*. Boston, Mass: Little Brown & Co; 1994:55–59.
18. Custer JR, Croup and related disorders. *Contemporary Pediatrics*. 1993:10:92–110.
19. Schmitt B. *Pediatric Telephone Advice*. Boston, Mass: Little Brown & Co; 1980:133–136.
20. Schmitt B. *Instructions for Pediatric Patients,* Boston Mass: Little Brown & Co; 1992:59.
21. Merenstein G, Kaplan D, Rosenberg A, eds. *Handbook of Pediatrics*. 17th ed. Appleton & Lange: Norwalk Conn; 1994: 518.

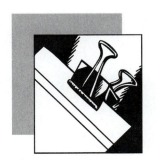

Part Three

Patient Information

Patricia A. Bunton
Richard D. Muma

Patient Information on...

■ Addison's Disease

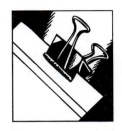

WHAT IS ADDISON'S DISEASE?

Addison's disease is a condition in which there is not enough hormone (cortisol) from the adrenal glands (located next to the kidneys) being released into the blood to circulate to other parts of the body.

WHAT CAUSES ADDISON'S DISEASE?

The most common cause is destruction of the adrenal glands by the body's own immune system.

HOW CAN I TELL IF I HAVE ADDISON'S DISEASE?

Addison's disease may cause a variety of symptoms. Some of the more common include weakness, tiredness, weight loss, loss of appetite, nausea, vomiting, diarrhea, and darkening of the skin.

HOW IS ADDISON'S DISEASE DIAGNOSED?

Diagnosis is based on low levels of cortisol in the blood. A computed tomographic (CT) scan of the adrenal glands may also be helpful in determining a more specific cause of the disease.

HOW IS ADDISON'S DISEASE TREATED?

Most commonly, daily doses of hydrocortisone are adequate to control the symptoms associated with Addison's disease.

IS THERE ANYTHING SPECIAL I NEED TO KNOW?

The body's need for cortisol is increased during infections, trauma, surgery, or anything that causes stress. Be sure to keep your health care provider informed if any of these conditions exist. It is advisable to carry a card or wear a bracelet giving information about your disease and need for hydrocortisone.

Provider _____

Phone Number _____

Additional Comments: _____

_____

_____

_____

_____

_____

_____

_____

Patient Information on...

■ AIDS and HIV

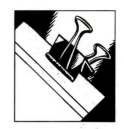

WHAT ARE HIV AND AIDS?

HIV (human immunodeficiency virus) is a virus that causes AIDS (acquired immunodeficiency syndrome). It is a serious disease that has caused thousands of deaths. There are many rumors and misbeliefs about HIV and AIDS. However, if one understands how it is spread, a plan can be developed to avoid it.

WHAT CAUSES HIV AND AIDS?

HIV is a virus that usually enters into the body through tears and breaks in the lining of the vagina and rectum (during sexual intercourse), after sharing IV drug needles, or is passed to an unborn child by an infected mother. Once infection takes place, HIV causes a breakdown in the immune system, rendering the body susceptible to other viruses, bacteria, fungi, parasites, and cancers. These organisms and cancers cause serious illnesses that are often deadly. When these illnesses develop or the immune system reaches a seriously low level, AIDS is diagnosed.

HOW CAN I TELL IF I HAVE HIV OR AIDS?

Initially most people have no symptoms. However, when the virus begins to progress, various symptoms may develop including headaches, fatigue, vaginal infections, swollen lymph glands, night sweats, fever, skin rashes, and sores in the mouth, nose, and anus. AIDS is the last stage of HIV infection and it is when serious illnesses occur like *Pneumocystis carinii* pneumonia, Kaposi's sarcoma, cervical cancer in women, and tuberculosis.

HOW IS HIV DIAGNOSED?

A special blood test can tell if you have HIV. Its name is the ELISA (enzyme-linked immunosorbent assay) test. If it is positive, a Western Blot blood test is done to confirm the ELISA test. You can and should have these tests done without using your name. The test detects antibodies the immune system makes, once it is exposed to HIV. However, after HIV enters the bloodstream there is a period of 6 weeks to 6 months before there are enough antibodies to make a positive test result. Therefore, you may need to get tested more than once.

HOW IS HIV TREATED?

Currently, HIV is treated by using various drugs including zidovudine (AZT, ZDV, or Retrovir), didanosine (ddI or Videx), zalcitabine (ddC or HiVid), and stavudine (D4T or Zerit). These and other drugs are currently being tested in combination with one another to determine if combination therapy is better.

IS THERE ANYTHING SPECIAL I NEED TO KNOW?

Precautions should be taken to prevent transmission to others by: (1) practicing safe sex; (2) using latex condoms with nonoxynol 9; (3) not sharing needles, razors, toothbrushes, and other personal hygiene items; and (4) not donating blood if you are HIV+ or engage in high risk behaviors.

For more information, contact the National AIDS Hotline at 1-800-342-AIDS.

Provider _____

Phone Number _____

Additional Comments: _____

_____

_____

_____

_____

_____

_____

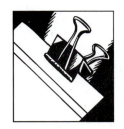

Patient Information on...

■ Alzheimer's Disease

WHAT IS ALZHEIMER'S DISEASE?

Alzheimer's disease is a condition in which there is persistent and progressive impairment of intellectual functioning (mostly memory). It affects about 2 million Americans. The incidence increases with age. Men and women are affected equally.

WHAT CAUSES ALZHEIMER'S DISEASE?

The cause of Alzheimer's disease is unknown but several factors have been suggested as possible causes including viruses and environmental toxins. The disease appears to be inherited in about 15%–20% of families, so Alzheimer's may be genetic.

HOW CAN I TELL IF I HAVE ALZHEIMER'S DISEASE?

Symptoms vary, but forgetfulness is the earliest sign. Inability to remember names and misplacing objects are common. As the condition progresses, it is more difficult to carry out tasks that require planning and judgment, as well as activities of daily living. There may be changes in mood, social withdrawal, and depression. In the latter stages, family members may not be recognized and verbal communication may stop.

HOW IS ALZHEIMER'S DISEASE DIAGNOSED?

A definite diagnosis of Alzheimer's can only be made by brain biopsy and by ruling out other causes of memory loss. A probable diagnosis can be made by a series of medical and psychologic tests.

HOW IS ALZHEIMER'S DISEASE TREATED?

Since there is currently no cure for Alzheimer's disease, treatment is directed toward improving the quality of life. A new drug called Cognex (tacrine hydrochloride) has been shown to improve thinking ability and slow the progression of the disease in some persons. Other medications may be given to treat specific symptoms like depression and anxiety.

IS THERE ANYTHING SPECIAL I NEED TO KNOW?

Caregivers must make numerous changes in the patient's surroundings to promote safety and reduce disorientation. Avoiding things that distract the patient and following strict schedules will reduce stress and anxiety.

For more information, contact the Alzheimer's Association at 1-800-621-0379.

Provider _____

Phone Number _____

Additional Comments:_____

_____

_____

_____

_____

_____

_____

_____

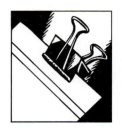

Patient Information on...
■ Angina Pectoris

WHAT IS ANGINA PECTORIS?

Angina pectoris is a severe constricting pain or discomfort in the center of the chest and associated with the heart. Approximately 3 million Americans have angina pectoris, also known as angina.

WHAT CAUSES ANGINA?

The arteries that carry oxygen-filled blood to the heart muscle (known as coronary arteries) become narrow as we age and the walls become irregular, which may allow for build-up of fat, cholesterol, and blood clots. When a coronary artery narrows, not allowing blood flow to a certain area of the heart, the heart develops ischemia (a deficiency of oxygenated blood) and the patient develops chest pain or angina.

HOW CAN I TELL IF I HAVE ANGINA?

People with angina may complain of chest discomfort, not necessarily chest pain. The description of this chest discomfort may include heaviness, squeezing, constricting, bursting, strangling, or burning. The location is usually in the middle part of the chest under the breast bone with radiation to the shoulders, neck, jaw, or arms. The discomfort or pain of angina usually lasts from 5–15 minutes and may be relieved with rest or the medication nitroglycerin. Pain lasting longer than 15 minutes may indicate a heart attack.

HOW IS ANGINA DIAGNOSED?

The diagnosis of angina is mostly made after the patient displays the typical features already described. Blood tests for cholesterol and lipids may aid in the diagnosis. An electrocardiogram (EKG or ECG) and an exercise stress test may also be used to evaluate the presence of angina pectoris.

HOW IS ANGINA TREATED?

The goal of therapy is to improve the quality of life of the patient with angina. Changing one's diet to include foods that are low in cholesterol, fat, and salt is very beneficial. If the person is overweight, a reducing diet should be instituted. Avoiding cigarettes may also improve the situation. Nitroglycerin should be carried by patients to take under the tongue when needed. The patient should seek medical care if the pain is not relieved with 2–3 tablets in 15 minutes. Angina that is no longer responsive to rest or medication should be further evaluated and in some cases patients may need balloon angioplasty or heart bypass surgery.

IS THERE ANYTHING SPECIAL I NEED TO KNOW?

Nitroglycerin should be stored in a cool, dark place. It usually causes a tingling sensation under the tongue and may cause headaches and flushing. If these symptoms do not occur, one may need a new prescription.

For more information contact the American Heart Association at 1-800-242-8721.

Provider _____

Phone Number _____

Additional Comments: _____

_____

_____

_____

_____

Patient Information on...
■ Anxiety

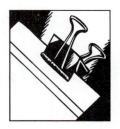

WHAT IS ANXIETY?

The term anxiety may be used in many ways. Some use it to name a physical or emotional response to fear or a threat. Others describe anxiety as a feeling of tension, excitement, nervousness, or worry. Still others describe anxiety as uncertainty and apprehension that leads to helplessness when an individual is unable to use coping alternatives effectively.

WHAT CAUSES ANXIETY?

Although the exact cause of anxiety is not known, there are a variety of theories as to its cause. There are several theories suggesting that anxiety is an emotional response to a situation in a person's life or environment. Others suggest a genetic or biological basis for anxiety. In addition, anxiety has been associated with some medical conditions or with the use or withdrawal of certain drugs or medications.

HOW CAN I TELL IF I HAVE ANXIETY?

Anxiety may range from mild to severe. Persons with mild anxiety are alert to themselves and to the environment and are able to learn and make decisions. In moderate anxiety, persons may begin to have a narrowed focus but are still capable of learning. At this level, anxiety may even be experienced as a motivating force. Severe anxiety causes disorganized thinking and decreases the ability to collect all the information needed to accurately assess a situation. Panic is the highest level of anxiety.

HOW IS ANXIETY DIAGNOSED?

The diagnosis of anxiety is based on characteristic symptoms. Medical and psychologic testing may also be helpful.

HOW IS ANXIETY TREATED?

Treatment is based on the degree of anxiety and how it affects one's daily life. Individual or family therapy may be recommended as well as the use of medications.

IS THERE ANYTHING SPECIAL I NEED TO KNOW?

It is important to recognize your own signs of high anxiety such as palpitations, fear, nervousness, anger, and irritability. Find new methods to cope with anxiety such as exercise and the use of relaxation techniques. Avoid the use of alcohol, caffeine, and drugs or medications that are not prescribed by your health care provider.

For more information, contact the National Mental Health Association at 1-800-969-6642.

Provider _____

Phone Number _____

Additional Comments: _____

_____

_____

_____

_____

_____

Patient Information on...

■ Asthma

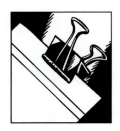

WHAT IS ASTHMA?

Asthma is defined as an obstructive airway disorder that is triggered by various factors leading to sudden shortness of breath. Asthma is the most common chronic disease in the United States, involving more than 5% of the population, of which two thirds are adults. In the past decade, the amount of disease in the US population has increased 60%.

WHAT CAUSES ASTHMA?

The cause of asthma is usually classified according to various factors. Conditions or factors that can cause an asthma attack include, but are not limited to, allergies (ragweed, cats, and peanuts), respiratory infections (common cold, bronchitis), exercise, certain emotions (anxiety), and the drug aspirin.

HOW CAN I TELL IF I HAVE ASTHMA?

An asthma attack is different in every person. However, attacks are usually described by the sudden presence of restlessness, anxiety, confusion, shortness of breath, wheezing, and a cough with thick mucus.

HOW IS ASTHMA DIAGNOSED?

In some cases, no tests will be ordered and the diagnosis will be made after a patient describes a history consistent with asthma (for example, sudden onset of shortness of breath and cough after exposure to an animal). Everyone, at some point, should have a chest x-ray, pulmonary function testing, arterial blood gas evaluation, and sputum (mucus) evaluation.

HOW IS ASTHMA TREATED?

The goals of management are to promote a normal life of the individual and to prevent future attacks (see below). Management of asthma includes prescription drugs like albuterol (Proventil and Ventolin) and metaproterenol (Alupent) inhalers and theophylline (Theo-Dur). These drugs work to open the lung air passages and are the most widely used. Side effects include nervousness and racing of the heart. Steroids and cromolyn sodium (Intal) are also used, mostly as a preventive measure.

IS THERE ANYTHING SPECIAL I NEED TO KNOW?

Yes! Factors such as cigarette smoke, dust, animals, certain foods, and stress trigger asthma attacks. Remove these factors from your life. If an attack occurs, use relaxation methods in order to remain calm and help slow the breathing pattern. If symptoms are not relieved from medication, call your health care provider or go to the nearest hospital facility.

For further information, contact the Asthma and Allergy Foundation of America at 1-800-727-8462.

Provider _____

Phone Number _____

Additional Comments: _____

_____

_____

_____

_____

_____

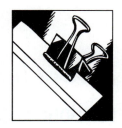

Patient Information on...
■ Asthma in Children

WHAT IS ASTHMA?

Asthma can be described as a chronic condition that suddenly leads to narrowing of the breathing tubes, shortness of breath, cough, and wheezing.

WHAT CAUSES ASTHMA?

The causes of asthma are usually classified according to various factors or conditions, which include, but are not limited to, allergies (ragweed, cats, and peanuts), respiratory conditions (common cold, bronchiolitis, cystic fibrosis, inhaling an object of some sort), exercise, certain emotions (anxiety), and the drug aspirin.

HOW CAN I TELL IF MY CHILD HAS ASTHMA?

An asthma attack is different in every child. However, attacks are usually described by the sudden presence of restlessness, anxiety, confusion, shortness of breath, wheezing, and a cough with thick mucus.

HOW IS ASTHMA DIAGNOSED?

In some cases, no tests will be ordered and the diagnosis will be made after a patient reveals a history consistent with asthma (for example, sudden onset of shortness of breath and cough after exposure to dust). Everyone, at some point, should have a chest x-ray, pulmonary function testing, arterial blood gas evaluation, and sputum (lung mucus) evaluation.

HOW IS ASTHMA TREATED?

The goals of the management are to promote a normal life of the child and to prevent future attacks (see below). Management of asthma includes drugs like albuterol (Proventil and Ventolin), metaproterenol (Alupent), and isoetharine inhalers. These drugs work to open the lung breathing tubes and are the most widely used. Side effects include nervousness and racing of the heart. Steroids and cromolyn sodium (Intal) are also used, mostly as a preventive measure.

IS THERE ANYTHING SPECIAL I NEED TO KNOW?

Factors such as cigarette smoke, dust, animals, certain foods, and stress trigger asthma attacks. Remove these from the child's life. If symptoms are not relieved from medication, call your health care provider or go to the nearest emergency room immediately.

For more information, contact the Asthma and Allergy Foundation of America at 1-800-727-8462.

Provider _____

Phone Number _____

Additional Comments: _____

_____

_____

_____

_____

_____

_____

Patient Information on...

■ Bone Fractures

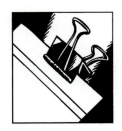

WHAT IS A FRACTURE?

A fracture is a break in the bone. Fractures are described in a variety of ways, depending on their location within the bone; their type, such as spiral, oblique, or comminuted; and the position of the fragments of the fractured bone, such as angulated or displaced.

WHAT CAUSES FRACTURES?

Most fractures are caused by trauma to the bone, either from a direct blow to the bone or from a twisting motion that causes the bone to break. However, occasionally a fracture, called a stress fracture, may occur when there is no history of injury. This type of fracture is more common in bones that are already weak from disease or the aging process.

HOW CAN I TELL IF I HAVE A FRACTURE?

Most persons will complain of some degree of discomfort or pain. There may be swelling and bruising in the affected area, as well as looking abnormal in shape. Movement of the involved area may be limited. If the blood vessels and nerves are damaged, the skin may be cool to the touch and a tingling sensation may be noted.

HOW ARE FRACTURES DIAGNOSED?

In most cases, fractures can be diagnosed from an x-ray. Occasionally, a fracture may be small enough or in a place difficult to see on x-ray and go undetected until the changes that occur with healing are seen on follow-up x-rays.

HOW ARE FRACTURES TREATED?

Immobilizing the fracture so that movement of the broken bone does not occur until healing is complete is the main method of treatment. This is done by placing a splint or cast on the affected area. Swelling is helped by elevation and ice on the fracture site. Pain medication may be prescribed and crutches may be needed to prevent weight bearing for fractures of the lower body.

IS THERE ANYTHING SPECIAL I NEED TO KNOW?

Most fractures will heal with either splinting or casting. However, if the fracture is severe and blood flow and nerves have been damaged, surgery may be required. Sometimes a cast or splint may be too tight and cause numbness or color change in the affected area. If this or any other change occurs that you have concerns about, call your health care provider immediately.

For more information, contact the National Rehabilitation Information Center at 1-800-346-2742.

Provider _____

Phone Number _____

Additional Comments: _____

_____

_____

_____

_____

_____

_____

_____

Patient Information on...

■ Breast Cancer

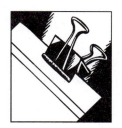

WHAT IS BREAST CANCER?

Breast cancer is a malignant tumor that invades healthy breast tissue and may spread to other organs, like the lungs, liver, bone, and brain. Unlike other cancers, breast cancer is primarily a disease of women. Each year 180,000 women develop breast cancer, resulting in about 46,000 deaths.

WHAT CAUSES BREAST CANCER?

The cause of breast cancer is unclear; however, some factors have been noted in relation to the disease. For example, women who have had mothers, sisters, or aunts with breast cancer are at increased risk. Other risk factors include age (more than 40 years old), excessive alcohol intake, and women who have never been pregnant.

HOW CAN I TELL IF I HAVE BREAST CANCER?

One should suspect breast cancer if there is nipple discharge, a painless breast mass, an area of skin thickening on the breast, or an "orange peel" appearance of the breast.

HOW IS BREAST CANCER DIAGNOSED?

A mammogram is the only method available to detect breast cancer before it is apparent by the patient or the patient's health care provider. However, the final diagnosis depends on the examination of involved breast tissue, usually after a biopsy.

HOW IS BREAST CANCER TREATED?

The treatment depends on how severe the tumor is and whether it has spread to other body organs. Depending on the type and severity, patients may or may not have their breast removed. Those in the early stages may have a lumpectomy (removal of the breast tumor) followed by radiation therapy. In the advanced stages, patients may have a mastectomy (removal of the breast) followed by radiation therapy, chemotherapy, or in some cases both.

IS THERE ANYTHING SPECIAL I NEED TO KNOW?

All women over age 40 should receive an annual breast exam from their health care provider. A mammogram is recommended every 1–2 years for all women beginning at age 50. It is also recommended that women perform monthly exams of their breasts beginning at the age of 20. Each month, 1–2 weeks after the menstrual period (or for postmenopausal women the same day each month) while bathing, place arms one at a time behind the head and: (1) Feel for lumps or changes in each breast and each armpit using a circular pattern. (2) Gently squeeze each nipple and look for a discharge. (3) Look for color changes of each breast.

For more information, contact the American Cancer Society at 1-800-227-2345.

Provider _____

Phone Number _____

Additional Comments: _____

_____

_____

_____

_____

_____

Patient Information on...
■ Chlamydia

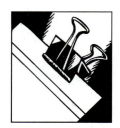

WHAT IS CHLAMYDIA?

Chlamydia is a sexually transmitted disease that is similar in its presentation to gonorrhea. In fact, chlamydia and gonorrhea are often diagnosed together. Infection may occur anywhere after sexual activity, but most commonly occurs on the cervix in women and inside the penis in men. Those who practice oral sex or have anal sex may also develop chlamydia in their throat or rectum.

WHAT CAUSES CHLAMYDIA?

Chlamydia is caused by an organism named *Chlamydia trachomatis*.

HOW CAN I TELL IF I HAVE CHLAMYDIA?

Signs and symptoms differ for men and women. Men commonly report an infection inside their penis (urethra), which causes painful urination, a yellow discharge, urinary frequency, and itching inside the penis. Women usually have no symptoms at all. If symptoms are present, they include a yellow vaginal discharge and bleeding and swelling of the cervix. In men, symptoms will develop 1–3 weeks after infection. Since women are often without symptoms, it is difficult to assess how long they are infected before being diagnosed.

HOW IS CHLAMYDIA DIAGNOSED?

Diagnosis is made after a patient displays the above signs and symptoms and after a culture of the discharge, or infected tissue, reveals the *Chlamydia trachomatis* organism.

HOW IS CHLAMYDIA TREATED?

Chlamydia is most widely treated with a 7 day course of doxycycline pills. This drug is well tolerated; however, if a patient is allergic to it, erythromycin can be used as an alternative.

IS THERE ANYTHING SPECIAL I NEED TO KNOW?

Yes! Chlamydia can be prevented by using latex condoms in combination with a spermaticide containing nonoxynol 9 when having sex. In addition, all sexual partners of an infected person should be tested for chlamydia. Finally, anyone with chlamydia should also be tested for syphilis, HIV, and gonorrhea.

For further information, contact the Centers for Disease Control and Prevention National Sexually Transmitted Diseases Hotline at 1-800-227-8922.

Provider _____

Phone Number _____

Additional Comments: _____

_____

_____

_____

_____

_____

_____

Patient Information on...

■ Colorectal Cancer

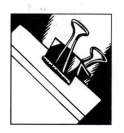

WHAT IS COLORECTAL CANCER?

Cancer of the colon and rectum are often referred to as colorectal cancer. It is a malignant tumor that invades healthy tissue of the colon and rectum but may spread to other organs, such as the liver. In the United States, colorectal cancer is second to lung cancer in causes of cancer-related death. A person has about a 1 in 20 lifetime risk of developing colorectal cancer. One's risk increases if related to someone diagnosed with colorectal cancer at a young age.

WHAT CAUSES COLORECTAL CANCER?

The exact cause of colorectal cancer is unknown; however, diet is often associated with this disease. For example, dietary fat, particularly animal fat from beef and pork, is associated with high risk, and dietary fiber, particularly grain fiber, is associated with low risk.

HOW CAN I TELL IF I HAVE COLORECTAL CANCER?

A persistent change in bowel habits should alert one to seek medical advice. Blood in the stools, persistent stomach discomfort, constipation with bouts of diarrhea, and constant fatigue should also alert one to seek a medical evaluation.

HOW IS COLORECTAL CANCER DIAGNOSED?

Several methods are used to aid in the diagnosis of colorectal cancer, which include a digital (finger) exam of the rectum, testing the stool for blood, a barium enema (an x-ray of the colon after receiving dye), and a lower endoscopy (using a camera on a tube to examine the colon).

HOW IS COLORECTAL CANCER TREATED?

About 85% of patients diagnosed with colorectal cancer have the tumor removed through surgery first. Those that have cancer in their rectum usually receive radiation therapy followed up with chemotherapy. Chemotherapy alone is used for cancer in other locations.

IS THERE ANYTHING SPECIAL I NEED TO KNOW?

The American Cancer Society recommends the following:

1. A yearly digital rectal exam starting at age 40.
2. A yearly stool check for blood beginning at age 50.
3. Every 3–5 years a lower endoscopy beginning at age 50.

For those who have a mother, father, brother, or sister with colorectal cancer diagnosed before the age of 55, a lower endoscopy, or barium enema every 5 years is urged. Some experts also recommend increases in dietary fiber, such as whole-grain breads, vegetables, and beans.

For further information, contact the American Cancer Society at 1-800-227-2345.

Provider _____

Phone Number _____

Additional Comments: _____

_____

_____

_____

_____

_____

_____

_____

Patient Information on...

■ Congestive Heart Failure

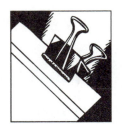

WHAT IS CONGESTIVE HEART FAILURE?

Congestive heart failure results when the heart can no longer pump an amount of blood adequate to meet the needs of the body.

WHAT CAUSES CONGESTIVE HEART FAILURE?

One of the most common causes of congestive heart failure in the United States is coronary artery disease. High blood pressure, diseases of the heart valves and heart muscle, and congenital heart defects (defects that newborns are born with) can also cause congestive heart failure.

HOW CAN I TELL IF I HAVE CONGESTIVE HEART FAILURE?

Symptoms depend on which side of the heart is affected. In left-sided heart failure, patients can have cough and shortness of breath when lying down or suddenly when sleeping. Any activity also causes shortness of breath. Right-sided heart failure commonly causes swelling of the feet, liver, and in some cases the abdominal area.

HOW IS CONGESTIVE HEART FAILURE DIAGNOSED?

Usually tests that determine cardiac function are ordered. The most common test is the echocardiogram. A chest x-ray and blood tests that test for cardiac damage and chemicals (electrolytes) in the blood may also be ordered.

HOW IS CONGESTIVE HEART FAILURE TREATED?

Management goals of congestive heart failure are to reduce the work load of the heart, improve heart performance, and control the excess amount of water and salt often found in congestive heart failure. Bed rest is also recommended in severe cases. Correcting underlying causes of congestive heart failure is the most important management feature. For example, if the patient has a problem with one of the heart valves, this valve needs to be fixed. In addition, drugs such as diuretics, angiotensin-converting enzyme (ACE) inhibitors, and digoxin may be given.

IS THERE ANYTHING SPECIAL I NEED TO KNOW?

The most important life-style change is limiting salt and liquids in the diet. Knowledge of one's weight is important and one should weigh three times a week. Any sudden increases in weight should be reported to a health care provider. Habits such as smoking should be stopped, if possible.

For more information contact the American Heart Association at 1-800-242-8721.

Provider _____

Phone Number _____

Additional Comments:_____

_____

_____

_____

_____

_____

Patient Information on...

■ COPD

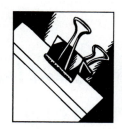

WHAT IS COPD?

Chronic obstructive pulmonary disease (COPD) includes a group of diseases that result in decrease of air flow in the lungs or of air moving out of the lungs. The term COPD is used to describe patients with at least two of the following diseases: chronic bronchitis, emphysema, and asthma. It is estimated that over 15 million Americans suffer from COPD. It is the fifth leading cause of death in the United States, and second only to heart disease as a cause of disability in adults under 65 years of age.

WHAT CAUSES COPD?

Several factors have been suggested as the cause of COPD. The primary cause is cigarette smoking, which accounts for 80%–90% of all cases. Other causes include exposure to dusts and gases, infection, and inherited genetic conditions.

HOW CAN I TELL IF I HAVE COPD?

Most individuals have a gradual increase in shortness of breath. Patients may also report the inability to walk as far, for example, without resting. They may also note mouth breathing, wheezing, a chronic cough, and an increase in mucous secretions from the lungs.

HOW IS COPD DIAGNOSED?

Since COPD includes a combination of diseases, the tests ordered will be different to diagnose each individual. In some cases, no tests will be indicated and the diagnosis will be made after a patient describes a history consistent with COPD. Everyone, at some point, should have a chest x-ray, pulmonary function testing, arterial blood gas evaluation, and sputum (mucus) evaluation.

HOW IS COPD TREATED?

Once a patient has been given the diagnosis of COPD, there is no cure available. However, instructions on the prevention of pulmonary infections (by getting influenza and pneumococcal vaccines), the performance of postural drainage (clearing mucus from the lungs), and eliminating smoking will slow the disease process. The most effective preventive measure against COPD is smoking cessation. In addition, other respiratory irritants (dust and chemicals) should be avoided. Certain medication, like bronchodilators (drugs that help open lung passages) may also be given.

IS THERE ANYTHING SPECIAL I NEED TO KNOW?

Yes! Understand how to treat signs and symptoms. If signs and symptoms are not relieved from medication, call a health care provider or go to the nearest emergency room. Also learn how to use relaxation and deep-breathing methods in order to remain calm and help slow the breathing pattern.

For further information, contact the American Lung Association at 1-800-586-4872.

Provider _____

Phone Number _____

Additional Comments: _____

_____

_____

_____

_____

_____

Patient Information on...

■ Croup

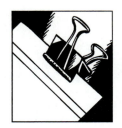

WHAT IS CROUP?

Croup is an inflammation or swelling of the voice box, or larynx. The voice becomes hoarse, due to swelling of the vocal cords. A harsh sounding "croupy" cough develops, which is often described as "brassy," "barking," or "seal-like." A coarse "crowing" sound can be heard when the child breaths in. This sound is called stridor. Stridor occurs as the opening between the vocal cords becomes more narrow due to swelling.

WHAT CAUSES CROUP?

Croup is usually caused by a viral infection and is part of a cold. Croup tends to occur more frequently in the fall and winter months, and the worst symptoms are seen in children under 3 years of age. Croup usually lasts for 5 to 6 days, and symptoms can change from mild to severe many times. If the croup happens to be caused by a virus called RSV, the illness can last as long as 10 days to 2 weeks. Sudden croup attacks do occur in well children.

HOW CAN I TELL IF CROUP IS SERIOUS?

Croup is usually a mild illness, but increased difficulty in breathing and sudden high fever indicate more serious illness. With mild croup, stridor is only present with crying or coughing, but as severity of illness increases, stridor occurs more often, even when the child is sleeping or relaxed.

Symptoms of worsening illness are:

1. Coughing attacks getting worse
2. More than 3 attacks of stridor
3. A fever of 103 to 104 degrees
4. Your child is not drinking much fluids

Danger symptoms requiring immediate medical attention:

1. Any sudden increase in stridor or croupy cough that concerns you
2. Increased difficult breathing and tugging-in or retractions between the ribs, below the ribs, or in the neck
3. Drooling
4. Difficulty in swallowing or talking
5. Lips turn blue or dusky
6. Your child can't sleep because of the croup
7. Warm mist won't clear up a sudden attack of stridor in 10 minutes

HOW IS CROUP DIAGNOSED?

Croup is usually diagnosed by the major symptoms of croupy cough, hoarseness, stridor and difficult breathing.

HOW IS CROUP TREATED?

Home Care for a Croupy Cough:

1. Mist—A cool vaporizer, running 24 hours a day provides added humidity that helps soothe the cough.
2. Fever—Acetaminophen may be given for fever over 102-103 degrees and also provides comfort. Tepid sponge baths also help reduce temperature.
3. Oral fluids—Encourage your child to drink plenty of clear liquids, in order to stay well hydrated and to keep mucous secretions thin rather than thick.
4. Close Observation—Croup can be a dangerous disease, so observe your child closely. Sleep in the same room during the illness.

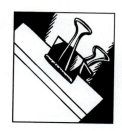

■ Croup *(continued)*

5. Provide rest—This helps children to relax, and reduces coughing spells.
6. Smoking—Don't smoke around your child. Smoking makes croup worse.
7. Contagiousness—Viral infections are contagious, so limit exposure to other children.

Care for Sudden Croup & Stridor Attacks: Sudden attacks of stridor and croup often improve with either warm or cool mist and reassurance. Warm steam from a shower in a closed bathroom often relieves the stridor. Take your child into the foggy bathroom for 10 minutes. Provide reassurance by holding and cuddling. Most children settle down and then rest comfortably. A warm, wet washcloth held over the mouth may also help.

NOTE: If stridor continues, call for medical attention. If your child turns blue, passes out, or stops breathing, call emergency (911).

Provider _____

Phone Number _____

Additional Comments: _____

_____

_____

_____

_____

_____

Patient Information on...
■ Cushing's Syndrome and Disease

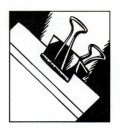

WHAT IS CUSHING'S?

Cushing's *syndrome* is a condition in which there is too much hormone (cortisol) being secreted from the adrenal gland (located next to the kidneys) and released into the blood. Cushing's *disease* also refers to an excess amount of cortisol being released from the adrenal gland, but it is caused by a defect in the brain. Cushing's *syndrome* may also be caused by taking steroids.

WHAT CAUSES CUSHING'S?

Approximately 85% of Cushing's cases are Cushing's *disease* and are caused by tumors of the pituitary gland (located in the brain). This defect in the pituitary gland sends a wrong message to the adrenal gland, which in turn releases too much hormone.

HOW CAN I TELL IF I HAVE CUSHING'S?

Since hormones affect many areas of the body, patients with Cushing's can have a variety of symptoms, some of which might include weight gain, weakness, high blood pressure, easy bruising, excessive body hair, darkening of the skin, and "stretch marks." Women may have abnormal periods and men may not be able to have an erection.

HOW IS CUSHING'S DIAGNOSED?

Urine and blood cortisol levels are used to make the diagnosis. A computed tomographic (CT) scan may be done to look for tumors in the brain and adrenal glands that may be affecting the release of the hormones.

HOW IS CUSHING'S TREATED?

Most commonly, surgery is required to remove tumors of the pituitary gland. Occasionally, adrenal tumors are treated with radiation or removed through surgery.

IS THERE ANYTHING SPECIAL I NEED TO KNOW?

Cushing's can cause several complications such as diabetes and high blood pressure. Infections are also more common. Therefore, it is very important to keep all appointments with the health care provider, so that these problems can be watched for.

Provider _____

Phone Number _____

Additional Comments: _____

_____

_____

_____

_____

_____

Patient Information on...

■ Cystitis

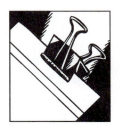

WHAT IS CYSTITIS?

Cystitis is an infection located in the bladder. It is more common in women than men. Persons who are at risk for cystitis include sexually active women, pregnant women, women who use barrier contraceptives such as diaphragms, men with prostatic obstruction, persons with urinary catheters, and diabetics.

WHAT CAUSES CYSTITIS?

In most cases, cystitis is caused by the bacterium *Escherichia coli*. This bacterium lives in the intestines, where it helps with the digestive process. If it gets into the bladder, however, it can cause cystitis.

HOW CAN I TELL IF I HAVE CYSTITIS?

The most common complaints are frequent urination, a feeling of urgency to urinate, pain with urination, discomfort in the lower abdomen, and blood in the urine.

HOW IS CYSTITIS DIAGNOSED?

Diagnosis is based on symptoms and on tests done on a sample of urine.

HOW IS CYSTITIS TREATED?

If the cystitis is caused by a bacterium, the treatment is antibiotics that are taken for a variable amount of time, depending on the severity and length of the infection and on the condition of the patient.

IS THERE ANYTHING SPECIAL I NEED TO KNOW?

There are several things that can be done to prevent cystitis. Drinking plenty of fluid is important, especially acid fluids such as cranberry juice. Women should wipe themselves from front to back and should avoid using vaginal deodorants and bubble bath. Women should urinate immediately after intercourse. Be sure to take all medication as prescribed by the health care provider.

Provider _____

Phone Number _____

Additional Comments: _____

_____

_____

_____

_____

_____

Patient Information on...
■ Depression

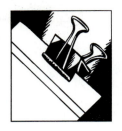

WHAT IS DEPRESSION?

Depression is an emotion characterized by feelings of sadness, low spirits, disappointment, frustration, and gloominess. Depression can be associated with the normal grief process, with menopause in middle-aged women, and with poor health. Depression has also been associated with single parenthood, lack of the necessities of life, and unemployment.

WHAT CAUSES DEPRESSION?

There are a variety of ideas as to what causes depression. Some have suggested that it results from a chemical imbalance in the body. Others believe that depression is associated with feelings of low self-esteem and anger that is directed inward. Symptoms of depression can occur during times of illness, and certain medications can contribute to the development of depression.

HOW CAN I TELL IF I AM DEPRESSED?

There are a variety of symptoms that can suggest depression and not every person who is depressed will have all the symptoms of depression. In general, there is a decrease in appetite, weight loss, and a change in normal sleep patterns. There may be a loss of energy, feelings of worthlessness or guilt, decreased ability to think or concentrate, and loss of interest in or pleasure from things that were enjoyed in the past. In severe cases, depression may lead to thoughts of suicide.

HOW IS DEPRESSION DIAGNOSED?

Diagnosis is based on symptoms and on the results of medical and psychologic tests.

HOW IS DEPRESSION TREATED?

The main methods of treatment include individual or family therapy and the use of medications. In addition, it is important to get adequate rest, exercise, and eat balanced meals. Avoid alcohol, caffeine, and any medications that are not prescribed by your health care provider.

IS THERE ANYTHING SPECIAL I NEED TO KNOW?

Depression is a common emotional condition. Asking for help is a sign of strength and the first step toward recovery. Medications given for depression may take from 1 to 3 weeks to take effect so don't quit taking them because they don't seem to be working. Dry mouth is a common side effect of medications and may be relieved with gum or hard candy.

For more information, contact the National Foundation for Depressive Illness at 1-800-248-4344 or the National Mental Health Association at 1-800-969-6642.

Provider _____

Phone Number _____

Additional Comments: _____

_____

_____

_____

_____

_____

_____

Patient Information on...

■ Diabetes Mellitus

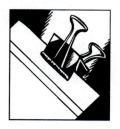

WHAT IS DIABETES MELLITUS?

Diabetes mellitus is a condition in which the blood sugar level is too high. There are two main types: type I, in which insulin is required (insulin-dependent) and type II, in which insulin is not required (non–insulin-dependent). Diabetes affects about 8 million people in the United States, the majority of whom have type II.

WHAT CAUSES DIABETES MELLITUS?

Elevated blood sugar in type II is the result of the cells of the body being resistant to insulin, which is needed to help the cells use sugar for energy. Therefore, the sugar stays in the blood. Also, the pancreas, which produces insulin, no longer responds adequately to sugar intake. Elevated sugar in type I is the result of no insulin being produced by the pancreas.

HOW CAN I TELL IF I HAVE DIABETES MELLITUS?

The most common symptoms are thirst, hunger, and frequent urination. Other symptoms may include tiredness or problems with infections, such as a sore on the skin that does not heal, or frequent vaginal yeast infections in women. Visual changes may also occur.

HOW IS DIABETES MELLITUS DIAGNOSED?

Two fasting blood sugar levels of over 140 mg/dL are needed to make the diagnosis.

HOW IS DIABETES MELLITUS TREATED?

Diabetes can sometimes be controlled by a proper diet and exercise. Medications may also be prescribed if needed. Insulin injections are required for those with type I diabetes and may be used for type II diabetes if other treatments fail to maintain normal blood sugar levels.

IS THERE ANYTHING SPECIAL I NEED TO KNOW?

Patients with diabetes must assume a major role in the medical management of this condition. It is very important to follow your health care provider's instructions on diet, exercise, and medications so that complications from diabetes can be avoided. Be sure to report any changes in your medical condition to your health care provider as soon as possible.

For more information, contact the American Diabetes Association at 1-800-232-3472.

Provider _____

Phone Number _____

Additional Comments: _____

_____

_____

_____

_____

_____

_____

_____

Patient Information on...
■ Diverticulosis

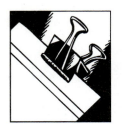

WHAT IS DIVERTICULOSIS?

Diverticulosis is a condition in which there is an outpouching that forms at a weak place in the large intestine (colon). There may be one or more pouches that form. If the pouches become infected, the condition is called diverticulitis.

WHAT CAUSES DIVERTICULOSIS?

This condition is part of the aging process. However, lack of adequate fiber in the diet may be a contributing factor.

HOW CAN I TELL IF I HAVE DIVERTICULOSIS?

Diverticulosis is usually without symptoms; however, abdominal pain may be present, and rarely, there may be blood in the stool. If there is infection (diverticulitis), pain may be more severe and diarrhea and fever may be present.

HOW IS DIVERTICULOSIS DIAGNOSED?

The diagnosis is made by x-rays or scans of the abdomen. In some cases, a scope may be passed into the lower part of the colon through the rectum so that the colon can be seen.

HOW IS DIVERTICULOSIS TREATED?

A diet that is high in fiber may reduce the symptoms. Hospitalization may be necessary if bleeding occurs. In rare cases, surgery is required if bleeding does not stop on its own. If infection is present, antibiotics may be given.

IS THERE ANYTHING SPECIAL I NEED TO KNOW?

Increasing the amount of fiber in the diet may be helpful in reducing symptoms and in preventing further problems.

Provider _____

Phone Number _____

Additional Comments: _____

_____

_____

_____

_____

_____

_____

_____

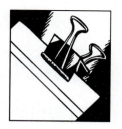

Patient Information on...

■ Endocarditis

WHAT IS ENDOCARDITIS?

Endocarditis is inflammation of the inner lining of the heart. There are two types: infective and noninfective.

WHAT CAUSES ENDOCARDITIS?

Infective endocarditis is caused by bacteria. These bacteria can enter the blood stream during surgical and dental procedures and with use of intravenous drugs. Noninfective endocarditis is usually caused by a blood clot within the heart. Risk factors for the development of endocarditis include a history of rheumatic fever, a defect in the heart and heart valves, and artificial heart valves.

HOW CAN I TELL IF I HAVE ENDOCARDITIS?

Symptoms of endocarditis include fatigue, fever, muscle aches, weight loss, and decreased appetite. Classically patients will have fever, anemia, and a new murmur (an extra heart sound). Another finding that may be seen includes hemorrhages, or blood, under the nails.

HOW IS ENDOCARDITIS DIAGNOSED?

If endocarditis is suspected, tests like a complete blood count (CBC), erythrocyte sedimentation rate (ESR), and blood cultures will be required. An electrocardiogram (EKG) or echocardiogram, and a chest x-ray will also be ordered.

HOW IS ENDOCARDITIS TREATED?

Treatment with antibiotics should begin immediately when the diagnosis is made. Examples include cefazolin sodium (Ancef) and penicillin. The length of treatment depends on the severity of the infection, but the drug is usually given for up to 6 weeks.

IS THERE ANYTHING SPECIAL I NEED TO KNOW?

Persons with the named risk factors should be given antibiotics before any dental, upper respiratory, genital, or urinary tract procedure. An example is amoxicillin 3 grams orally 1 hour before the procedure and 1.5 grams 6 hours after the procedure.

For more information, contact the American Heart Association at 1-800-242-8721.

Provider _____

Phone Number _____

Additional Comments: _____

_____

_____

_____

_____

_____

_____

_____

Patient Information on...

■ Genital Herpes

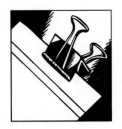

WHAT IS GENITAL HERPES?

Genital herpes is a sexually transmitted disease and the most common cause of genital blisters and ulcers. These sores may appear on the penis, scrotum, anus, and rectal area, outside and inside the vagina, cervix, and throat.

WHAT CAUSES GENITAL HERPES?

Genital herpes is caused by a virus called herpes simplex. There are two subtypes to this virus called herpes simplex virus-1 (HSV-1) and herpes simplex virus-2 (HSV-2). Either of these may cause genital herpes; however, HSV-2 is usually the cause.

HOW CAN I TELL IF I HAVE GENITAL HERPES?

Genital herpes presents as groups of small blisters, which over several days collapse and turn into ulcers. The blisters and ulcers tend to be very painful and may become secondarily infected with bacteria. Prior to the appearance of herpes, patients may experience burning, tingling, or itching at the site of infection.

HOW IS GENITAL HERPES DIAGNOSED?

Diagnosis is usually made after patients present with the typical sores as described above. However, the blisters and ulcers can be cultured.

HOW IS GENITAL HERPES TREATED?

Herpes simplex is a chronic disease for which there is no cure available. Active sores are treated with a 10-day course of acyclovir (Zovirax). Recurrent lesions are treated in the same manner. If a person is prone to frequent recurrences, prolonged therapy with acyclovir is recommended. Acyclovir is well tolerated, without any significant side effects.

IS THERE ANYTHING SPECIAL I NEED TO KNOW?

Genital herpes can be prevented by using latex condoms and avoiding sexual contact with those who are infected. It is also important to remember that infected individuals, or those who still have blisters present, can transmit the disease. In addition, any person found to be infected with herpes should be counseled and tested for HIV.

For further information, contact the Centers for Disease Control and Prevention National Sexually Transmitted Diseases Hotline at 1-800-227-8922.

Provider _____

Phone Number _____

Additional Comments: _____

_____

_____

_____

_____

_____

Patient Information on...

■ Genital Warts

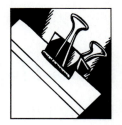

WHAT ARE GENITAL WARTS?

Genital warts, or condyloma acuminata, are viral growths that are sexually transmitted. Infection occurs, after sexual activity, usually on the vagina and penis. Those who practice oral or anal sex may also develop them in the mouth and on the anal-rectal area.

WHAT CAUSES GENITAL WARTS?

Genital warts are caused by human papilloma virus.

HOW CAN I TELL IF I HAVE GENITAL WARTS?

Genital warts appear as soft, fleshy growths that resemble the vegetable cauliflower. The most common sites involved are the vulva (outside the vagina), around the rectum and anus, penis, vagina, cervix, and the throat. Genital warts may get so big that they may interfere with sexual intercourse, urination, and bowel movements.

HOW ARE GENITAL WARTS DIAGNOSED?

Diagnosis is usually made after a person seeks medical help with growths as described above; however, a biopsy may also be taken.

HOW ARE GENITAL WARTS TREATED?

Treatments may include the following:

1. Freezing the warts with liquid nitrogen.
2. Applying an acidlike preparation that dissolves the warts.
3. Removal of the warts with a laser.
4. Injecting interferon into the warts.
5. Removal of warts with surgery.

IS THERE ANYTHING SPECIAL I NEED TO KNOW?

Genital warts can be prevented by using a latex condom and by avoiding sexual contact with infected persons. Warts may not appear for years after exposure and may come back after treatment. In addition, all persons diagnosed with genital warts should be counseled and tested for HIV.

For further information, contact the Centers for Disease Control and Prevention National Sexually Transmitted Diseases Hotline at 1-800-227-8922.

Provider _____

Phone Number _____

Additional Comments: _____

_____

_____

_____

_____

_____

Patient Information on...
■ Glomerulonephritis

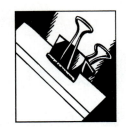

WHAT IS GLOMERULONEPHRITIS?

The kidney acts as a filter by eliminating wastes through the production of urine. The glomerulus is a part of the kidney that is responsible for making urine and maintaining a proper fluid balance within the body. Glomerulonephritis is inflammation of the glomerulus. It can occur at any age but is more common in children ages 2–12.

WHAT CAUSES GLOMERULONEPHRITIS?

Most commonly, glomerulonephritis occurs 6–20 days after a skin (eg, impetigo) or throat infection caused by group A streptococcus.

HOW CAN I TELL IF I HAVE GLOMERULONEPHRITIS?

The majority of patients will have an abrupt onset of blood in the urine (smokey-colored), swelling (especially in the face), and increased blood pressure. Other symptoms include tiredness, flank discomfort, weight gain, less urine output, and low-grade fever.

HOW IS GLOMERULONEPHRITIS DIAGNOSED?

Diagnosis is based on symptoms and on the results of urine and blood tests. Occasionally, a biopsy of the kidney may be necessary.

HOW IS GLOMERULONEPHRITIS TREATED?

Most of the time glomerulonephritis will resolve on its own in 1 to 3 weeks. Other measures that may be used include a salt-restricted diet, high blood pressure medication, water pills, and temporary kidney dialysis. Antibiotics may be given for the strep infection.

IS THERE ANYTHING SPECIAL I NEED TO KNOW?

While this condition may cause a temporary decrease in urine output, normal urine production will resume for most people within weeks. Blood in the urine may be noticed for months after the condition is diagnosed. It is important to take all prescribed medication for strep infections to prevent this condition from occurring.

For more information, contact the National Kidney Foundation at 1-800-622-9010.

Provider _____

Phone Number _____

Additional Comments: _____

_____

_____

_____

_____

_____

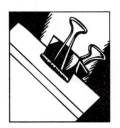

Patient Information on...

■ Gonorrhea

WHAT IS GONORRHEA?

Gonorrhea is a sexually transmitted disease. Infection may occur anywhere after sexual activity but most commonly occurs on the cervix in women and inside the penis in men after intercourse. Those who practice oral sex or have anal sex may also develop gonorrhea in their throat or rectum.

WHAT CAUSES GONORRHEA?

Gonorrhea is caused by an organism named *Neisseria gonorrhoeae*.

HOW CAN I TELL IF I HAVE GONORRHEA?

Signs and symptoms differ for men and women. Men commonly report an infection inside their penis (urethra), which causes painful urination and a yellow discharge. Women may have no symptoms at all. If symptoms are present, they may include a yellow vaginal discharge, vaginal itching, or painful urination. For both men and women, symptoms will develop 2–7 days after infection.

HOW IS GONORRHEA DIAGNOSED?

Diagnosis is made after a patient complains of the above signs and symptoms and examination of the discharge reveals the *Neisseria gonorrhoeae* organism.

HOW IS GONORRHEA TREATED?

The treatment of choice for uncomplicated gonorrhea is a shot of ceftriaxone and a week's supply of doxycycline pills. Both drugs are well tolerated and very effective. Doxycycline is given to make sure another organism (*Chlamydia trachomatis*) is also treated, since it is transmitted in the same way and often present at the same time.

IS THERE ANYTHING SPECIAL I NEED TO KNOW?

Yes! Gonorrhea can be prevented by using latex condoms in combination with a spermaticide containing nonoxynol 9 when having sex. In addition, all sexual partners of an infected person should be tested for gonorrhea. Finally, anyone with gonorrhea should also be tested for syphilis and HIV.

For further information, contact the Centers for Disease Control and Prevention National Sexually Transmitted Diseases Hotline at 1-800-227-8922.

Provider _____

Phone Number _____

Additional Comments: _____

_____

_____

_____

_____

_____

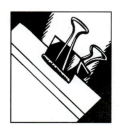

Patient Information on...

■ Headaches

WHAT IS A HEADACHE?

The term *headache* literally means a pain in the head. It is one of the most common reasons that a person seeks medical care. There are several types, including tension headache, migraine headache, and cluster headache. Infrequently, headaches may be a symptom of a more serious disease.

WHAT CAUSES HEADACHES?

Tension headaches are thought to be caused by contraction of the muscles around the skull. These headaches are worse during times of stress, depression, and anxiety. Migraine headaches are thought to be caused by a cycle of spasm and relaxation of the blood vessels in the head. Although the exact cause of cluster headaches is unknown, they, too, are thought to be associated with changes in the blood vessels of the head. More serious causes of headaches include tumors, blood clots, and infections.

HOW CAN I TELL IF I HAVE HEADACHES?

It is not difficult to tell if you have a headache, but it may be difficult to determine which type of headache you have, so that proper treatment can be given. Tension headaches are usually a dull ache and may feel like a tight band around the head. Migraine headaches cause a moderate to severe throbbing-type pain and may be associated with nausea and vomiting. Cluster headaches cause severe pain and have an explosive onset. Headaches caused by serious disease are progressively worse and are associated with changes in the neurologic system.

HOW ARE HEADACHES DIAGNOSED?

A good medical history and physical exam will be sufficient in diagnosing most types of headaches. In some cases, x-rays or scans of the head and sinuses may be necessary.

HOW ARE HEADACHES TREATED?

Treatment depends on the type of headache. Most headaches can be controlled or diminished by proper medication and behavioral changes to reduce stress.

IS THERE ANYTHING SPECIAL I NEED TO KNOW?

Maintaining good health by eating a well-balanced diet, getting adequate exercise and rest, and avoiding alcohol, caffeine, and tobacco can go a long way in preventing and minimizing the effects of most headaches. However, if the headaches get progressively worse and are associated with other symptoms, be sure to see your health care provider.

For more information, contact the National Headache Foundation at 1-800-843-2256.

Provider _____

Phone Number _____

Additional Comments: _____

_____

_____

_____

_____

_____

Patient Information on...

■ Heart Attack

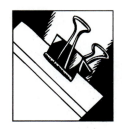

WHAT IS A HEART ATTACK?

Acute myocardial infarction (MI), more commonly known as a heart attack, is the major cause of death in the United States. A heart attack occurs when a coronary artery (artery that supplies blood and oxygen to the heart muscle) becomes clogged, not allowing blood and oxygen to reach an area of the heart. When this happens, the heart may stop pumping.

WHAT CAUSES HEART ATTACKS?

Clogging of the coronary arteries that leads to a heart attack can be caused by plaque formations in the arteries (usually a result of prolonged elevations of cholesterol), coronary artery spasms, and blood clots.

HOW CAN I TELL IF I HAVE HAD A HEART ATTACK?

The patient having a heart attack usually has chest pain that is described as a heavy pressure or squeezing sensation and that radiates to the jaw and upper arms. The longer the pain continues, the more damage to the heart. Some patients may also note shortness of breath, anxiety, nausea, vomiting, fatigue, and increased sweating.

HOW IS A HEART ATTACK DIAGNOSED?

The electrocardiogram (ECG) is the most important test but may not show any changes in the early stages. Certain blood tests, known as cardiac enzymes (CK-MB) can also help diagnose a heart attack.

HOW IS A HEART ATTACK TREATED?

Individuals are almost always admitted to the hospital for treatment. Oxygen and narcotics or intravenous nitroglycerin are often used to decrease the pain and discomfort. Streptokinase and tissue plasminogen (t-PA) may be used to increase or preserve blood flow to the injured area of the heart.

IS THERE ANYTHING SPECIAL I NEED TO KNOW?

As part of improving the function of the heart, there are several changes that need to be incorporated into one's life after a heart attack has occurred. These include:

1. Preparing and eating foods low in fat and salt
2. Exercising in moderation
3. Lowering stress level
4. Lowering blood pressure
5. Lowering cholesterol
6. Lowering fat levels
7. Avoiding smoking

For more information, contact the American Heart Association at 1-800-242-8721.

Provider _____

Phone Number _____

Additional Comments: _____

_____

_____

_____

_____

_____

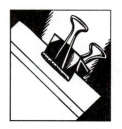

Patient Information on...

■ Hepatitis

WHAT IS HEPATITIS?

Hepatitis literally means "inflammation of the liver." It may be caused by a number of different viruses or by ingestion of certain drugs or toxins.

WHAT SPECIFICALLY CAUSES HEPATITIS?

There are five viruses that cause hepatitis (type A, B, C, D, and E). These viruses are transmitted through contact with another person who has the virus. Contacts with the virus can be made through sexual encounters, through poor hygiene practices, or by using contaminated needles or blood products. Some drugs, such as acetaminophen (Tylenol), when taken in large doses, may cause hepatitis. Wild mushrooms and alcohol are toxins that can also cause hepatitis.

HOW CAN I TELL IF I HAVE HEPATITIS?

Persons with hepatitis may complain of tiredness, decreased appetite, nausea, stomach pain, and fever. Jaundice (yellowing of the skin) may occur, as well as a darkening of the color of the urine. Some cases of hepatitis may be so mild that there are either no symptoms or the symptoms may be thought to be caused by a cold or the flu.

HOW IS HEPATITIS DIAGNOSED?

Diagnosis is based on symptoms, physical exam findings, and blood tests for the specific hepatitis viruses and liver function. If hepatitis persists, a liver biopsy may need to be done.

HOW IS HEPATITIS TREATED?

Most cases of hepatitis are treated with bed rest. When needed, medications for nausea are given as well as IV fluids. More serious cases of hepatitis may require changes in the diet, daily injections of interferon, or a liver transplant.

IS THERE ANYTHING SPECIAL I NEED TO KNOW?

There is a vaccine to prevent hepatitis B infection. Talk to your health care provider about how to get it. Hepatitis can be prevented by using good hygiene (washing hands after using the bathroom), and by practicing safe sex (use condoms). IV drug users should not share needles.

For more information, contact the American Liver Foundation at 1-800-223-0179.

Provider _____

Phone Number _____

Additional Comments:_____

_____

_____

_____

_____

_____

_____

_____

Patient Information on...

■ Hernias

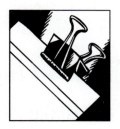

WHAT IS A HERNIA?

A hernia is a rupture or protrusion of a structure through the wall that normally surrounds it. Hernias can be of many different types such as an inguinal hernia, umbilical hernia, or hiatal hernia. A person can be born with a hernia or it can be acquired. In most cases, hernias are not life-threatening.

WHAT CAUSES HERNIAS?

In most cases, hernias are caused by a weakness in the wall of muscle or tissue that surrounds a structure. At times, the weakness is there at birth; at other times, it may occur following surgery or from heavy lifting or straining.

HOW CAN I TELL IF I HAVE A HERNIA?

Symptoms may vary depending on where the hernia is located and how serious it is. In general, there will be discomfort or pain at the affected site, which at times may radiate to surrounding areas. Also, there may be a noticeable bulge or enlargement at the location of the hernia.

HOW ARE HERNIAS DIAGNOSED?

Some hernias may be diagnosed from the medical history and physical exam, while others may require x-rays or scans to determine the type and location of the hernia.

HOW ARE HERNIAS TREATED?

Some hernias may resolve without treatment. However, others may require surgery. Your health care provider will be able to recommend the treatment that is best for your particular type of hernia.

IS THERE ANYTHING SPECIAL I NEED TO KNOW?

While most hernias are not life-threatening, if the blood supply is cut off or the hernia presses on the nerves, more serious problems may occur. If you think you have a hernia, do not strain unnecessarily, do not lift heavy objects, and do not do anything that causes discomfort. See your health care provider for proper evaluation and treatment.

Provider _____

Phone Number _____

Additional Comments: _____

_____

_____

_____

_____

_____

_____

_____

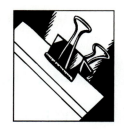

Patient Information on...
■ Hiatal Hernia

WHAT IS A HIATAL HERNIA?

A hiatal hernia is a condition in which part of the stomach moves upward into the chest through an opening in the diaphragm. This opening naturally allows the esophagus to be connected to the stomach, but in this condition it becomes large enough to allow the stomach to slip upward through it.

WHAT CAUSES A HIATAL HERNIA?

The cause of hiatal hernias is unknown.

HOW CAN I TELL IF I HAVE A HIATAL HERNIA?

Most cases of hiatal hernia produce no symptoms. However, if gastric juices flow backward into the esophagus, there may be complaints of heartburn or a bitter taste in the mouth or throat.

HOW IS A HIATAL HERNIA DIAGNOSED?

The diagnosis is based on symptoms and is confirmed by x-rays or by looking through a tube that is passed into the stomach.

HOW IS A HIATAL HERNIA TREATED?

If symptoms are present, medications such as antacids (Maalox) or those that help clear acids from the stomach may be given (cimetidine [Tagamet] and ranitidine [Zantac]). Not eating before going to bed and elevating the head of the bed on 6-inch blocks may help. If symptoms are severe and other treatments have not helped, surgery may be an alternative.

IS THERE ANYTHING SPECIAL I NEED TO KNOW?

In addition to other treatments, avoiding fatty foods, alcohol, chocolate, and cigarettes may be helpful. Weight loss is recommended for those who are overweight.

Provider _____

Phone Number _____

Additional Comments: _____

_____

_____

_____

_____

_____

_____

Patient Information on...

■ Hypertension (High Blood Pressure)

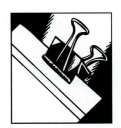

WHAT IS HYPERTENSION?

Hypertension is the sustained elevation of blood pressure. Hypertension is called the "silent killer" because there are often no early warning signs or symptoms until it reaches advanced stages. This is the most common cardiovascular disorder, affecting about one out of four Americans. Uncontrolled hypertension, over a long period of time, can damage the eyes, heart muscle, kidneys, and cause strokes.

WHAT CAUSES HYPERTENSION?

In most cases hypertension has no known cause. When this is the case, medical professionals call it essential hypertension. In a small number of people, hypertension is caused by kidney disorders. When this is the case it is called secondary hypertension.

HOW CAN I TELL IF I HAVE HYPERTENSION?

There may not be any noticeable symptoms or signs of hypertension. However, some patients may complain of headaches or nose bleeds.

HOW IS HYPERTENSION DIAGNOSED?

Taking the blood pressure is the primary way to diagnose hypertension. Elevated blood pressures (any reading 140/90 and above) should be confirmed on at least two separate office visits before a diagnosis of hypertension can be made.

HOW IS HYPERTENSION TREATED?

The most important goal in the treatment of hypertension is to keep the blood pressure under control and prevent damage to the eyes, heart, and kidneys. Controlled blood pressure will also help prevent strokes. If the hypertension is secondary, the underlying problem needs to be corrected (for example, if the cause is a kidney disease, it needs to be treated). Patients may be prescribed diuretics, beta blockers, calcium channel blockers, or angiotensin-converting enzyme (ACE) inhibitors to lower blood pressure.

IS THERE ANYTHING SPECIAL I NEED TO KNOW?

Several life-style changes for the hypertensive patient may help to control blood pressure. Exercise and weight loss should be addressed if indicated. Avoidance of smoking and dietary salt is also recommended.

For more information contact the American Heart Association at 1-800-242-8721.

Provider _____

Phone Number _____

Additional Comments: _____

_____

_____

_____

_____

_____

_____

Patient Information on...

■ Hyperthyroidism

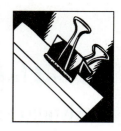

WHAT IS HYPERTHYROIDISM?

Hyperthyroidism is a condition in which the thyroid gland produces too much thyroid hormone. An excess of thyroid hormone can produce changes in the skin, the eyes, the heart, the nerves and muscles, and other parts of the body as well as behavior. It is a common disorder, especially among women between the ages of 20 and 40.

WHAT CAUSES HYPERTHYROIDISM?

There are many causes of hyperthyroidism. The most common cause is Grave's disease in which there is enlargement and increased activity of the thyroid gland, leading to excess amounts of thyroid hormone.

HOW CAN I TELL IF I HAVE HYPERTHYROIDISM?

The affects of hyperthyroidism vary among individuals, but symptoms such as nervousness, heat intolerance, increased sweating, tiredness, weakness, muscle cramps, frequent bowel movements, or weight change may be noted. There may also be heart palpitations (racing of the heart) or chest pain. Women may have irregular periods.

HOW IS HYPERTHYROIDISM DIAGNOSED?

Diagnosis is based on symptoms and by measuring thyroid hormone levels in the blood. A thyroid scan may also be helpful.

HOW IS HYPERTHYROIDISM TREATED?

There are three main methods of treatment: medications, removal of part of the thyroid gland by surgery, or by destroying part of the gland with radioactive iodine.

IS THERE ANYTHING SPECIAL I NEED TO KNOW?

Physical and mental problems caused by hyperthyroidism may persist even after treatment, especially those associated with the eye, heart, and behavior. Other members of the family may need to be screened for hyperthyroidism.

For more information contact the American Thyroid Association at 1-718-882-6047.

Provider _____

Phone Number _____

Additional Comments: _____

_____

_____

_____

_____

_____

_____

_____

_____

Patient Information on...

■ Hypothyroidism

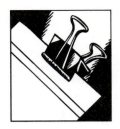

WHAT IS HYPOTHYROIDISM?

Hypothyroidism is a condition in which too little thyroid hormone is released by the thyroid gland. Lack of thyroid hormone may affect virtually all body functions and may range from mild to severe. It is more common in the elderly and in women.

WHAT CAUSES HYPOTHYROIDISM?

Hypothyroidism may be caused by failure of the thyroid gland to release enough thyroid hormone or it may be caused by lack of hormones from other glands in the body that stimulate the thyroid gland to release thyroid hormone.

HOW CAN I TELL IF I HAVE HYPOTHYROIDISM?

Hypothyroidism may be so mild that it may go undetected or it may cause any of a number of symptoms, some of which might be weakness, tiredness, muscle and joint aching, cold intolerance, constipation, dry skin, weight change, thinning of hair and nails, and puffiness of the face and eyelids.

HOW IS HYPOTHYROIDISM DIAGNOSED?

Hypothyroidism is diagnosed by clinical symptoms and by measuring thyroid hormone levels in the blood.

HOW IS HYPOTHYROIDISM TREATED?

Most of the symptoms of hypothyroidism will improve within 2 weeks of beginning a daily dose of thyroid hormone, and will resolve within 3–6 months.

IS THERE ANYTHING SPECIAL I NEED TO KNOW?

It is very important to take the prescribed amount of thyroid hormone as directed by your health care provider and to keep regular appointments so that the condition can be monitored. Some drugs can affect thyroid blood tests, so be sure to make your health care provider aware of all medication you are taking.

For more information contact the American Thyroid Association at 1-718-882-6047.

Provider _____

Phone Number _____

Additional Comments: _____

_____

_____

_____

_____

_____

_____

_____

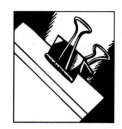

Patient Information on...
■ Irritable Bowel Syndrome

WHAT IS IRRITABLE BOWEL SYNDROME?

Irritable bowel syndrome (IBS) is a group of symptoms that include abdominal pain, alternating diarrhea and constipation, and abdominal bloating. Some may experience nausea and lack of appetite. This syndrome affects all age groups but is more common in young women.

WHAT CAUSES IRRITABLE BOWEL SYNDROME?

Although there is no specific cause, there are certain factors that seem to play a role in the symptoms that occur with IBS. There is thought to be an increase in the speed at which food moves through the intestines, leading to diarrhea. Symptoms may be caused by certain foods, such as those with lactose (dairy products) and caffeine, as well as low- or high-fiber foods. Anxiety or stress may also play a role in producing symptoms.

HOW CAN I TELL IF I HAVE IRRITABLE BOWEL SYNDROME?

The symptoms of IBS are intermittent and vary from person to person and from time to time. Crampy abdominal pain that follows a meal or a time of stress is a common complaint. Pain is relieved after a bowel movement, which can alternate between constipation and diarrhea. There may be abdominal bloating, so that clothes feel tight. Nausea and vomiting are occasionally seen.

HOW IS IRRITABLE BOWEL SYNDROME DIAGNOSED?

The initial step in diagnosing IBS is to exclude other causes for the symptoms. To do this, abdominal x-rays may be done as well as tests on blood and stool samples.

HOW IS IRRITABLE BOWEL SYNDROME TREATED?

Treatment consists of avoiding foods that cause symptoms. For some, increasing the amount of fiber in the diet is beneficial, as is decreasing the amount of fat intake. Measures to help reduce stress and anxiety are helpful. Medications are also available to slow the movement of food through the intestines.

IS THERE ANYTHING SPECIAL I NEED TO KNOW?

While there is no cure for IBS, understanding those factors that increase the symptoms can go a long way in dealing with this condition.

Provider _____

Phone Number _____

Additional Comments: _____

_____

_____

_____

_____

_____

Patient Information on...

■ Kidney Stones

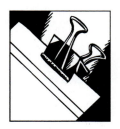

WHAT ARE KIDNEY STONES?

Kidney stones are formed by the accumulation of crystals that do not dissolve well in liquids. The stones may block the flow of urine and lead to pain and blood in the urine. Kidney stones are more common in men than in women.

WHAT CAUSES KIDNEY STONES?

The exact cause is not known, but there are some things that encourage the formation of stones such as frequent urinary tract infections, an abnormal structure within the kidney, and some dietary factors such as excessive intake of protein. Not enough fluid intake and certain medications may also lead to stone formation.

HOW CAN I TELL IF I HAVE KIDNEY STONES?

Sometimes the only symptom is blood in the urine. However, when the stones block the flow of urine, there may be a sudden onset of pain that increases over time. The pain typically radiates to the groin and is colicky in nature. Nausea and vomiting may be present as well as problems with urination.

HOW ARE KIDNEY STONES DIAGNOSED?

Diagnosis is based on symptoms as well as the fact that most stones are visible on x-rays of the kidney. Other tests may be done on urine and blood to help confirm the diagnosis.

HOW ARE KIDNEY STONES TREATED?

Some stones may pass on their own. High-frequency sound waves may be used to break up the stones into smaller pieces so that they can be passed. At times, surgery may be required to remove the stones. Once the stones have been analyzed, treatment may include changes in diet and medication.

IS THERE ANYTHING SPECIAL I NEED TO KNOW?

The best way to prevent stone formation is to drink plenty of fluids. It is also important to follow the instructions of the health care giver concerning diet and medication.

For more information, contact the National Kidney Foundation at 1-800-622-9010.

Provider _____

Phone Number _____

Additional Comments: _____

_____

_____

_____

_____

_____

_____

_____

_____

Patient Information on...

■ Lung Cancer

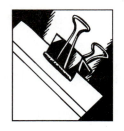

WHAT IS LUNG CANCER?

Lung cancer, a malignant tumor, is a disease of modern times. Although the number of cases has increased over the last six decades, it was not until recently that scientific studies linked smoking, especially cigarette smoking, to the rising death rate attributed to lung cancer. The American Cancer Society projects that almost 200,000 new cases of lung cancer will be diagnosed over the next year.

WHAT CAUSES LUNG CANCER?

Cigarette smoking is the most important cause of lung cancer in both men and women in the United States.

HOW CAN I TELL IF I HAVE LUNG CANCER?

The symptoms of lung cancer depend on its severity, type, and extent. Initial symptoms may include a persistent dry cough, a cough that produces blood, weight loss, shortness of breath, and chest pain.

HOW IS LUNG CANCER DIAGNOSED?

Lung cancer is diagnosed through a chest x-ray, a lung computed tomographic (CT) scan, and a biopsy of the lung mass. Since lung cancer is known to spread to other organs, all patients with suspected lung cancer should also receive a complete blood count and liver function tests.

HOW IS LUNG CANCER TREATED?

If possible, removal of the lung tumor is the preferred treatment choice. However, in most cases the tumor is too far advanced and surgery is not possible. Radiation therapy and chemotherapy are used when surgery is not an option. Lung cancer patients must be observed closely and receive periodic tests that monitor the side effects of chemotherapy (anemia, low blood counts) and whether the cancer is worsening.

IS THERE ANYTHING SPECIAL I NEED TO KNOW?

Since smoking has been identified as the primary cause of lung cancer, if one smokes, a strong consideration should be given to stop. A prescription of nicotine gum or a nicotine patch may be helpful and may facilitate smoking cessation. If one has never smoked, encouragement should be given to never start. Some experts also agree that smokers should have a periodic chest x-ray to rule out the presence of cancer.

For further information, contact the American Cancer Society at 1-800-227-2345.

Provider _____

Phone Number _____

Additional Comments: _____

_____

_____

_____

_____

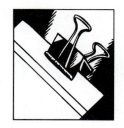

Patient Information on...

■ Menopause

WHAT IS MENOPAUSE?

Menopause is the cessation of menses, or the last menstrual period in a woman's life. The median age at menopause is 50 to 51 years.

WHAT CAUSES MENOPAUSE?

At around 40 years of age ovarian function begins to change and ovulation (discharge of an egg from the ovary) decreases and eventually stops. A decrease in the hormone called estrogen also occurs at this time. With decreased estrogen levels, women are at risk for developing osteoporosis and heart disease.

HOW CAN I TELL IF I AM GOING THROUGH MENOPAUSE?

Although there is wide variety of symptoms among women, the hot flash is usually the first sign of menopause. Hot flashes are frequently accompanied by sweating, sleep distur-bances, vaginal dryness, thinning of the skin, hair shedding, changes in nail texture, and mood changes.

HOW IS MENOPAUSE DIAGNOSED?

Menopause is usually diagnosed after the typical signs and symptoms occur in women after the age of 40. Hormone blood levels may be drawn in some cases to confirm the diagnosis.

HOW IS MENOPAUSE TREATED?

Because the signs and symptoms of menopause result from declining estrogen production, estrogen replacement will cor-rect most of the changes. Some women also need to take an-other hormone, progestin, to prevent the development of uterine cancer while on estrogen.

IS THERE ANYTHING SPECIAL I NEED TO KNOW?

Menopausal women must have regular Pap smears and mammograms. They must also practice a healthy life-style with attention to diet, particularly to adequate calcium intake to help prevent osteoporosis.

Provider _____

Phone Number _____

Additional Comments: _____

_____

_____

_____

_____

_____

_____

Patient Information on...

■ Murmurs

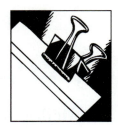

WHAT ARE MURMURS?

A murmur is an extra heart sound that usually develops from a damaged portion of the heart or heart valve. Some murmurs, however, may develop in individuals without heart disease. Examples include athletes and babies. In these cases the murmur is not harmful.

WHAT CAUSES MURMURS?

Murmurs may be caused by disorders in the body that alter the function of the heart. Anemia and pregnancy are examples. Other causes include defects in the heart valves or the circulation of blood within the heart. Murmurs can be heard through a stethoscope and have a "blowing" sound.

HOW CAN I TELL IF I HAVE A MURMUR?

Most patients are not aware that they have a murmur. However, some people may initially complain of fatigue, shortness of breath, chest pain, blackouts, or swelling in the legs and feet.

HOW ARE MURMURS DIAGNOSED?

Several tests may be done to diagnose a murmur. Two tests, an echocardiogram and heart catheterization, are used to aid in the demonstration of murmurs. A chest x-ray and electrocardiogram (ECG) may be used to identify complications caused by a murmur (examples include congestive heart failure and an enlarged heart).

HOW ARE MURMURS TREATED?

The management of a murmur is to prevent and treat complications that may arise. For example, patients with mitral regurgitation are at risk for developing endocarditis under certain situations. In these cases, antibiotics are given before dental and surgical procedures to prevent endocarditis. Some patients will require heart valve replacement.

IS THERE ANYTHING SPECIAL I NEED TO KNOW?

Patients with murmurs usually do not have any major lifestyle changes if their condition is mild. However, murmurs can worsen over time. With the worsening of murmurs, patients need to be reminded of symptoms that might be present including chest pain, shortness of breath, blackouts, and swelling in the legs and feet.

For more information contact the American Heart Association at 1-800-242-8721.

Provider _____

Phone Number _____

Additional Comments: _____

_____

_____

_____

_____

• _____

_____

_____

Patient Information on...
■ Osteoarthritis

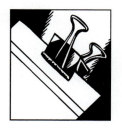

WHAT IS OSTEOARTHRITIS?

Osteoarthritis is a disorder of the joints that causes pain and loss of movement. It is the most common type of arthritis and affects almost all persons over the age of 60. It may develop in any joint, but it most commonly affects the hips, knees, feet, spine, and hands.

WHAT CAUSES OSTEOARTHRITIS?

This type of arthritis is thought to be caused by "wear and tear" from normal everyday activity, which leads to destruction of joints. However, obesity, injury to a joint, and frequent use of joints are factors that increase the risk of developing osteoarthritis.

HOW CAN I TELL IF I HAVE OSTEOARTHRITIS?

Most people notice pain in a joint during times of activity, which goes away with rest. Stiffness may occur and it may take more energy to move the joint. As the condition worsens, joints may not move as far as they once did, swelling may occur, and joint deformity may be noted.

HOW IS OSTEOARTHRITIS DIAGNOSED?

Diagnosis is based on symptoms and x-ray of joints. Narrowing of joint spaces and bone spurs are common findings. Blood tests are normal in osteoarthritis.

HOW IS OSTEOARTHRITIS TREATED?

Osteoarthritis cannot be cured, but pain can be relieved with aspirin or anti-inflammatory drugs. Ibuprofen (Advil) is a good example. Joint function may be helped by a special exercise program prescribed by your health care provider. Surgical repair of the joint may be an option in severe cases.

IS THERE ANYTHING SPECIAL I NEED TO KNOW?

It is important to maintain a balance of rest, exercise, and medication. If you are overweight, talk to your health care provider about a weight reduction plan. Most importantly, do not take any medications that are not prescribed by your health care provider, including over-the-counter drugs. Medications for osteoarthritis can cause stomach and intestinal bleeding, so notify your provider immediately if this should occur.

For more information, contact the Arthritis Foundation at 1-800-283-7800.

Provider _____

Phone Number _____

Additional Comments: _____

_____

_____

_____

_____

_____

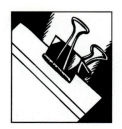

Patient Information on...

■ Osteoporosis

WHAT IS OSTEOPOROSIS?

Osteoporosis is a condition of decreased bone mass that results in thin, fragile bone that breaks easily. Osteoporosis affects more than 20 million people in the United States, and its incidence is on the rise because of an increase in the population over the age of 65. Most cases of osteoporosis occur in women.

WHAT CAUSES OSTEOPOROSIS?

Osteoporosis is associated with a number of factors, the most common being old age and the length of time since menopause in women. As individuals grow older, their bones normally become thinner and more brittle. After menopause, women have less estrogen, which helps prevent bone loss. Thus in older women, advancing age and a lack of estrogen leads to weakened bones. Smoking and decreased physical activity also contribute to the development of osteoporosis.

HOW CAN I TELL IF I HAVE OSTEOPOROSIS?

Early in the disease most patients have no symptoms. If signs and symptoms are present, they may include a gradual loss in height due to broken bones of the spine. Patients may also break bones in their arms and hips.

HOW IS OSTEOPOROSIS DIAGNOSED?

Unfortunately, the diagnosis of osteoporosis is most often made late in the disease, when bones are broken. However, bone density can be measured to determine early development of osteoporosis.

HOW IS OSTEOPOROSIS TREATED?

The primary focus should be directed toward prevention of bone loss before the development of symptoms and prevention of further bone loss once disease is present. In women, estrogen therapy is the main medication used to prevent the development of osteoporosis. Other drugs, including calcitonin, etidronate, and vitamin D are also used in management.

IS THERE ANYTHING SPECIAL I NEED TO KNOW?

Life-style changes include ensuring adequate amounts of calcium either through diet or calcium tablets, regular weight-bearing exercise (example, walking), and avoiding smoking and alcohol.

For more information contact the National Osteoporosis Foundation at 1-800-223-9994.

Provider _____

Phone Number _____

Additional Comments: _____

_____

_____

_____

_____

_____

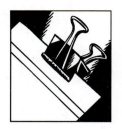

Patient Information on...

■ Pancreatitis

WHAT IS PANCREATITIS?

Pancreatitis is an infection of the pancreas. The pancreas is located in the upper part of the abdomen. It produces fluids that aid in digestion of food and also makes insulin.

WHAT CAUSES PANCREATITIS?

Drinking excessive amounts of alcohol is one of the most common causes of pancreatitis. Other causes include gallstones, injury to the stomach area, ingestion of certain drugs such as water pills (diuretics) and some antibiotics, and viral infections.

HOW CAN I TELL IF I HAVE PANCREATITIS?

Stomach pain that goes into the back is the most common symptom of pancreatitis. Nausea, vomiting, and a fever may also occur. If the condition continues for a long time, diarrhea and weight loss may be noted.

HOW IS PANCREATITIS DIAGNOSED?

Diagnosis is based on symptoms and on an elevated amylase or lipase levels detected in the blood.

HOW IS PANCREATITIS TREATED?

Treatment consists of "putting the pancreas to rest" by not eating or drinking anything. This requires that fluids be given through an IV to prevent dehydration. Pain medication is usually necessary. Pancreatitis usually improves within 1 week.

IS THERE ANYTHING SPECIAL I NEED TO KNOW?

It is important to avoid whatever is causing the problem. If that is alcohol, do not drink. If the pancreatitis is caused by a specific drug, don't take that drug again. Be sure to follow your health care provider's instructions.

Provider _____

Phone Number _____

Additional Comments: _____

_____

_____

_____

_____

_____

_____

_____

Patient Information on...

■ Pediatric Allergic Rhinitis

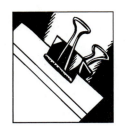

WHAT IS ALLERGIC RHINITIS?

Allergic rhinitis, often referred to as a "runny" nose in response to an allergy, is a very common condition among children. The rhinitis may occur when seasons change or persist throughout the year.

WHAT CAUSES ALLERGIC RHINITIS?

Typical causes for seasonal allergic rhinitis include pollens from trees, grasses, and weeds. Causes that may occur throughout the year include air pollution, cigarette smoke, mold spores, animal dander, perfumes, chemicals, dust mites, feathers, and roaches.

HOW CAN I TELL IF MY CHILD HAS ALLERGIC RHINITIS?

Symptoms and signs of allergic rhinitis include sneezing, itching of the nose, ear, roof of mouth, and throat, clear "runny" nose, stuffiness of the nose, drainage from the nose into the throat that causes coughing, and constant "sniffing." Because of this, the child may be unable to breathe through his or her nose and breathe through the mouth. He or she may snore at night.

HOW IS ALLERGIC RHINITIS DIAGNOSED?

The signs and symptoms described above are usually all that is needed to make a diagnosis. However, a microscopic examination of the mucus from the nose will help confirm the presence of allergic rhinitis.

HOW IS ALLERGIC RHINITIS TREATED?

Medications include antihistamines and decongestants (Dimetapp), cromolyn sodium (Intal), and steroids. They may be used alone or in combination, depending on the severity.

IS THERE ANYTHING SPECIAL I NEED TO KNOW?

Avoidance of known causes of symptoms is the most effective means of managing allergic rhinitis, but it is not always practical. There are, however, vacuum cleaners that are much better at removing substances that trigger allergic rhinitis. The child's room should be as allergy-free as possible including the removal of carpets, drapes, stuffed animals, feather pillows, plants, and animals. Bedding should be washed regularly and dried on high heat to kill dust mites.

For more information, contact the Asthma and Allergy Foundation of America at 1-800-727-8462.

Provider _____

Phone Number _____

Additional Comments: _____

_____

_____

_____

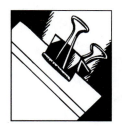

Patient Information on...

■ Pediatric Anemia

WHAT IS ANEMIA?

Anemia in children is a very common condition that can be treated by eating correctly and taking vitamins. By definition, anemia refers to a condition of fewer red blood cells (RBCs) in the body than is considered normal. A child may become anemic when there are not enough RBCs made in the body, when RBCs are destroyed, or when there is uncontrolled bleeding.

WHAT CAUSES ANEMIA?

The most common cause of anemia in children is not enough iron in the diet. Lead poisoning can also lead to anemia and is seen in children who live in older homes and eat sweet-tasting paint chips containing lead. Children may also develop anemia from a lack of vitamin B_{12}, folic acid, or as a result of sickle cell disease.

HOW CAN I TELL IF ANEMIA IS PRESENT?

Most children who develop anemia have persistent fatigue, weakness, and become pale in color.

HOW IS ANEMIA DIAGNOSED?

A simple blood test called a complete blood count (CBC) can be done first to screen for anemia. Depending on the result, further blood tests may be required.

HOW IS ANEMIA TREATED?

Treatment depends on the cause. Changes in diet may be needed. For example, foods high in iron like peas, spinach, and meat can be added to the diet of a child with iron-deficiency anemia. Most likely, the child will also need an oral iron supplement.

IS THERE ANYTHING SPECIAL I NEED TO KNOW?

Infants who rely on milk for vitamins, particularly iron, need to be on iron-fortified formula or have some other way of receiving enough iron. An example is an oral iron supplement. Usually breast-fed babies do not need any additional vitamins if the mother eats well and takes her vitamins.

Provider _____

Phone Number _____

Additional Comments: _____

_____

_____

_____

_____

_____

_____

_____

_____

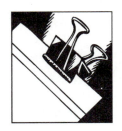

Patient Information on...

■ Pediatric Gastroenteritis

WHAT IS GASTROENTERITIS?

Gastroenteritis in children is a common illness which causes diarrhea and vomiting. It starts as a sudden increase in bowel movements or "stools," which are more soft or loose. As diarrhea increases, stools become more frequent, watery, and may be green in color. Breast-fed infants normally have watery, yellow, "seedy" looking stools after most feedings, every 2 to 4 hours, and diarrhea is determined only by increased number of stools. Some children also vomit or "throw up."

WHAT CAUSES GASTROENTERITIS?

The most common cause of gastroenteritis in children is viral infection that affects the stomach and intestines. It can sometimes be caused by bacteria or parasite infections, or other factors such as a change in diet.

HOW CAN I TELL IF GASTROENTERITIS IS SERIOUS?

Dehydration, or loss of body fluids, is the most important problem to treat, especially in the infant and very young child. Symptoms are reduced or no tears when crying, reduced or no urination or dark urine, dry lips and mouth.

HOW IS GASTROENTERITIS DIAGNOSED?

A history of the illness and careful examination of the child for dehydration are done first. Stool cultures for infection and blood tests for evaluating infection or dehydration may be necessary.

HOW IS GASTROENTERITIS TREATED?

Diet treatment of dehydration caused by diarrhea and vomiting is the major therapy. Depending on stool culture results, antibiotic medication may also be used. Diet treatment begins with replacing fluid losses, and is called oral rehydration therapy (ORT). When fluid losses have been replaced, a slow return to a bland and then to regular diet is started. The diet depends on severity of diarrhea, dehydration, and age.

Infants Under 1 Year

Frequent but very small amounts of clear fluids by mouth are offered. Commercially available oral electrolyte solutions such as Pedialyte, Rehydralyte, Infalyte, or Ricelyte are recommended for the first 24 hours. If your baby is on cow's milk formula, a slow introduction of half strength formula may be started. If diarrhea does not improve or becomes worse, a soy formula may be recommended instead. If your baby has been taking solid foods, slowly begin feeding banana, apple, cooked carrot, rice, toast, and lean meat. Improvement is gradual and takes about a week.

Children Over 1 Year

Milk and milk products should be eliminated for 1 week. Electrolyte solutions and other clear fluids can be offered, along with additional foods such as noodles, soft cooked fruits and vegetables, bland soups, cultured yogurt, soft boiled eggs or crackers.

Other Considerations:

Diarrhea is contagious and hand-washing after diaper or toilet care prevents spread. Diaper rash from diarrhea can be treated by keeping the skin clean and dry and applying protective ointments, such as zinc oxide paste or petroleum jelly.

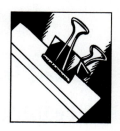

■ Pediatric Gastroenteritis *(continued)*

IS THERE ANYTHING SPECIAL I NEED TO KNOW?

It is important to provide all the fluid your child wants in order to correct dehydration. Clear fluids alone should be used for the first 24 hours only because they do not contain needed calories. Avoid high sugar solutions as the only fluids. Do not use boiled skim milk or broth because they are too high in salt. Do not use over the counter diarrhea medications because they are not effective in children.

Provider _____

Phone Number _____

Additional Comments: _____

_____

_____

_____

_____

_____

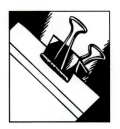

Patient Information on...

■ Pediatric Jaundice

WHAT IS JAUNDICE?

Jaundice is a condition described as yellowness of the skin, whites of the eyes, and other parts of the body, including some body fluids.

WHAT CAUSES JAUNDICE?

Jaundice can be caused by a blockage of bile passageways in the liver, malfunctioning liver cells, breast feeding, and the destruction of red blood cells.

HOW CAN I TELL IF MY CHILD HAS JAUNDICE?

As stated above, the skin, whites of the eyes, or other body parts become yellow.

HOW IS JAUNDICE DIAGNOSED?

Jaundice is diagnosed after a person develops a yellowish discoloration. The diagnosis of the cause of jaundice depends on several factors. Initially a blood sample is drawn for measurement of the bilirubin level and, depending on the results, further blood tests may be needed.

HOW IS JAUNDICE TREATED?

The cause determines the management of jaundice. If the problem is thought to be from breast feeding, using formula for 2 to 3 days will correct the problem. Infants who have jaundice after birth may need to be placed under a "bili light." Blood transfusions may be necessary for those infants with hemolytic anemia (which results when the mother's blood is different from the infant's).

IS THERE ANYTHING SPECIAL I NEED TO KNOW?

Most of the time, jaundice can be treated easily. It is important to make sure that infants who have jaundice drink large amounts of fluid because they run the risk of becoming dehydrated.

Provider _____

Phone Number _____

Additional Comments: _____

_____

_____

_____

_____

_____

_____

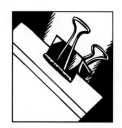

Patient Information on...

■ Pediatric Otitis Media

WHAT IS OTITIS MEDIA?

Otitis media is an infection of the middle ear (eardrum and the little bones behind the drum). This infection is so common that almost every child, by the time they are 3 years of age, has experienced at least one infection. Most experience more. In fact, it is so common that if you suspect your child is ill, otitis media should be considered as one of the causes.

WHAT CAUSES OTITIS MEDIA?

Three bacteria commonly infect the ear: *Streptococcus pneumoniae*, *Haemophilus influenzae*, and *Moraxella catarrhalis*.

HOW CAN I TELL IF MY CHILD HAS OTITIS MEDIA?

After infection develops, most young children have ear pain, tug at their ears, develop a fever, and become very irritable. Prior to the development of otitis media, patients usually have had a viral upper respiratory illness or an allergy.

HOW IS OTITIS MEDIA DIAGNOSED?

The above signs and symptoms along with an abnormal ear exam (example, bulging of the eardrum) usually confirm the diagnosis. Patients may also need tests to determine the eardrum mobility (tympanogram).

HOW IS OTITIS MEDIA TREATED?

Because many bacteria are resistant, erythromycin-sulfamethoxazole (Pediazole) has been the drug of choice. Trimethoprim-sulfamethoxazole (Bactrim) has also been used, as has amoxicillin, but these drugs are less effective because of bacterial resistance. Most common side effects include allergic reactions and stomach and intestinal discomfort.

IS THERE ANYTHING SPECIAL I NEED TO KNOW?

It is very important that all medication is taken as directed. If only some of the medication is taken, the infection may not be cleared and extra medication will be needed.

Provider _____

Phone Number _____

Additional Comments: _____

_____

_____

_____

_____

_____

_____

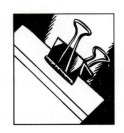

Patient Information on...

■ Pediatric Sinusitis

WHAT IS SINUSITIS?

Sinusitis is an infection of the sinuses caused by bacteria which usually occurs after a viral upper respiratory illness.

WHAT CAUSES SINUSITIS?

Three bacteria commonly infect the sinuses: *Streptococcus pneumoniae, Haemophilus influenzae,* and *Moraxella catarrhalis.*

HOW CAN I TELL IF MY CHILD HAS SINUSITIS?

Sinusitis in children usually has a different presentation from that of adults. Children may have a yellow-colored runny nose discharge, fever, swelling around their eyes, and painful sinuses, or "common cold" symptoms that linger for 1–2 weeks.

HOW IS SINUSITIS DIAGNOSED?

The presence of the above signs and symptoms are all that is necessary to diagnose most cases. Other cases require sinus x-rays and cultures of nasal mucus.

HOW IS SINUSITIS TREATED?

Because many bacteria are drug-resistant, erythromycin-sulfamethoxazole (Pediazole) has been the drug of choice.

Trimethoprim-sulfamethoxazole (Bactrim) has also been used as well as amoxicillin, but these drugs have become less effective because of resistance. Most common side effects include allergic reactions and stomach and intestinal discomfort.

IS THERE ANYTHING SPECIAL I NEED TO KNOW?

It is very important that all medication be taken as directed. If only some of the medication is taken, the infection may not be cleared and extra medication will be needed.

Provider _____

Phone Number _____

Additional Comments: _____

_____

_____

_____

_____

_____

_____

_____

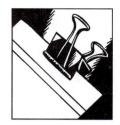

Patient Information on...

■ Peptic Ulcer Disease

WHAT IS PEPTIC ULCER DISEASE?

Peptic ulcer disease is a condition in which there is either too much acid production in the esophagus (swallowing tube), stomach, or first part of the small intestine, or there is a breakdown in the defenses that protect these areas, or both. These factors lead to the formation of an ulcer, which is a "craterlike" indention.

WHAT CAUSES PEPTIC ULCER DISEASE?

There are many factors that contribute to the formation of ulcers, one of which is overproduction of acid, which may be stimulated by stress or certain foods. Certain bacteria, alcohol, and some drugs like aspirin and anti-inflammatories (example, ibuprofen [Advil]) may break down the protective defenses. Smoking is thought to contribute to or delay healing of ulcers.

HOW CAN I TELL IF I HAVE PEPTIC ULCER DISEASE?

A mild to moderate aching or burning-type pain in the stomach is the most common symptom. The pain may come several hours after eating a meal and is usually relieved by eating or taking antacids. When an ulcer bleeds, there can be blood when vomiting (vomit will have a coffee-ground consistency) or blood in a bowel movement, which makes it a tarry color.

HOW IS PEPTIC ULCER DISEASE DIAGNOSED?

Peptic ulcer disease is diagnosed by the symptoms and by x-rays or by looking through a scope that is passed into the stomach.

HOW IS PEPTIC ULCER DISEASE TREATED?

Medications are the main method of treatment for peptic ulcer disease. Antacids (Maalox) may be given to neutralize the acids in the stomach, or medications may be given to block the production of acids by the stomach (cimetidine [Tagamet] and ranitidine [Zantac]). Antibiotics may be given to kill bacteria that may be contributing to ulcer formation. Rarely will surgery be required.

IS THERE ANYTHING SPECIAL I NEED TO KNOW?

Changes in life-style such as avoiding alcohol, not smoking, and avoiding aspirin or anti-inflammatory medications, like ibuprofen, can be helpful. Be sure to take medications as prescribed by your health care provider and report any signs of bleeding immediately.

Provider _____

Phone Number _____

Additional Comments: _____

_____

_____

_____

_____

_____

_____

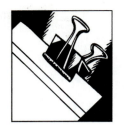

Patient Information on...

■ Pericarditis

WHAT IS PERICARDITIS?

Pericarditis is defined as inflammation of the membrane surrounding the heart (pericardial sac). The pericardial sac holds the heart in place and protects it from organisms and infection from other areas of the chest.

WHAT CAUSES PERICARDITIS?

The cause of pericarditis is usually unknown. However, certain viruses, bacteria, fungi, tumors, and autoimmune disorders have been known to trigger an attack.

HOW CAN I TELL IF I HAVE PERICARDITIS?

The most common symptom is chest pain. It is typically described as a sharp, midchest pain that radiates to the left shoulder and worsens with deep breaths or while lying down. It is also relieved by sitting up and leaning forward. Fever and muscle aches may be present as well.

HOW IS PERICARDITIS DIAGNOSED?

The diagnosis is made after a sound, called a rub, is heard while listening over the heart with a stethoscope. A chest x-ray, electrocardiogram (ECG), and blood tests may also be ordered to aid in the diagnosis.

HOW IS PERICARDITIS TREATED?

If the cause of pericarditis is known, treatment should be started. For example, if the cause is a bacterial infection antibiotics should be given. However, if the cause is viral or unknown, management consists only of pain and anti-inflammatory medications.

IS THERE ANYTHING SPECIAL I NEED TO KNOW?

Pericarditis may lead to a serious condition known as cardiac tamponade. In this condition, fluid collects rapidly in the pericardial sac, restricting the heart from pumping effectively. Symptoms of tamponade will occur acutely and require immediate correction, which includes cutting a window into the pericardial sac.

For more information, contact the American Heart Association at 1-800-242-8721.

Provider _____

Phone Number _____

Additional Comments: _____

_____

_____

_____

_____

_____

Patient Information on...

■ Pneumonia

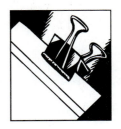

WHAT IS PNEUMONIA?

Pneumonia is an infection involving the lung tissue. As a result of the infection, fluid collects in the involved tissue, which prevents gas exchange and causes shortness of breath. If untreated this condition can be fatal. In fact, pneumonia is the most serious respiratory infection and a major cause of death in the United States. Overall, it is the fifth leading cause of death. More than 1 million cases of pneumonia are diagnosed each year, affecting persons of all ages. The development of pneumonia occurs throughout the year, with a higher rate during the winter months.

WHAT CAUSES PNEUMONIA?

Pneumonia can be caused by numerous organisms, such as viruses, bacteria, fungi, and parasites.

HOW CAN I TELL IF I HAVE PNEUMONIA?

Depending on the organism causing the infection, the symptoms vary. Some patients experience few symptoms, whereas other are seriously ill. High fever, chest pain, shaking chills, and a cough with mucus is common in most cases. However, some cases of pneumonia produce a dry cough.

HOW IS PNEUMONIA DIAGNOSED?

The diagnosis of pneumonia is suspected after a patient presents with the typical signs and symptoms (see above). A chest x-ray usually confirms the presence of pneumonia. Examination of lung secretions (mucus) is also routinely done to aid in the diagnosis.

HOW IS PNEUMONIA TREATED?

Pneumonias caused by bacteria, fungi, and parasites are treated with specific antibiotics. Penicillin and erythromycin are common choices. Viral pneumonias are not usually treated with medications unless a secondary bacterial infection is suspected or a patient has pneumonia caused by herpes. It is important to remember that antibiotics are not without side effects, particularly penicillin. Many patients are allergic to penicillin and experience a rash, shortness of breath, or severe allergic reaction when they take it. Erythromycin is usually well tolerated, but it may cause stomach discomfort.

IS THERE ANYTHING SPECIAL I NEED TO KNOW?

It is important that you take all medication as prescribed even if symptoms are resolved. In addition, smoking can cause recovery to be delayed. Consider cutting back or stopping if you smoke. Finally, if you are 65 or older, you should have a pneumococcal and a viral influenza vaccine.

For further information, contact the American Lung Association at 1-800-586-4872.

Provider _____

Phone Number _____

Additional Comments: _____

_____

_____

_____

_____

_____

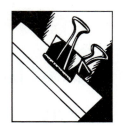

Patient Information on...
■ Pregnancy

WHAT GENERAL INFORMATION SHOULD I KNOW?

Seeking medical evaluation early in pregnancy is very important. Evaluation of the mother and unborn baby helps prevent miscarriages, premature births, birth defects, and medical complications that may occur in the mother.

HOW CAN I TELL IF I AM PREGNANT?

One should suspect pregnancy if your menstrual periods stop. In these cases, a pregnancy test should be done. There are many tests that can be purchased, or one can be ordered by a health care provider. One may also experience fatigue, nausea, vomiting, breast tenderness and distention, and frequent urination.

HOW IS PREGNANCY DIAGNOSED?

There are different signs that indicate pregnancy. Some can be determined by the patient, others need assistance from a health care provider. The signs include a bluish discoloration of the vagina and cervix, skin discoloration under the eyes and over the nose, uterine (womb) enlargement, uterine contractions, movement of the baby, and a positive pregnancy test. One must remember, however, a positive pregnancy test does not always mean there is viable pregnancy. Pregnancy tests can still be positive after a recent miscarriage.

HOW SHOULD PREGNANCY BE MANAGED?

A complete medical history and physical exam should be done soon after one learns of her pregnancy. Extensive tests should be ordered to test for cervical diseases, sexually transmitted diseases, anemia, blood type, Rh factor, German measles, urinary tract infections, hepatitis, and sickle cell disease (African Americans only). Later in the pregnancy, tests will be done to rule-out spinal deformities in the baby and diabetes in the mother. In women who are over the age of 35, amniocentesis may be done to rule out genetic defects. All pregnant women should start prenatal vitamins soon after becoming pregnant or before, if possible.

IS THERE ANYTHING SPECIAL I NEED TO KNOW?

All patients should be aware of "danger signals" that may indicate a problem. These include: (1) vaginal bleeding; (2) vaginal leaking of fluid before due date; (3) severe stomach pain; (4) swelling of the face and hands and persistent swelling of the feet and ankles; (5) severe headaches not relieved with acetaminophen (Tylenol); and (6) decreased movement of the baby. Pregnant women should also consult their health care provider before taking any medication, as some may adversely effect their pregnancy and baby. Acetaminophen (Tylenol) is safe for minor aches and pains. Alcohol, tobacco products, and illegal drugs should also be avoided. Finally, proper rest, a well-balanced diet, and the avoidance of potentially harmful activity should be maintained.

Provider _____

Phone Number _____

Additional Comments: _____

_____

_____

_____

_____

_____

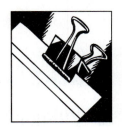

Patient Information on...

■ Prostate Cancer

WHAT IS PROSTATE CANCER?

Prostate cancer is a malignant tumor that invades healthy prostatic tissue and may spread to other organs, like the bone and liver. Unlike other cancers, prostate cancer is a disease of men. In addition, this cancer is more likely to occur in older men. The number of prostate cancer cases reported has increased markedly. The American Cancer Society estimates that there will be an 18% increase in cases over the next year.

WHAT CAUSES PROSTATE CANCER?

Four factors have been cited as possible causes of prostate cancer. These include genetics, exposure to environmental toxins, chronic prostate infections, and male hormones.

HOW CAN I TELL IF I HAVE PROSTATE CANCER?

Many patients with prostate cancer have no symptoms at all. Others may have complaints of frequent urination, especially at night, or dribbling. The majority of cases are discovered when a mass is found on a routine rectal examination.

HOW IS PROSTATE CANCER DIAGNOSED?

After a nodule is found, either through a rectal exam or ultrasound, the mass is biopsied. A tumor marker known as prostate-specific antigen (PSA) is a blood test also used to evaluate prostate cancer.

HOW IS PROSTATE CANCER TREATED?

The type of treatment depends on the severity of the tumor and whether it has spread. For example, early stages of disease are treated by removal of the tumor, followed by radiation therapy. Advanced stages may be managed with female hormones, removing both testicles, and chemotherapy in some cases.

IS THERE ANYTHING SPECIAL I NEED TO KNOW?

The American Cancer Society and the National Cancer Institute recommend a yearly digital (finger) rectal examination beginning at age 40.

For further information, contact the American Cancer Society at 1-800-227-2345.

Provider _____

Phone Number _____

Additional Comments: _____

_____

_____

_____

_____

_____

_____

Patient Information on...
■ Pulmonary Embolism

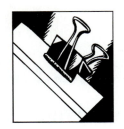

WHAT IS PULMONARY EMBOLISM?

Pulmonary embolism is a condition that results when an embolus (blood clot, air bubble, or pieces of tissue) begins to travel inside the blood vessels and lodges in the lung blood vessels. This leads to a disruption in the supply of blood to the lung tissue and usually to inadequate oxygen availability. In the United States, it is estimated that pulmonary emboli contribute to 100,000 deaths per year and about one half of these deaths occur within 2 hours after an embolus develops.

WHAT CAUSES PULMONARY EMBOLISM?

More than 95% of emboli are from blood clots that arise from the deep leg veins. These clots develop after periods of inactivity, such as prolonged bed rest or sitting for long periods of time, following major abdominal or hip surgery, in obesity, and with the use of birth control pills.

HOW CAN I TELL IF I HAVE PULMONARY EMBOLISM?

The most common symptom is sudden, sharp, one-sided chest pain accompanied by shortness of breath and cough. Other classic findings include fever, anxiety, sweating, nausea, vomiting, and feeling faint.

HOW IS PULMONARY EMBOLISM DIAGNOSED?

The diagnosis of pulmonary embolism should be suspected in any person who displays the above findings. Pulmonary angiography (an x-ray of the pulmonary vessels after dye is injected) is the "gold standard" test. However, a ventilation-perfusion lung scan is frequently done because it is safer and also very accurate.

HOW IS PULMONARY EMBOLISM TREATED?

General management of pulmonary embolism includes giving the patient oxygen, medication (streptokinase or urokinase) that will dissolve the clot, and medication that will prevent clots from forming (heparin and coumadin).

IS THERE ANYTHING SPECIAL I NEED TO KNOW?

Medication like streptokinase, urokinase, heparin, and coumadin can cause excessive bleeding and hemorrhage. If any of these conditions occur, one's health care provider should be informed. Do not take drugs that promote bleeding like aspirin or ibuprofen (Motrin, Advil) while taking medication for pulmonary embolism. Foods rich in vitamin K such as green, leafy vegetables; cauliflower; tomatoes; fish; liver; cheese; egg yolks; and fats from red meat also promote clotting and should be avoided. Prolonged sitting, crossing legs, and constrictive clothing (girdles) should also be avoided. However, when indicated, elastic stockings may be worn to prevent clots from developing.

For more information, contact the American Lung Association at 1-800-586-4872.

Provider _____

Phone Number _____

Additional Comments: _____

_____

_____

_____

_____

_____

_____

Patient Information on...
■ Pyelonephritis

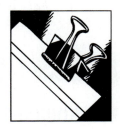

WHAT IS PYELONEPHRITIS?

Pyelonephritis is a urinary infection involving the kidney. It is more common in women and the elderly. Persons who are at risk for pyelonephritis include pregnant women, diabetics, those with a history of kidney stones or recurrent bladder infections, those with catheters, or those who are hospitalized.

WHAT CAUSES PYELONEPHRITIS?

In most cases, pyelonephritis is caused by the bacterium *Escherichia coli*. This bacterium lives in the intestines, where it helps with the digestive process. However, if it gets into the bladder and then moves up into the kidney, it can cause pyelonephritis.

HOW CAN I TELL IF I HAVE PYELONEPHRITIS?

Persons with pyelonephritis usually have a sudden onset of fever, chills, pain in the lower back and sides, aches, and tiredness. Other symptoms include frequent urination, painful urination, nausea, vomiting, and dehydration.

HOW IS PYELONEPHRITIS DIAGNOSED?

Diagnosis is based on symptoms and on the results of urine and blood tests. Occasionally, pictures of the kidney may be taken to see if there is something blocking the flow of urine through the kidney.

HOW IS PYELONEPHRITIS TREATED?

Antibiotics are the treatment for pyelonephritis. These may be given by mouth or through an IV, depending on the severity of the infection. Dehydration may also be treated with IV fluids.

IS THERE ANYTHING SPECIAL I NEED TO KNOW?

It is important to prevent bladder infections, as these can progress to kidney infections. To decrease the chance of getting a bladder infection, women should wipe themselves from front to back and should avoid using vaginal deodorants and bubble bath. Women should also urinate immediately after intercourse. Antibiotics may need to be taken for at least 2 weeks, so be sure to take all medication prescribed by your health care provider.

For more information, contact the National Kidney Foundation at 1-800-622-9010.

Provider _____

Phone Number _____

Additional Comments: _____

_____

_____

_____

_____

_____

_____

_____

Patient Information on...
■ Rheumatoid Arthritis

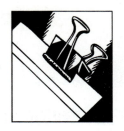

WHAT IS RHEUMATOID ARTHRITIS?

Rheumatoid arthritis is a chronic inflammatory disease that most commonly affects the joints but can affect the eyes, heart, lungs, nerves, and other areas of the body. Symptoms vary from mild to a severe form with progressive deformity of joints. Women are affected more often than men.

WHAT CAUSES RHEUMATOID ARTHRITIS?

The cause is unknown, but some experts believe that the symptoms are caused by an inflammatory response that destroys normal tissue, possibly as a reaction to a virus.

HOW CAN I TELL IF I HAVE RHEUMATOID ARTHRITIS?

Most patients complain of joint pain with movement and stiffness that is worse in the morning or after periods of inactivity. Joint swelling may also be noted. Most commonly the fingers, wrists, knees, ankles, and toes are involved. Other symptoms include generalized body discomfort, tiredness, and weight loss.

HOW IS RHEUMATOID ARTHRITIS DIAGNOSED?

Diagnosis is based on symptoms, joint deformities noted on x-rays, and blood tests. A blood test that is positive for rheumatoid factor is suggestive of rheumatoid arthritis but can be present in other diseases as well.

HOW IS RHEUMATOID ARTHRITIS TREATED?

A variety of methods may be used including exercise, splinting of joints, physical therapy, and medications such as aspirin or anti-inflammatory drugs such as ibuprofen (Advil). Stronger medications may be needed for severe disease and occasional use of steroids may be helpful. Surgery may be done in severe cases.

IS THERE ANYTHING SPECIAL I NEED TO KNOW?

A balance of gentle exercise, rest, and diet is important. Avoid overuse of joints, especially if this increases pain. Do not take any over-the-counter medications without first asking your health care provider.

For more information, contact the Arthritis Foundation at 1-800-283-7800.

Provider _____

Phone Number _____

Additional Comments: _____

_____

_____

_____

_____

_____

_____

Patient Information on...

■ Seizure Disorders

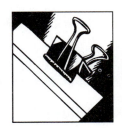

WHAT IS A SEIZURE DISORDER?

A seizure disorder is a condition in which parts of the brain become overexcited, resulting in sudden and sometimes violent contractions or convulsive movements of groups of muscles. The condition is also called epilepsy. Seizures may be classified into three types: partial, generalized, and unclassified.

WHAT CAUSES A SEIZURE DISORDER?

Seizures can be described as a primary disorder, in which there is no known cause. These are possibly related to genetic makeup. Seizures can also be caused by abnormal conditions such as head trauma, birth defects, infections, tumors, or diseases of the blood vessels in the brain.

HOW CAN I TELL IF I HAVE A SEIZURE DISORDER?

Most seizures consist of three phases: the aura, in which the person may experience unusual tastes or smells, or complain of dizziness, headache, or difficulty with speech; the ictal phase, which is the seizure itself; and the postictal phase, which consists of confusion, loss of memory of the event, and sleepiness.

HOW IS A SEIZURE DISORDER DIAGNOSED?

Along with the medical history and physical exam, several blood tests are usually done. One of the most helpful tests measures brain waves. It is called an electroencephalogram (EEG). A computed tomographic (CT) scan or a magnetic resonance imaging (MRI) scan of the head may also be done.

HOW IS A SEIZURE DISORDER TREATED?

Treatment consists of medications (phenytoin [Dilantin], carbamazepine [Tegretol], and phenobarbital) that are selected according to the type of seizure activity. Most persons will need to remain on medication for life.

IS THERE ANYTHING SPECIAL I NEED TO KNOW?

Persons with seizure disorders must have safety as a priority. Activities must be planned so that injury will be prevented in case a seizure should occur. Always use seat belts when traveling. Pad counter and furniture edges. Be sure to have someone along when participating in potentially hazardous activities such as swimming. Wear a medical alert bracelet at all times.

For more information, contact the Epilepsy Information Service at 1-800-642-0500.

Provider _____

Phone Number _____

Additional Comments: _____

_____

_____

_____

_____

_____

Patient Information on...
■ Seizure Disorders in Children

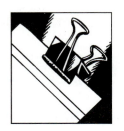

WHAT ARE SEIZURES?

Seizures are sudden jerking movements that may only involve certain body parts or may cause jerking movements over the entire body. Seizures may also be associated with sensation and emotional changes. When seizures occur, the person experiencing them is not aware of them nor can he or she control them.

WHAT CAUSES SEIZURES?

Most seizures are caused by high fevers, structural problems of the brain (example, abnormal development of the brain or tumors of the brain), and abnormal body chemicals already in the body or taken at some point. There are some people who have seizures for no apparent reason.

HOW CAN I TELL IF MY CHILD HAS SEIZURES?

One should be concerned about seizures if sudden uncontrolled jerking movements occur. A classic presentation of seizures in children includes a blank stare without any response. Typically this seizure (petit mal) is brought to attention by the child's teacher after the teacher notices brief periods of not paying attention in class.

HOW ARE SEIZURES DIAGNOSED?

To determine the exact cause, tests to rule out diseases that may cause seizures, chemical imbalances, or birth defects must be done first. These include blood tests, x-rays of the brain, and an electroencephalogram (EEG). An EEG measures brain wave activity and can give clues as to the cause of the seizure.

HOW ARE SEIZURES TREATED?

There are many drugs that are used to treat seizures (examples, phenobarbital, phenytoin, valproic acid, carbamazepine, and ethosuximide). Most are well tolerated but have to be monitored closely to determine if the dosage is correct. If not, seizures may occur unexpectedly. If a seizure occurs, the person having the seizure should be allowed to seize. Remove any surrounding objects that may harm him or her. It is not recommended to place any objects in the individual's mouth or extend the neck.

IS THERE ANYTHING SPECIAL I NEED TO KNOW?

All medication should be taken as directed to prevent seizures. In addition, emotional disturbances like anxiety, depression, anger, feelings of guilt and inadequacy often occur as a reaction to the seizures in the parents of the affected child as well as in the child old enough to understand. These thoughts are normal, but counseling should be sought to prevent serious problems like depression or suicide.

Provider _____

Phone Number _____

Additional Comments: _____

_____

_____

_____

_____

_____

_____

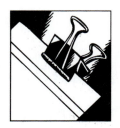

Patient Information on...
■ Skin Cancer

WHAT IS SKIN CANCER?

Skin cancer is the most common type of cancer in the United States. Over 500,000 cases are newly diagnosed each year. Of those cases, about 9,000 will result in death. Skin cancer is a preventable disease. With the right education and screening, a major impact could be made to reduce the number of cases and deaths.

WHAT CAUSES SKIN CANCER?

The exact cause is unknown; however, exposure to ultraviolet radiation from the sun and tanning beds increases one's chance of getting skin cancer. This is particularly true for lighter-skinned individuals. The three main types of skin cancer include basal cell carcinoma, squamous cell carcinoma, and melanoma. The last two, if not removed, run the risk of spreading to other body organs.

HOW CAN I TELL IF I HAVE SKIN CANCER?

Changes in the skin, particularly an ulcer that does not heal or a mole the begins to change colors, especially on the face, ears, lips, chest, and trunk should alert one that skin cancer is a possibility.

HOW IS SKIN CANCER DIAGNOSED?

To make a diagnosis it is necessary to biopsy the suspected area of skin.

HOW IS SKIN CANCER TREATED?

Usually when a biopsy is performed it is necessary to remove the entire lesion. Hence, removal of the lesion also remains the treatment of choice, especially before it spreads to other body organs. Radiation therapy is sometimes recommended for basal cell carcinoma and squamous cell carcinoma when removal is not possible.

IS THERE ANYTHING SPECIAL I NEED TO KNOW?

Yes! Prevention of skin cancer can be accomplished through regular screening (examining the skin) and most importantly through avoiding prolonged sun exposure (between hours of 10 AM and 2 PM) and tanning beds. If you are required to be in the sun, many brands of sunscreens are available and should be used. A sunscreen with a minimum SPF (sun protective factor) of 15 should be used on the body and 25–30 on the face. Ideally, sunscreens should be applied 30 minutes before expected sun exposure and reapplied after sweating or swimming. Waterproof sunscreens are available and do not need to be reapplied as often. If a tan is necessary, bronzing gels are available that provide the appearance of a tan. The effect is both safe and immediate.

For further information, contact the American Cancer Society at 1-800-227-2345.

Provider _____

Phone Number _____

Additional Comments: _____

_____

_____

_____

_____

_____

_____

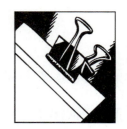

Patient Information on...
■ Strains and Sprains

WHAT ARE STRAINS AND SPRAINS?

A strain is a soft-tissue injury that results from stretching of a muscle, tendon, or ligament. A sprain is similar to a strain but involves the soft tissues of a joint. These types of injuries commonly occur during exercise and athletic competition.

WHAT CAUSES STRAINS AND SPRAINS?

Strains are usually due to exertion or overuse of muscles and connecting tendons and ligaments. Strains may affect any muscle group and usually cause minimal discomfort and disability. Sprains can affect any joint but most commonly occur at the ankle when it is turned inward, leading to injury of the ligaments on the outside of the ankle.

HOW CAN I TELL IF I HAVE A STRAIN OR SPRAIN?

Most strains or sprains will result in some degree of discomfort, from mild to severe pain. Movement of the joint may be limited and there may be swelling and bruising. The affected part may look abnormal in shape and size. Walking may be difficult when the knees or ankles are involved.

HOW ARE STRAINS AND SPRAINS DIAGNOSED?

Most strains and sprains can be diagnosed from the history and physical exam. An x-ray may be done to determine the degree of soft-tissue injury or to look for fractures.

HOW ARE STRAINS AND SPRAINS TREATED?

The basic treatment for any strain or sprain consists of:

1. Elevating the injured area.
2. Placing an ice pack on the site for 20 minutes every 4 hours.
3. Compressing the injury by wrapping it with an Ace wrap or splint.
4. Avoiding bearing weight on the injured site.

Anti-inflammatory medications (ibuprofen [Advil and Motrin]) and naproxen sodium (Aleve) are helpful in reducing pain, swelling, and inflammation.

IS THERE ANYTHING SPECIAL I NEED TO KNOW?

While most strains and sprains will completely resolve with time, some injuries may require additional treatment such as physical therapy. A slow, progressive return to activity is best. More serious injuries may cause discomfort and swelling for a long period of time and require follow-up with a specialist.

For more information, contact the National Rehabilitation Information Center at 1-800-346-2742.

Provider _____

Phone Number _____

Additional Comments: _____

_____

_____

_____

_____

_____

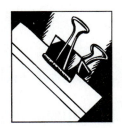

Patient Information on...

■ Strokes

WHAT IS A STROKE?

A stroke is a condition in which part of the brain does not get enough blood supply and oxygen. It is the third leading cause of death in the United States and a frequent cause of physical and mental disability. Strokes are more common after age 60 and in those who have high blood pressure.

WHAT CAUSES STROKES?

Strokes are caused by either blood clots in the brain associated with hardening of the arteries or by bleeding in the brain associated with high blood pressure and rupture of small vessels.

HOW CAN I TELL IF I HAVE A STROKE?

Specific symptoms of stroke are determined by the location and size of the affected area in the brain. Most commonly there is difficulty with speech, movement of the legs and arms, and problems with vision (usually noticed more on one side of the body). Some strokes are preceded by one or more episodes of mild stroke-like symptoms that go away within 24 hours.

HOW ARE STROKES DIAGNOSED?

Diagnosis requires a careful history and physical examination along with numerous laboratory tests. A computed tomographic (CT) scan or magnetic resonance imaging (MRI) scan of the head is helpful in determining the location and type of stroke.

HOW ARE STROKES TREATED?

Treatment in the early stages is directed at maintaining the functioning of the body and preventing further damage. Medications for high blood pressure and irregular heart rhythms may be given, as well as those to prevent further formation of blood clots. Long-term treatment consists of reducing risk factors and various therapies that will help regain as much function as possible.

IS THERE ANYTHING SPECIAL I NEED TO KNOW?

Since there is no cure for stroke, life-style changes that reduce the risk of stroke are especially important. These include treatment of hypertension, avoiding the use of tobacco, weight loss for those overweight, and regular exercise.

For more information, contact the National Stroke Association at 1-800-787-6537.

Provider _____

Phone Number _____

Additional Comments: _____

_____

_____

_____

_____

_____

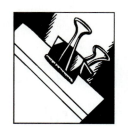

Patient Information on...

■ Substance Use and Abuse

WHAT IS SUBSTANCE USE AND ABUSE?

Substance users and abusers refers to those who use a drug, medication, or a toxin habitually or are addicted to it. In addition to affecting the person who abuses a substance, drug and alcohol abuse affect the family, the community, and society. It is estimated that the current levels of substance abuse in the United States contribute to at least 75,000 deaths and costs about 152 billion dollars a year.

WHAT CAUSES SUBSTANCE USE AND ABUSE?

There are several theories as to what causes substance abuse. Some say that it is a complex interplay between biologic, psychologic, and environmental factors. Those who treat substance use and abuse suggest that either the physical trait or a predisposition to substance abuse is inherited. More research needs to be done to understand the causes of this complex issue.

WHAT SYMPTOMS ARE ASSOCIATED WITH SUBSTANCE USE AND ABUSE?

Symptoms vary among individuals, depending on the substance used, the amount and frequency of use, and the tolerance the person has for the substance. In general, symptoms include disturbances of perception, attention, thinking, judgment, body movement, and ability to relate to others. Symptoms can last for hours or days.

HOW IS SUBSTANCE USE AND ABUSE DIAGNOSED?

There are criteria for the diagnosis of specific substance use and abuse disorders. In general, *intoxication* with a sub-

stance refers to the effects on the central nervous system that are reversible once the substance is no longer in use, whereas *abuse* refers to a repeated pattern of use that leads to significant impairment or distress.

HOW IS SUBSTANCE USE AND ABUSE TREATED?

There are a variety of treatments ranging from brief intervention, which focuses on increasing a person's awareness of the problem, to treatment of a life-threatening physical or psychologic crisis, which may require hospitalization. Other methods of treatment include individual or group counseling, and support groups such as Alcoholics Anonymous (AA).

IS THERE ANYTHING SPECIAL I NEED TO KNOW?

Substance use and abuse affects all aspects of life, including physical and emotional health, family relationships, economic security, and employment. By taking the first step, which is to recognize the problem, those affected can learn new, healthy ways of living and relating.

For more information, contact the Center for Substance Abuse Treatment at 1-800-662-4357.

Provider _____

Phone Number _____

Additional Comments: _____

_____

_____

_____

_____

_____

Patient Information on...

■ Syphilis

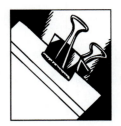

WHAT IS SYPHILIS?

Syphilis is a sexually transmitted disease. It is capable of infecting virtually any organ throughout the body. The infection enters through breaks in skin and through body openings, like the mouth, penis, vagina, and rectum.

WHAT CAUSES SYPHILIS?

Syphilis is caused by the organism *Treponema pallidum*.

HOW CAN I TELL IF I HAVE SYPHILIS?

Patients are seen in different stages. Initially after infection patients may have a painless ulcer at the site of infection (primary syphilis). If not treated, the disease will progress and patients will develop a rash, usually on the palms and soles (secondary syphilis). If still untreated, patients will go through a period without symptoms (latent syphilis). After this period patients may develop very serious conditions of their heart or brain (tertiary syphilis).

HOW IS SYPHILIS DIAGNOSED?

Several methods are used, however, an RPR (rapid plasma reagin) or VDRL (Venereal Disease Research Laboratory) blood test is usually the initial test done to determine infection.

HOW IS SYPHILIS TREATED?

The management of syphilis clearly depends on staging. Primary, secondary, or early latent disease of less than 1 year's duration require a single injection of penicillin G. If the duration is greater than 1 year, three weekly injections of penicillin G are required. With tertiary syphilis, IV penicillin is required. There is no good alternative to penicillin if a patient has an allergy to the drug; therefore, desensitization is recommended.

IS THERE ANYTHING SPECIAL I NEED TO KNOW?

Syphilis can be prevented by using latex condoms and avoiding sexual contact with those who are infected. It is important to remember that infected individuals who have no symptoms can still transmit the disease. In addition, any person found to be infected with syphilis should be counseled and tested for HIV.

For further information, contact the Centers for Disease Control and Prevention National Sexually Transmitted Diseases Hotline at 1-800-227-8922

Provider _____

Phone Number _____

Additional Comments: _____

_____

_____

_____

_____

_____

Patient Information on...

■ Systemic Lupus Erythematosus

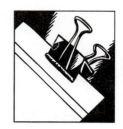

WHAT IS SYSTEMIC LUPUS ERYTHEMATOSUS?

Systemic lupus erythematosus (SLE) is an autoimmune disorder that can affect any part of the body and cause a variety of symptoms. Although it can occur at any age, it usually begins between 15 and 25 years of age and is more common in women.

WHAT CAUSES SLE?

The cause is not entirely clear, but it is thought that substances called antibodies, which usually help the body fight against infection, begin to destroy various parts of the body instead. This leads to damage of the vessels, nerves, muscles, and other parts of the body.

HOW CAN I TELL IF I HAVE SLE?

The symptoms vary depending on what part of the body is involved and may come and go throughout the course of the disease. The most common complaints are fever, weakness, and general discomfort. Facial rashes, joint pain, and difficulty breathing may also occur.

HOW IS SLE DIAGNOSED?

Diagnosis is difficult because there is no single test that can confirm the disease. A variety of tests that require blood and urine samples may be done. Other tests include those used to evaluate the heart and lungs.

HOW IS SLE TREATED?

SLE cannot be cured. Treatment is determined by how severe the symptoms are. Rashes may require only the use of sunscreen and joint pain may be treated with anti-inflammatory drugs. Ibuprofen (Motrin, Advil) is an example. Severe symptoms may require the use of steroids prescribed by a health care provider.

IS THERE ANYTHING SPECIAL I NEED TO KNOW?

It is especially important to take care of your health, including adequate amounts of exercise and rest, eating a balanced diet, and avoiding stress and sunlight. Pregnancy can increase the symptoms, so discuss options with your health care provider.

For more information, contact the Lupus Foundation at 1-800-558-0121.

Provider _____

Phone Number _____

Additional Comments: _____

_____

_____

_____

_____

_____

_____

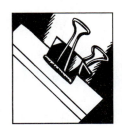

Patient Information on...
■ Testicular Cancer

WHAT IS TESTICULAR CANCER?

Testicular cancer is a malignant tumor that invades healthy testicles but may spread to other body organs, usually the intestines and liver. Testicular cancer is uncommon in comparison to other cancers such as those of the breast and lung. Approximately 5000 cases occur annually in the United States. Although uncommon, testicular cancer is the most common solid tumor in men aged 15–35.

WHAT CAUSES TESTICULAR CANCER?

The cause of testicular cancer is unclear; however, several factors have been noted in relation to the disease. For example, undescended testes (testes which have not dropped into the scrotum) that are not corrected in early childhood have been correlated with an increased development of testicular cancer. In addition, a higher rate of development has also been reported in twins, suggesting the presence of genetic factors.

HOW CAN I TELL IF I HAVE TESTICULAR CANCER?

The most common alerting sign of a testicular tumor is a painless and firm testicular mass. However, testicular cancer may also cause pain, especially if there is swelling of the testicle.

HOW IS TESTICULAR CANCER DIAGNOSED?

If testicular carcinoma is suspected, surgery is indicated; this should include removal of the involved testicle and biopsy of the mass on the testicle.

HOW IS TESTICULAR CANCER TREATED?

The treatment depends on how severe the tumor is and whether it has spread to other body organs. Depending on the type and the severity, patients will either get radiation therapy, chemotherapy, or in some cases both.

IS THERE ANYTHING SPECIAL I NEED TO KNOW?

Yes! Just as women are taught at an early age to examine their breasts, boys and men must also learn to examine their testes.

Each month, boys (starting at age 15 and continuing through adulthood) should:

1. Examine their testes while showering.
2. While showering, feel their testes for any swelling, small rocklike masses, or any new change in the size.
3. Notice any pain or heaviness of the testes.

Normally the testes are soft and spongy without any firm masses or swelling.

For further information, contact the American Cancer Society at 1-800-227-2345.

Provider _____

Phone Number _____

Additional Comments:_____

_____

_____

_____

_____

_____

_____

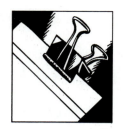

Patient Information on...

■ The Prevention of HIV

WHAT IS HIV?

HIV (human immunodeficiency virus) is a virus that causes AIDS (acquired immunodeficiency syndrome). It is a serious disease that has caused thousands of deaths. There are many rumors and misbeliefs about HIV. However, if one understands how it is spread, a plan can be developed to avoid it.

HOW IS HIV TRANSMITTED?

HIV usually enters the body through tears and breaks in the lining of the vagina and rectum (during sexual intercourse), after sharing IV drug needles, or is passed on to an unborn child by an infected mother. There is NO evidence that HIV can be transmitted by shaking hands, hugging, kissing, sitting next to a person with HIV or AIDS, sneezing, coughing, donating blood, sharing eating or writing utensils, telephones, water fountains, toilet seats, or working or attending school together.

WHO IS AT RISK FOR DEVELOPING HIV INFECTION?

Individuals at increased risk for developing HIV infection include those who:

1. Have had one sexual experience with an HIV-infected person.
2. Have multiple sexual partners.
3. Are prostitutes.
4. Are intravenous drug users sharing needles.

HOW CAN I TELL IF I HAVE HIV?

Initially most people have no symptoms. However, when the virus begins to progress, various symptoms may develop including headaches, fatigue, vaginal infections, swollen lymph glands, night sweats, fever, skin rashes, and sores in the mouth, nose, and anus.

HOW IS HIV DIAGNOSED?

A special blood test can tell if you have HIV. Its name is the ELISA (enzyme-linked immunosorbent-assay) test. If it is positive, a Western Blot blood test is done to confirm the ELISA test. You can and should have these tests done without using your name. The test detects antibodies the immune system makes, once it is exposed to HIV. However, after HIV enters the bloodstream there is a period of 6 weeks to 6 months before there are enough antibodies to make a positive test result. Therefore, one may need to get tested more than once.

IS THERE ANYTHING SPECIAL I NEED TO KNOW?

Yes! Special precautions should be taken to prevent transmission to one's self and others by:

1. Practicing safe sex;
2. Using latex condoms with nonoxynol 9;
3. Not sharing needles, razors, toothbrushes and other personal hygiene items; and
4. Not donating blood if you are HIV+ or engage in high risk behavior.

For further information, contact the National AIDS Hotline at 1-800-342-AIDS.

Provider _____

Phone Number _____

Additional Comments:_____

_____

_____

_____

_____

Patient Information on...

■ Tonsillitis and Pharyngitis in Children

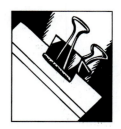

WHAT ARE TONSILLITIS AND PHARYNGITIS?

Tonsillitis is an infection of the tonsils and pharyngitis is an infection of the throat. Often these conditions are seen together and are treated the same way. Along with ear infections, tonsillitis and pharyngitis represent the most common illnesses seen in children.

WHAT CAUSES TONSILLITIS AND PHARYNGITIS?

Most infections are caused by viruses; however, a bacterium named *Streptococcus* occurs in 15%–40% of pharyngitis cases. Diphtheria bacteria and *mycoplasma*, although uncommon, may also cause infection. Common viral causes include Epstein-Barr virus (which causes mononucleosis), echovirus, and coxsackievirus.

HOW CAN I TELL IF MY CHILD HAS TONSILLITIS AND PHARYNGITIS?

The classical signs and symptoms of tonsillitis and pharyngitis are a sore throat, fever, and redness and pus of the throat and tonsils. In addition, the tonsils are usually enlarged and tender. Although it is uncommon today, pharyngitis caused by *Streptococcus* may lead to scarlet and rheumatic fever.

HOW ARE TONSILLITIS AND PHARYNGITIS DIAGNOSED?

Most cases are diagnosed after a child displays the typical signs and symptoms. In some cases, a rapid strep screen and a throat culture are done.

HOW ARE TONSILLITIS AND PHARYNGITIS TREATED?

Depending on the cause, the treatment varies. Since most infections are caused by viruses, only medication to relieve symptoms is necessary. If *Streptococcus* is identified, penicillin is given. For those that are allergic to penicillin, erythromycin can be used. Both antibiotics are well tolerated; however, allergic reactions and stomach upset may occur.

IS THERE ANYTHING SPECIAL I NEED TO KNOW?

All medication should be taken as directed and the course completed in order to prevent recurrent infections.

Provider _____

Phone Number _____

Additional Comments: _____

_____

_____

_____

_____

_____

_____

_____

_____

_____

Patient Information on...
■ Tuberculosis

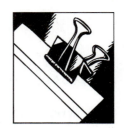

WHAT IS TUBERCULOSIS?

Tuberculosis refers to an infection of body organs by a mycobacterium organism. The organism mostly infects the lungs. In this case, the disease is often referred to as pulmonary tuberculosis. Tuberculosis is an ancient infection that has plagued humans throughout recorded history. Although improved working conditions, housing, nutrition, and modern treatment have resulted in a decline in the number of deaths, tuberculosis still remains a worldwide problem.

WHAT CAUSES TUBERCULOSIS?

In humans, the microorganism *Mycobacterium tuberculosis* is primarily responsible for causing tuberculosis.

HOW CAN I TELL IF I HAVE TUBERCULOSIS?

For individuals who develop tuberculosis, the symptoms vary depending on the extent of the disease. The most common symptom is a dry cough that eventually leads to a cough with white to yellow mucus. Blood may also be found in the mucus. Chest pain, fever, night sweats, fatigue, and weight loss may also be present.

HOW IS TUBERCULOSIS DIAGNOSED?

The infection can be detected, in most cases before any symptoms are present, by getting a skin test. The tuberculin purified protein derivative (PPD) skin test remains the best test for detecting tuberculosis infection. To detect whether there is active disease, one must get more specific tests. The chest x-ray is the most commonly used test to determine if there is disease in the lungs. Certain blood tests, cultures, and biopsies may also be required to isolate active disease in the blood, lung secretions (mucus), bone marrow, and skin.

HOW IS TUBERCULOSIS TREATED?

Once tuberculosis is proven to be present, patients are given a combination of drugs (isoniazid [INH], rifampin, pyrazinamide, and ethambutol) for 6–9 months. The number of drugs is determined by the severity of the disease. Numbness and tingling and liver problems may occur during treatment. Regular follow-up appointments with a clinician are recommended.

IS THERE ANYTHING SPECIAL I NEED TO KNOW?

Yes! This disease is on the upswing and in order to effectively fight it and its reoccurrence, everyone must take all medications as directed. Also, since tuberculosis is spread by coughing and sneezing, it is necessary to cover one's mouth and nose with a mask during active infection (usually 2 weeks). If anyone is around a tuberculosis patient, they also should wear a mask and be tested for infection. Finally, tuberculosis is a curable disease if all medications are taken!

For more information, contact the American Lung Association at 1-800-586-4872.

Provider _____

Phone Number _____

Additional Comments: _____

_____

_____

_____

_____

_____

Patient Information on...
■ Upper Respiratory Infections

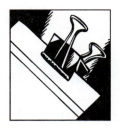

WHAT ARE UPPER RESPIRATORY INFECTIONS

Upper respiratory infections (URIs), or the common cold, are the most common type of infections seen in the doctor's office. Pharyngitis (infection of the throat), laryngitis (infection of the voice-box), tracheitis (infection of the windpipe), and sinusitis (infection of the sinuses) are classified as URIs. Ear infections are also common.

WHAT CAUSES URIs?

Infections involving the throat, voice box, and trachea are usually caused by viruses, whereas sinus infections are mostly caused by bacteria.

HOW CAN I TELL IF I HAVE A URI?

In general most people will experience fever and fatigue at some point during the infection. A sore throat is the usual symptom when pharyngitis is present. Laryngitis usually causes hoarseness, and tracheitis causes a tickle sensation in the chest and pain when breathing in and out. A cough may be present with all of these conditions, especially if there is mucous drainage in the involved areas. Sinusitis usually produces painful sinuses and headaches around the eyes, cheeks, or temples. There may also be discolored or foul-smelling mucus draining from the nose.

HOW ARE URIs DIAGNOSED?

The diagnosis is usually made when a patient exhibits the typical findings listed above. Some may require throat cultures, blood counts, and sinus x-rays, depending on the symptoms.

HOW ARE URIs TREATED?

If the infection is caused by bacteria, antibiotics are usually given for 7–10 days. In severe cases, especially sinusitis, treatment may last up to 30 days. No treatment is given for infections caused by viruses. In any case, patients should be given supportive treatment consisting of decongestants (Dimetapp), aspirin, or acetaminophen (Tylenol) as indicated for congestion and fever.

IS THERE ANYTHING SPECIAL I NEED TO KNOW?

If given antibiotics, one must take all that are prescribed, even if symptoms resolve before the medication is gone. Also, cigarette smoke, dusts, and pollution irritate all these infections and may slow the healing process.

For more information, contact the American Lung Association at 1-800-586-4872.

Provider _____

Phone Number _____

Additional Comments: _____

_____

_____

_____

_____

_____

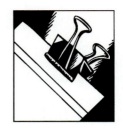

Patient Information on...

■ Urinary Incontinence

WHAT IS URINARY INCONTINENCE?

Urinary incontinence literally means there is an uncontrollable loss of urine. Urine loss may range from a few drops to very large amounts. It is estimated that 8 to 12 million Americans suffer from this disorder.

WHAT CAUSES URINARY INCONTINENCE?

There are numerous causes of urinary incontinence including stool impaction, decreased ability to move about (bedridden), weakened muscles in the pelvis that control the urge to urinate, prolonged use of urinary catheters (tubes), and some neurologic disorders (seizures).

HOW CAN I TELL IF I HAVE URINARY INCONTINENCE?

A sudden uncontrollable loss of urine indicates that one has urinary incontinence.

HOW IS URINARY INCONTINENCE DIAGNOSED?

A complete medical history and physical examination is necessary to make the diagnosis. A urine sample, blood tests, and x-rays may also be required.

HOW IS URINARY INCONTINENCE TREATED?

Exercises to strengthen the muscles that control the urge to urinate can be instituted in mild cases. Medications are primarily used in more advanced cases. Surgery may prove to be necessary if these measures fail.

IS THERE ANYTHING SPECIAL I NEED TO KNOW?

Sufferers need to realize this condition is not a part of growing old and that treatment truly exists. Seeking help from qualified medical personnel can in most cases prove helpful in relieving symptoms and in most cases provide complete resolution.

For more information contact: The Simon Foundation at 1-800-237-4666.

Provider _____

Phone Number _____

Additional Comments: _____

_____

_____

_____

_____

_____

Patient Information on...
■ Vaginitis

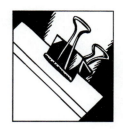

WHAT IS VAGINITIS?

Vaginitis is an inflammation of the vagina. Nearly every woman at some time in her life experiences an infection of the vagina. During pregnancy and usually once a month (after periods) there is an increase in vaginal secretions. This normal vaginal discharge has no odor, but some women may mistake this for a vaginal infection.

WHAT CAUSES VAGINITIS?

Most vaginal infections are caused by bacteria, fungi (yeast), and protozoa (*Trichomonas*).

HOW CAN I TELL IF I HAVE VAGINITIS?

Depending on the cause of the infection, most patients report some form of unusual discharge, which may be thick, thin, cheesy, yellow, green, or foul-smelling. The patient may also report itching and burning inside and outside her vagina.

HOW IS VAGINITIS DIAGNOSED?

To obtain a diagnosis, the patient must undergo a pelvic examination to view and examine the vagina and cervix. The most important part of the pelvic exam is testing the discharge for bacteria, fungi, and protozoa.

HOW IS VAGINITIS TREATED?

Treatment consists of medication that may be taken for 7 days, depending on the severity of the infection. Drugs such as metronidazole, ampicillin, and miconazole may be used.

IS THERE ANYTHING SPECIAL I NEED TO KNOW?

During pregnancy, vaginitis is more likely to occur. Tell your health care provider if you are pregnant, as some types of antibiotics cannot be given to pregnant women. Also, sexual partners of those with vaginitis should be treated in some cases. Ask your health care provider if your sexual partner should be treated. To prevent yeast infections from developing, remember to dry the outside vaginal area thoroughly after a shower, bath, or swim. Change out of a wet bathing suit or damp workout clothes as soon as possible. A dry area is less likely to encourage the growth of yeast. Wear cotton underwear, avoid tight-fitting clothes, wipe from the front to the rear (away from the vagina), and don't douche unless your health care practitioner tells you to do so. Douching may disturb the normal vaginal bacterial balance. Remember, all medications should be taken as prescribed.

Provider _____

Phone Number _____

Additional Comments: _____

_____

_____

_____

_____

_____

_____

_____

Appendix I

Anatomical Diagrams for Use in Patient Teaching

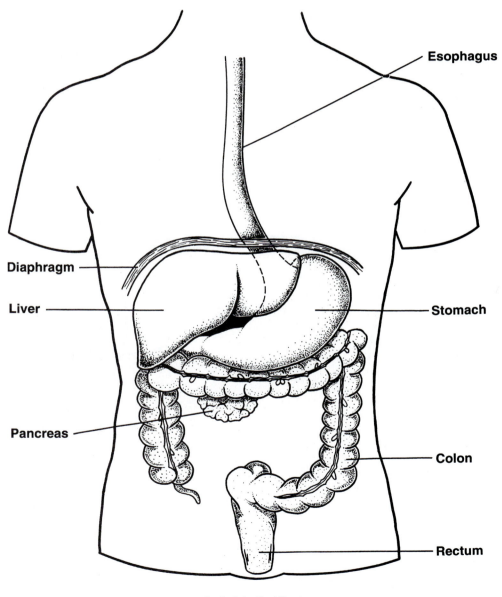

Esophagus

Diaphragm

Liver

Stomach

Pancreas

Colon

Rectum

Gastrointestinal Tract

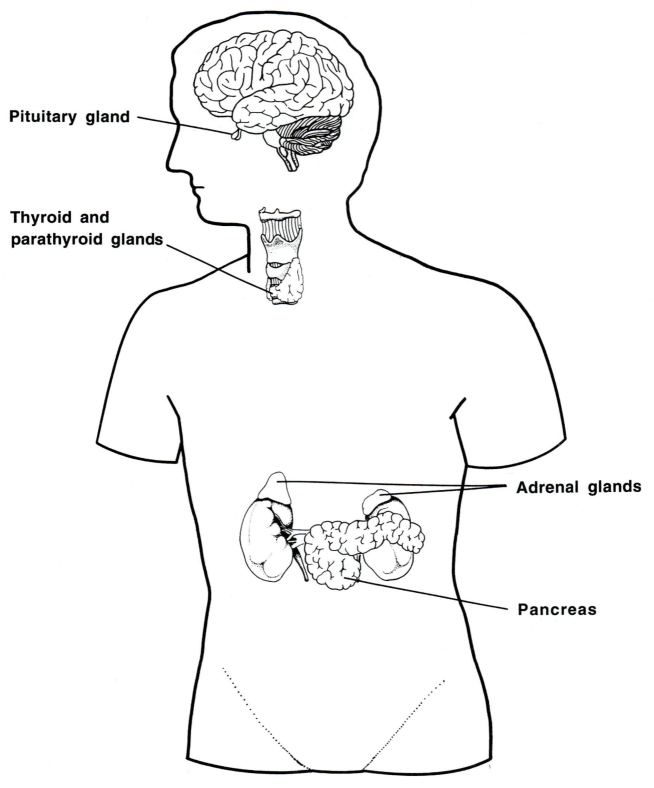

Pituitary gland

**Thyroid and
parathyroid glands**

Adrenal glands

Pancreas

Endocrine Glands

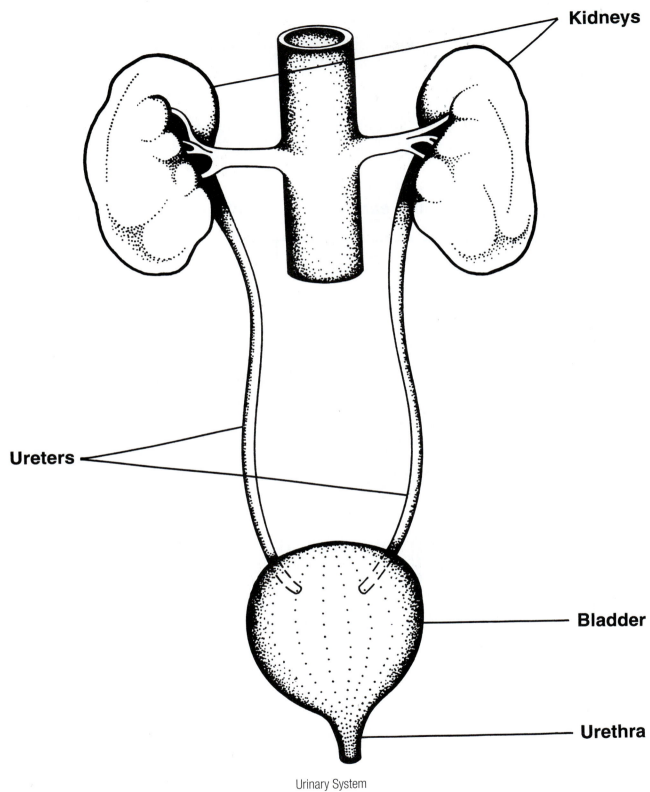

Kidneys

Ureters

Bladder

Urethra

Urinary System

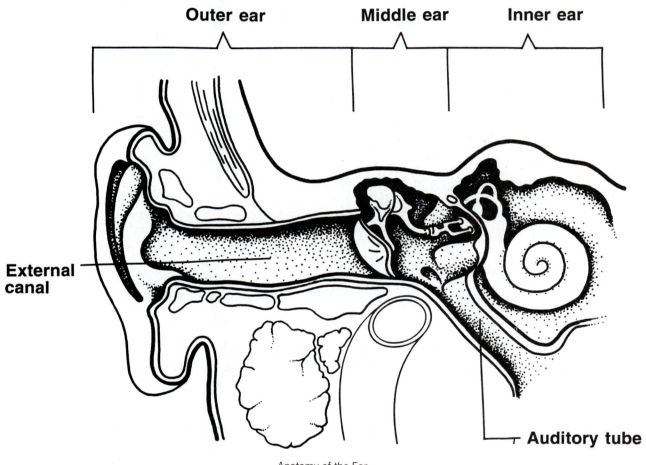

Anatomy of the Ear

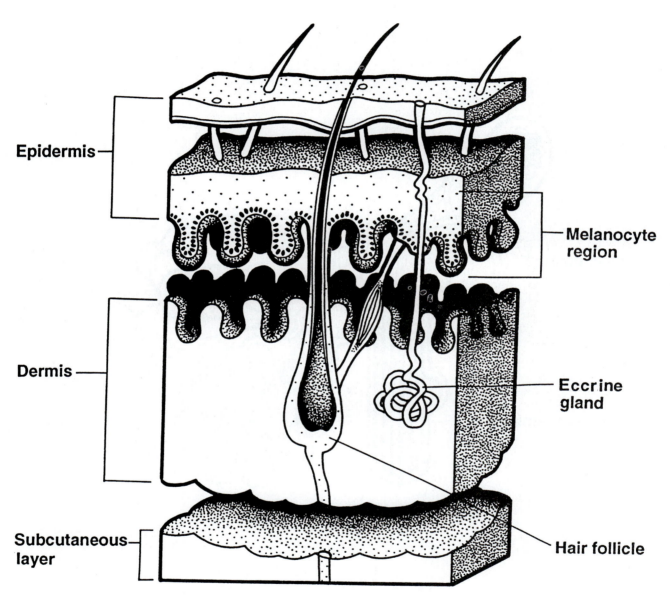

Epidermis

Melanocyte region

Dermis

Eccrine gland

Subcutaneous layer

Hair follicle

Skin Anatomy

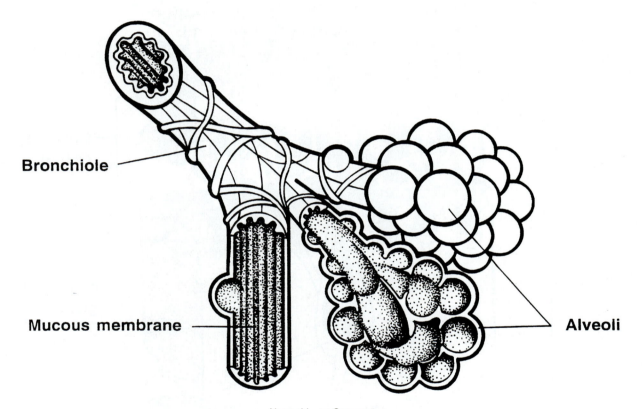

Bronchiole

Mucous membrane

Alveoli

Normal Lung Segment

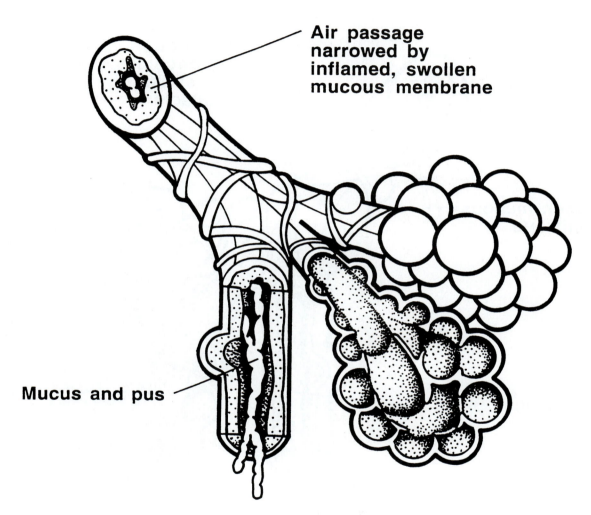

Air passage narrowed by inflamed, swollen mucous membrane

Mucus and pus

Lung segment demonstrating Chronic Bronchitis

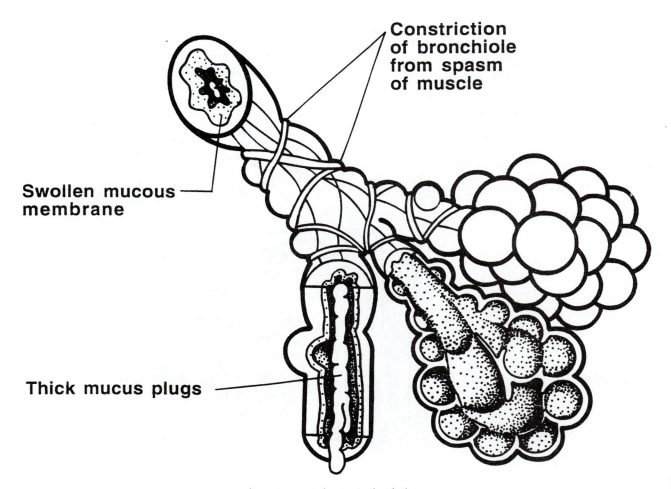

**Constriction
of bronchiole
from spasm
of muscle**

**Swollen mucous
membrane**

Thick mucus plugs

Lung segment demonstrating Asthma

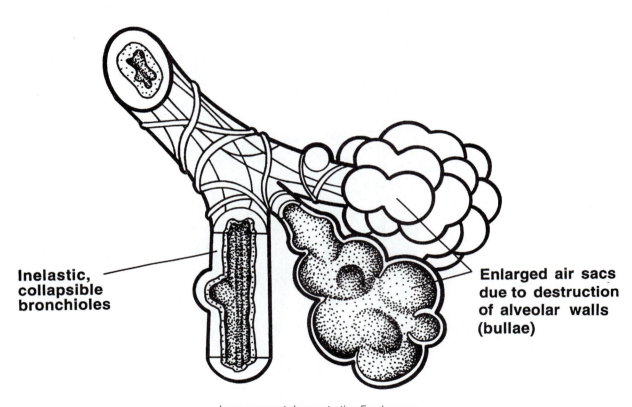

Inelastic, collapsible bronchioles

Enlarged air sacs due to destruction of alveolar walls (bullae)

Lung segment demonstrating Emphysema

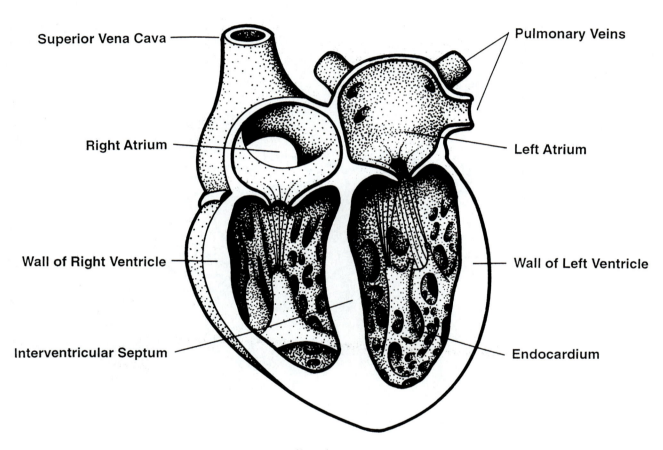

Superior Vena Cava

Pulmonary Veins

Right Atrium

Left Atrium

Wall of Right Ventricle

Wall of Left Ventricle

Interventricular Septum

Endocardium

Heart Anatomy

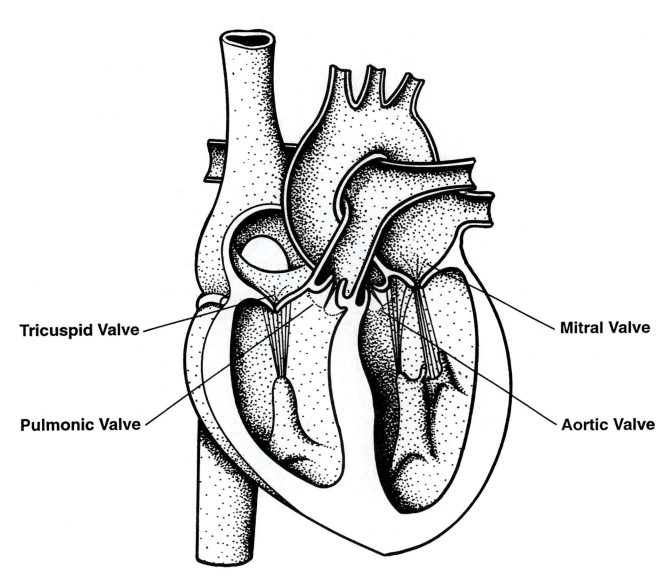

Tricuspid Valve

Pulmonic Valve

Mitral Valve

Aortic Valve

Heart Valves

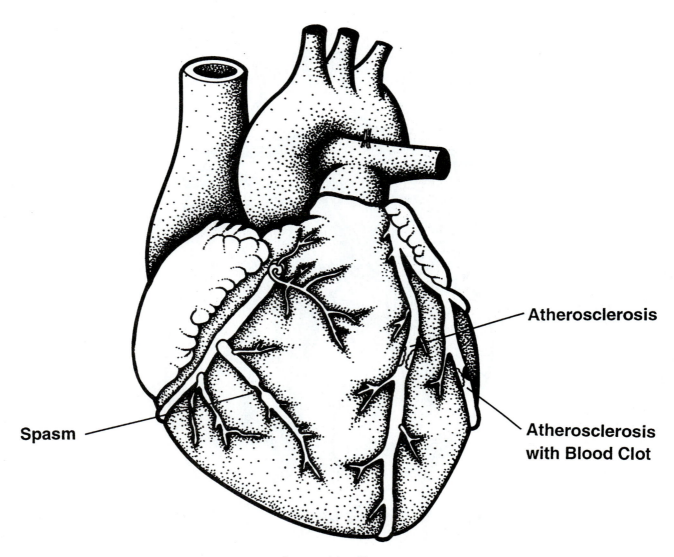

Atherosclerosis

Spasm

**Atherosclerosis
with Blood Clot**

Coronary Artery Disease

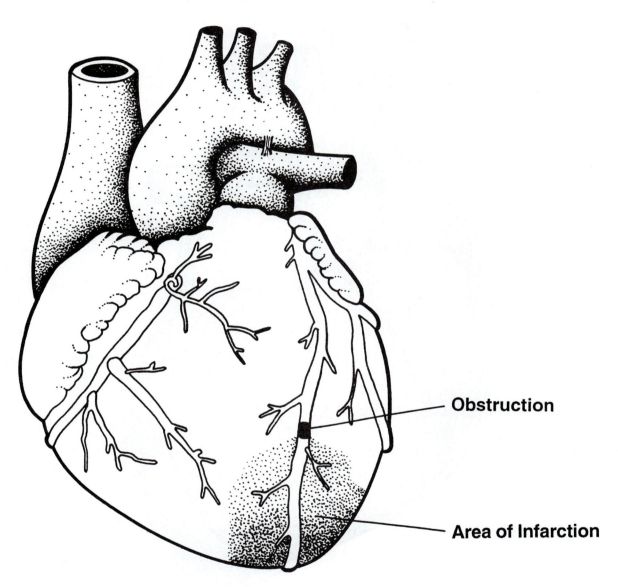

Obstruction

Area of Infarction

Myocardial Infarction (Heart Attack)

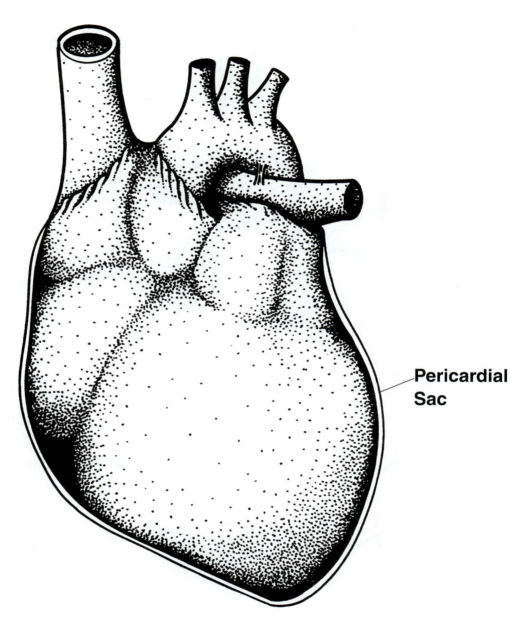

**Pericardial
Sac**

Pericardial Sac

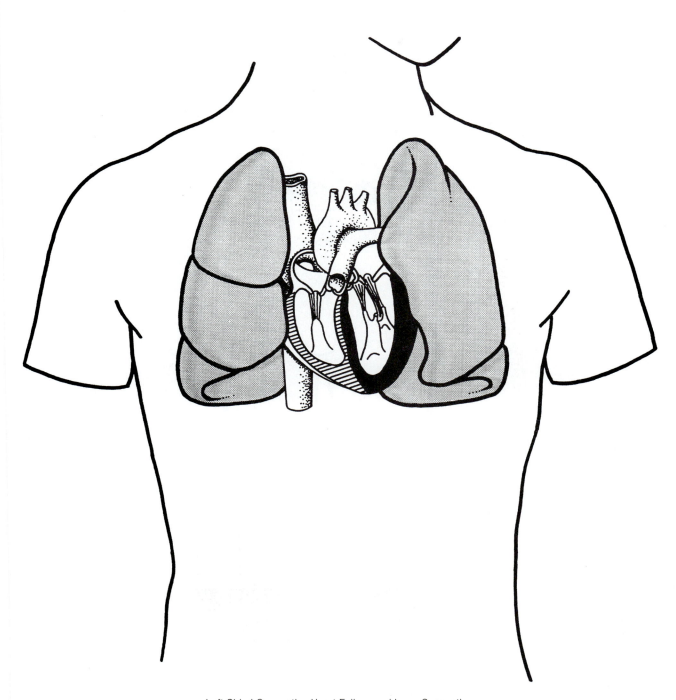

Left Sided Congestive Heart Failure and Lung Congestion

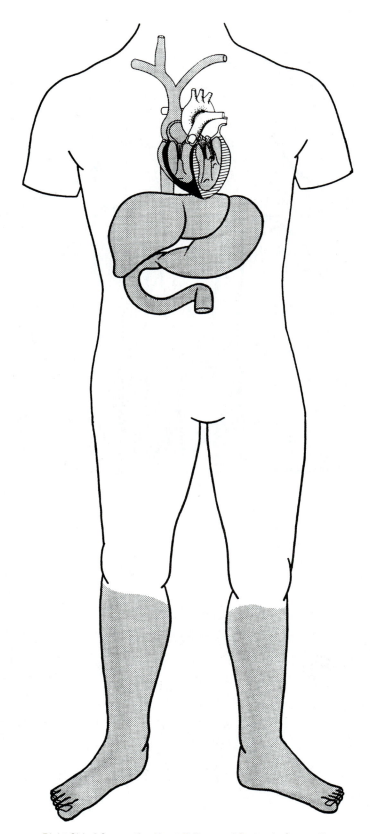

Right Sided Congestive Heart Failure and Systemic Congestion

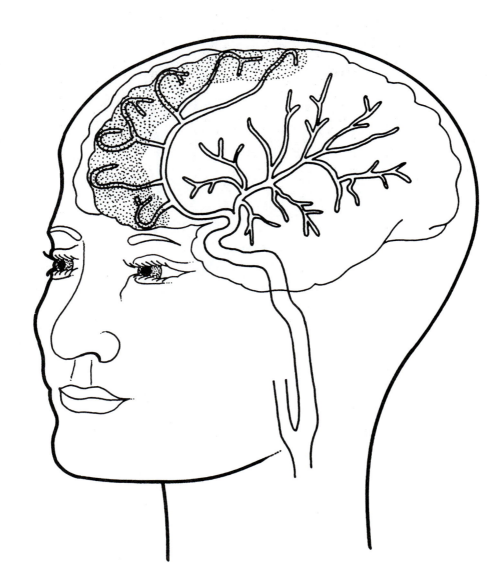

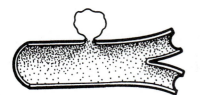

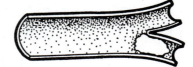

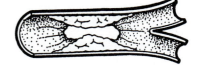

Stroke from hemorrhage

Stroke from blood clot (thrombus)

Stroke from clogged artery and clot

Different types of Stroke

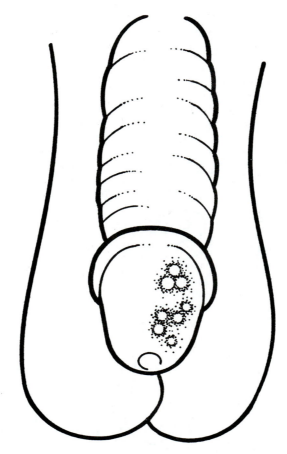

Genital Herpes of the Penis

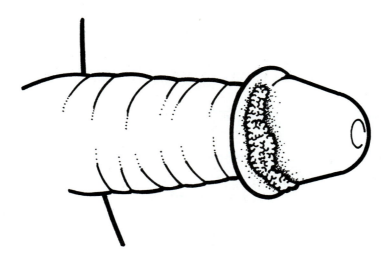

Venereal Wart of the Penis

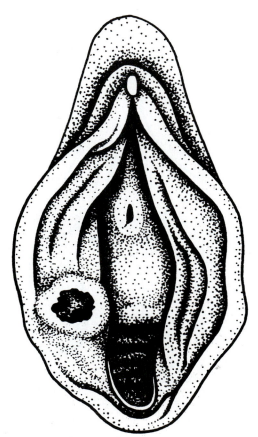

Syphilitic Chancre of the Vagina

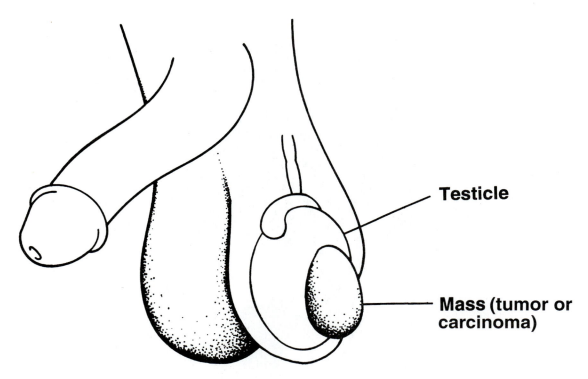

Testicle

Mass (tumor or carcinoma)

Testicular Carcinoma

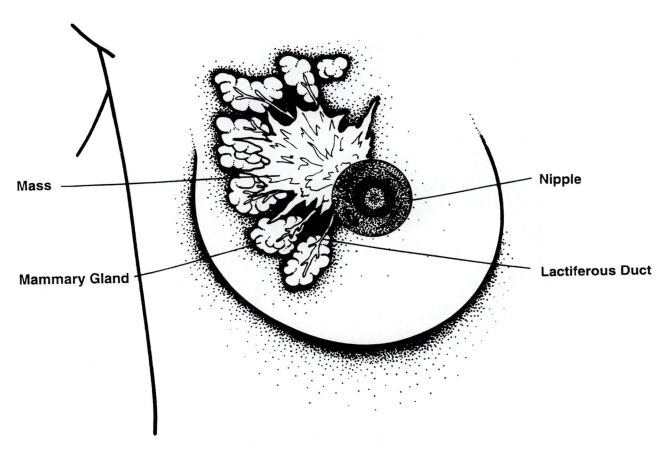

Mass

Mammary Gland

Nipple

Lactiferous Duct

Cancer of the Breast

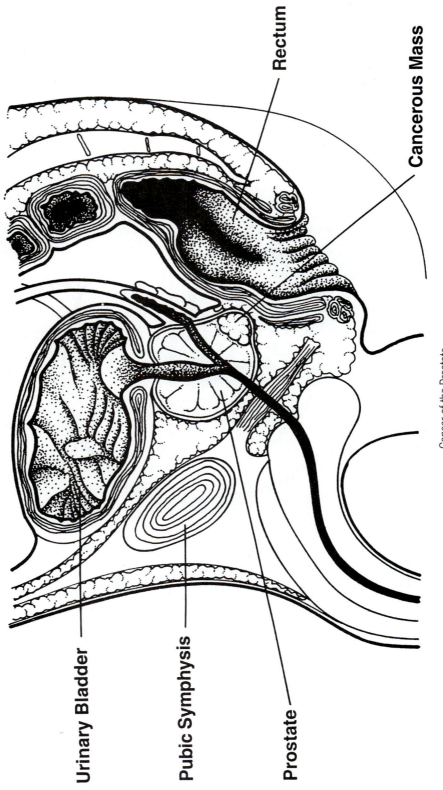

Cancer of the Prostate

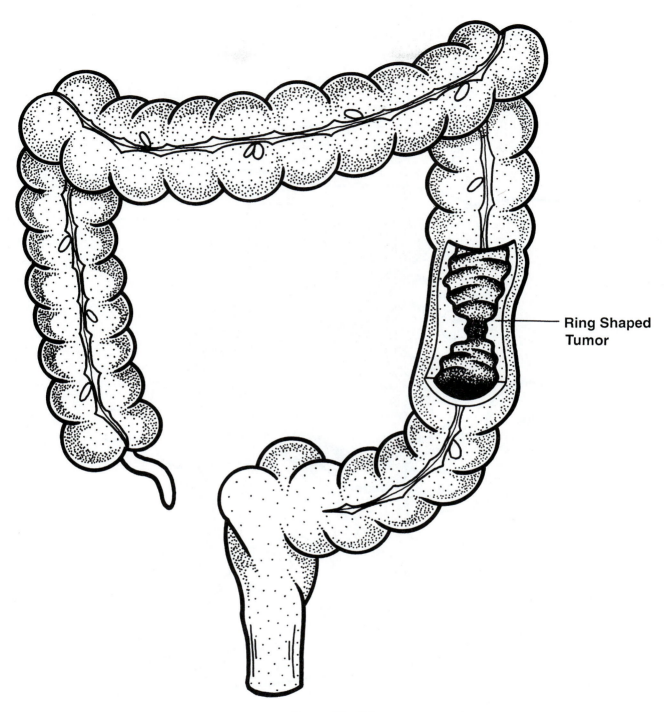

Ring Shaped Tumor

Cancer of the Colon

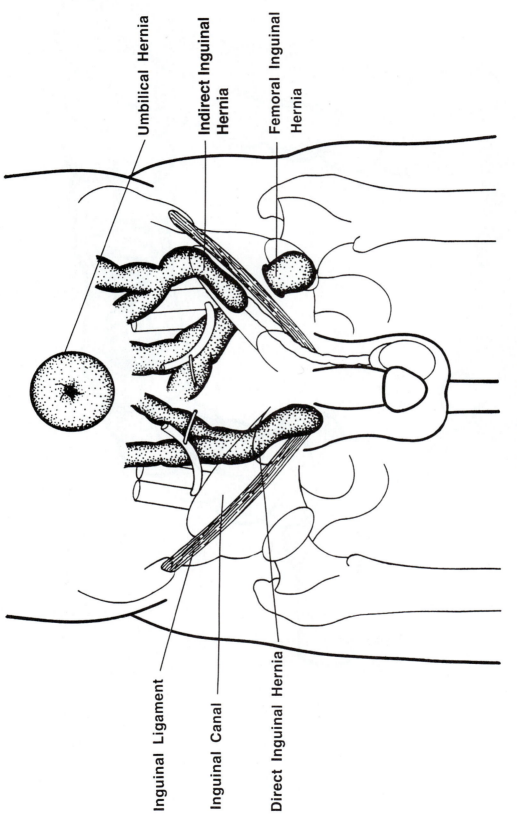

Umbilical Hernia

Indirect Inguinal Hernia

Femoral Inguinal Hernia

Inguinal Ligament

Inguinal Canal

Direct Inguinal Hernia

Different Types of Hernias

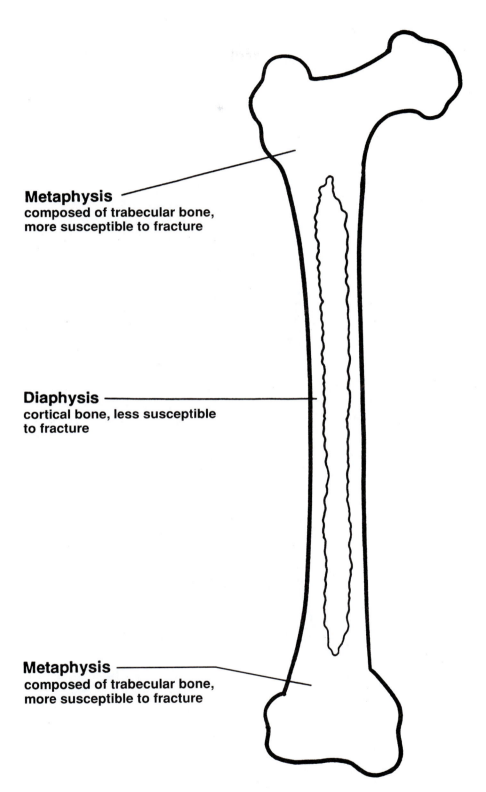

Metaphysis
**composed of trabecular bone,
more susceptible to fracture**

Diaphysis
**cortical bone, less susceptible
to fracture**

Metaphysis
**composed of trabecular bone,
more susceptible to fracture**

Femoral Bone

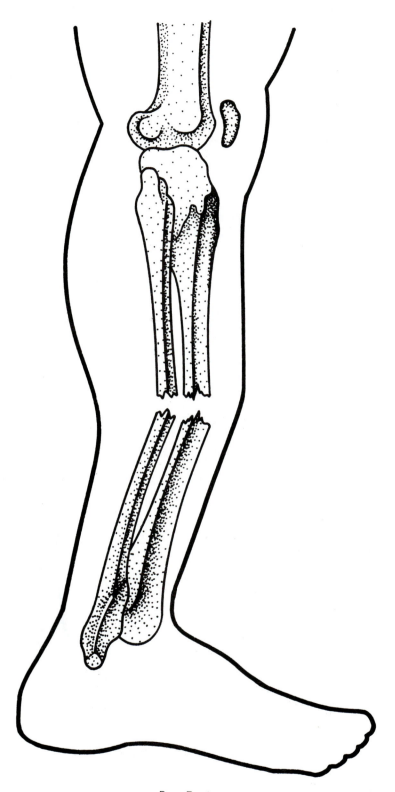

Bone Fractures

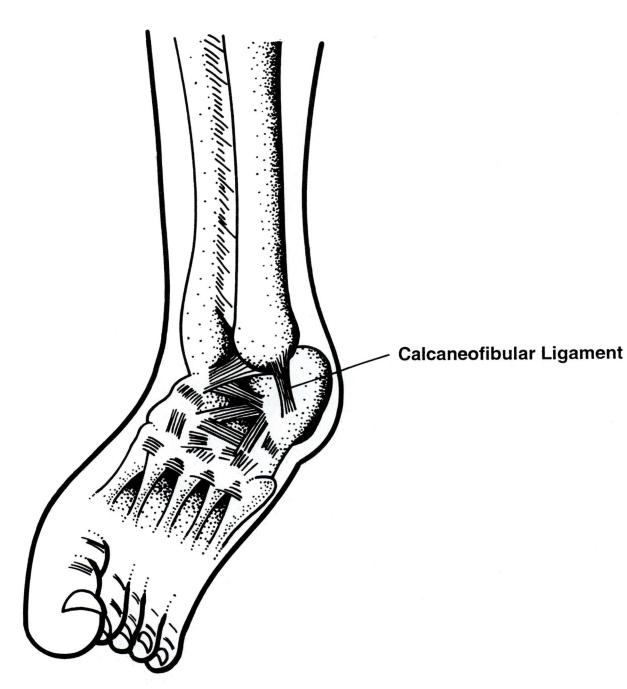

Calcaneofibular Ligament

Sprained Ankle

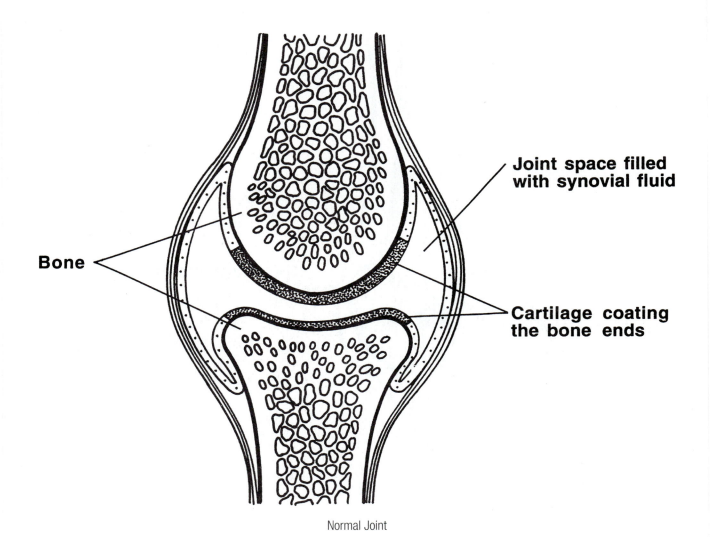

**Joint space filled
with synovial fluid**

Bone

**Cartilage coating
the bone ends**

Normal Joint

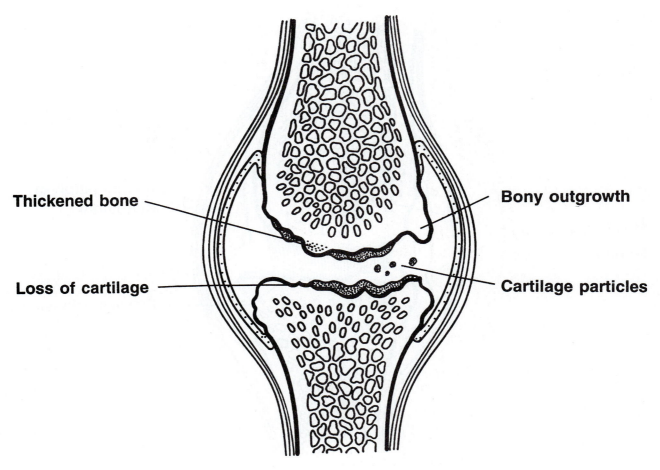

Thickened bone

Loss of cartilage

Bony outgrowth

Cartilage particles

Osteoarthritis

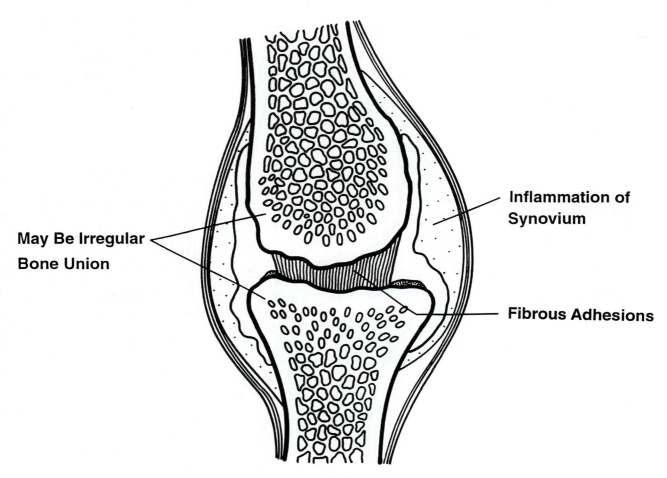

May Be Irregular Bone Union

Inflammation of Synovium

Fibrous Adhesions

Rheumatoid Arthritis

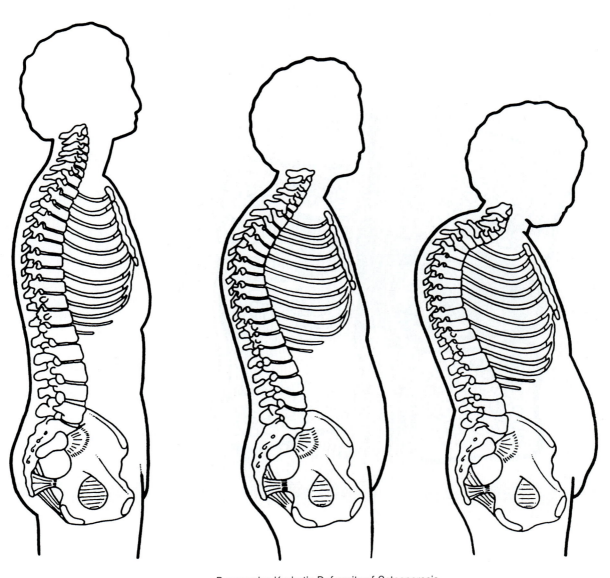

Progressive Kyphotic Deformity of Osteoporosis

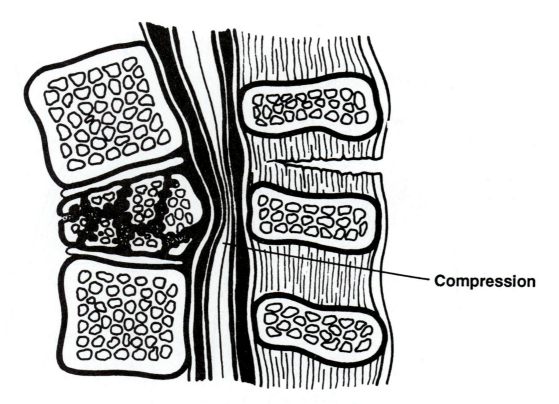

Compression

Wedge Shaped Compression Fracture of Osteoporosis

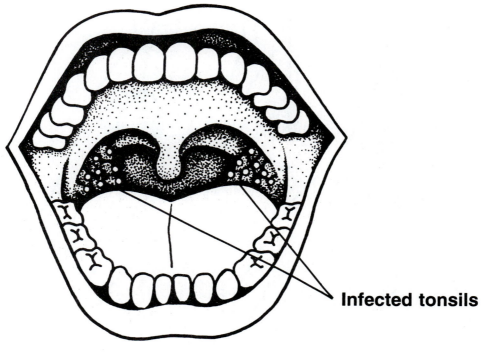

Infected tonsils

Tonsillitis

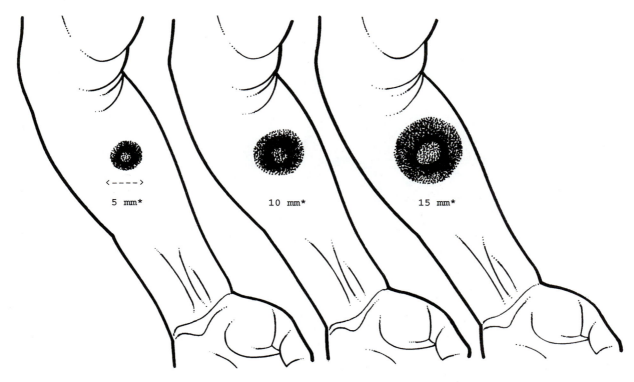

<--- -->
5 mm*   10 mm*   15 mm*

TB Skin Test

*Not to scale

Appendix II

Alternative Medicine

Richard D. Muma
Catherine S. Marsh

Introduction

In 1990, more than 1/3 of Americans used some form of alternative medical therapy, and they spent $13.7 billion on alternative treatments, more than half of the out-of-pocket expenditures for all conventional physicians' services in the U.S. during that time.[1] Such developments offer evidence of the mainstreaming of so-called alternative medicine.

Various types of alternative medicine, also known as complimentary medicine, has been used to treat ailments for centuries. Although not scientifically proven and controversial, doctors of traditional Chinese medicine have treated liver disease, back pain, and sinus problems with moxibustion, acupuncture, and herbs for at least 2,000 years. More recently, individuals with chronic disease processes, or those who perceived that they have been failed by traditional medicine, have been frequent users of a variety of therapies. Those individuals with AIDS, incurable cancer, and chronic musculoskeletal disorders have also been believers in alternative medicine. In a survey conducted in the United States by Eisenberg et al, one-third of their study population (n = 1539) reported using at least one unconventional therapy in the past year, and a third of these saw providers of unconventional therapy.[1] Chiropractic, massage, homeopathy, and acupuncture are the most common forms of therapy used.[1] Other therapies include moxibustion, relaxation, and herbal medicine.

The purpose of this section is not to discuss in detail the specific types of alternative medicine, but rather give the reader a general picture of alternative practices and why patients choose specific therapies. More importantly, this section is designed to raise the clinician's awareness of alternative medicine use by patients so that care and education can be optimized. Clinicians who are not aware of alternative medicine cannot help their patients decide which treatments work well together and which ones conflict with traditional western approaches.[2]

Why Patients Choose Unconventional Therapies

A substantial amount of unconventional therapy is used for minor medical conditions, health promotion, and disease prevention.[1] Most individuals use alternative approaches with traditional western medicine. A common reason for use, which seems to override other reasons, is that alternative modalities treat the whole person. Users also feel they are in control of the treatment and that their practitioners appear to be emotionally involved and concerned with their outcome. They also like that disease is viewed by alternative practitioners as positive rather than negative and that these same practitioners rely on their own intuition and less on diagnostic methods. Other reasons for use are feelings of unhappiness with allopathic medicine, including its limitations, side effects, and cost.

A reason for use also centers on the issue of control. An individual's desire to control what happens to him or her, particularly regarding his or her health, is likely to be realized with alternative approaches. By choosing alternative approaches, individuals are more likely to be satisfied because they selected it, unlike the allopathic approach, in which the therapy is sometimes predetermined. Other reasons clients give for selecting unconventional therapy include: inexpensive costs, noninvasive techniques, and its mind and body focus.

Types of Unconventional Therapies

There is no way that one can describe in detail all types of unconventional therapies in existence. What follows, however, is an abbreviated look at the most common therapies and some of their uses. In the January 1994 issue of *Self* magazine reports of a survey conducted in October of 1993 on alternative medicine were provided.[3] In that survey a number of therapies were identified by survey subjects. When asked the type of therapies used, the following were named:

Chiropractic	60%
Massage therapy	58%
Herbalism	42%
Relaxation techniques	40%

Holistic medicine	31%
Acupuncture	30%
Reflexology	24%
Biofeedback	9%
Osteopathy	6%
Macrobiotic diet	2%

Reasons for selection ranged from cervical disc rupture, chronic pain, to general wellness. Most survey respondents were satisfied with the therapy they chose and felt confident in their selection of alternative treatments for whatever ailments they may have had. Table 1 outlines selected unconventional therapies and includes some of their indications.

TABLE 1. SELECTED UNCONVENTIONAL THERAPIES[1–8]

Therapy	What Is It?	Use
Herbal Therapy	The essence of herbal therapy is the consumption of herbs to activate the body's own self-healing powers. Herbalists believe that the body can heal itself.	Healing, healthy life-style, pain relief
Chiropractic	A science of applied neurophysiologic diagnosis based on the theory that health and disease are life processes related to the function of the nervous system: irritation of the nervous system by mechanical, chemical, or psychic factors is the cause of disease; restoration and maintenance of health depend on normal function of the nervous system. Diagnosis is the diagnosis of these noxious irritants and treatment is their removal by the conservative method.	Back and neck pain, headaches, constipation, allergies, sinus problems, poor concentration, stomach and digestive problems
Massage/Touch	Involves systematically stroking, kneading, and pressing soft tissues of entire body to induce a state of total relaxation. The theory is if the body is totally relaxed it will heal itself.	Healing, reassurance, pain relief, muscle tension, stress, pleasure, warmth, and comfort
Imagery	Self-directed formation of mental images toward microbes, neoplastic cells, and viruses. These images are often described by patients as "armies of bodily cells killing off a disease, etc."	Immune disorders, cancers, various infections
Macrobiotics	Describes a life-style including a simple, balanced diet that promotes health and longevity. Macrobiotics advocates the use of traditional foods such as whole grains, beans, and locally grown vegetables as primary sources of food energy and nutrition. In addition, the diet includes soy foods, sea vegetables, whitefish, and shellfish. Whitefish and shellfish are substituted for red meat. Sea salts, rice syrup, and barley malt replace refined salt and sugar.	High blood pressure, high cholesterol, decreased energy, obesity.
Aromatherapy	Burning of trees, bushes, and small plants and using the aroma to treat various illnesses.	Back pain, high blood pressure, bronchitis, skin burns, yeast infections

(continued)

TABLE 1. SELECTED UNCONVENTIONAL THERAPIES[1-8] *(continued)*

Therapy	What Is It?	Use
Biofeedback	A techique whereby one seeks to consciously regulate a bodily function thought to be involuntary, as heartbeat, by using an instrument to monitor the function	High blood pressure, stress
Hypnosis	An artificially induced sleeplike condition in which an individual is extremely responsive to suggestion.	Smoking addiction, depression
Homeopathy	Use of substances that in healthy patients create symptoms like those of the disease being treated.	Various Diseases. Example: An itch might be treated with a preparation from poison oak
Acupuncture	The insertion of hair-thin needles, singly or in combination, into strategic points on the body to ease pain and treat a myriad of ailments caused by imbalances in the flow of chi, the life energy.	Sinus discomfort, neck pain, headaches, obesity, back pain, smoking addiction, arthritis, insomnia, impotence, nervousness
Moxibustion	Burning of herbs near (often through needles) or on the skin. This process stimulates the life force, chi.	Back and neck pain

Conclusion

The primary reason patients choose alternative, or unconventional therapy is that it allows them to be in control and participate in the healing process. For clinicians, an awareness and basic understanding of these modalities will enable them to better care for those individuals who choose such approaches. An open and nonjudgmental attitude toward unconventional therapy will improve patient-clinician rapport.

References

1. Eisenberg DM, Kessler RC, Foster C, et al. Unconventional medicine in the United States. *N Engl J Med* 1993;328: 246–252.

2. Harrison L. Unconventional wisdom. *New Physician*. 1993; (May–June):14–20.

3. Your answers on: alternative medicine. *Self*. 1994;(Jan):20.

4. Langone J. Acupuncture: new respect for an ancient remedy. *Discovery*. 1984;(Aug):70–73.

5. Kushi M. *The Macrobiotic Way*. Wayne, NJ: Avery Publishing Group; 1985:1–198.

6. Tenney L. *Today's Herbal Health*. Provo, Utah: Woodland Books; 1983.

7. Davis P. *Aromatherapy an A-Z*. Saffron Walden, England: CW Daniel Company Ltd.; 1988.

8. Lidell TS, Cooke CB, Porter A. *The Book of Massage*. New York, NY: Simon & Schuster; 1984.

Index

INSTRUCTIONS FOR USE OF DISK

In order to properly install the following program on your hard drive, you must follow the instructions listed below.

Please note, the command *<Enter>* requires that you hit the Enter key.

1. From a DOS prompt (C:\), type in the following:
   Cd <Enter>
   Md Test <Enter>
2. Insert the disk into Drive A or B
3. Type **A:** <Enter>   *or*   type **B:** <Enter>
4. At the A or B prompt, type the following:
   Copy Patiened.exe C:\Test <Enter>
5. Next, type in **C:** <Enter> (You will then be at the C:\ prompt)
6. Type the following:
   Cd <Enter>
   Cd Test <Enter>
   Patiened <Enter> (This will "expand" the file)

You now have access to all of the Patient Education Sheets that appear in the back of the book. They are contained in WordPerfect® files on your hard drive, in a directory called "Test." To access them in WordPerfect®, open that directory and click on the particular Patient Education Sheet in which you are interested.